W9-BHT-926

COMPREHENSIVE INTERVENTION WITH HEARING-IMPAIRED INFANTS AND PRESCHOOL CHILDREN

M. Suzanne Hasenstab
John S. Horner
University of Virginia
Charlottesville, Virginia

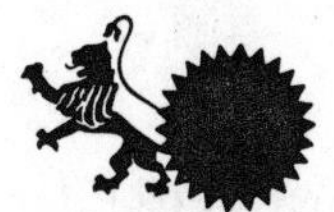

AN ASPEN PUBLICATION®
Aspen Systems Corporation
Rockville, Maryland
London
1982

Library of Congress Cataloging in Publication Data

Hasenstab, Suzanne.
Comprehensive intervention with hearing-impaired infants and preschool children.

Includes bibliographies and indexes.
1. Hearing disorders in children.
2. Language disorders in children.
3. Education, Preschool.
I. Horner, John S.
II. Title.
RF291.5.C45H28 618.92'855 81-14989
ISBN: 0-89443-384-9 AACR2

Library of Congress Catalog Card Number: 81-14989
ISBN: 0-89443-384-9

Printed in the United States of America

1 2 3 4 5

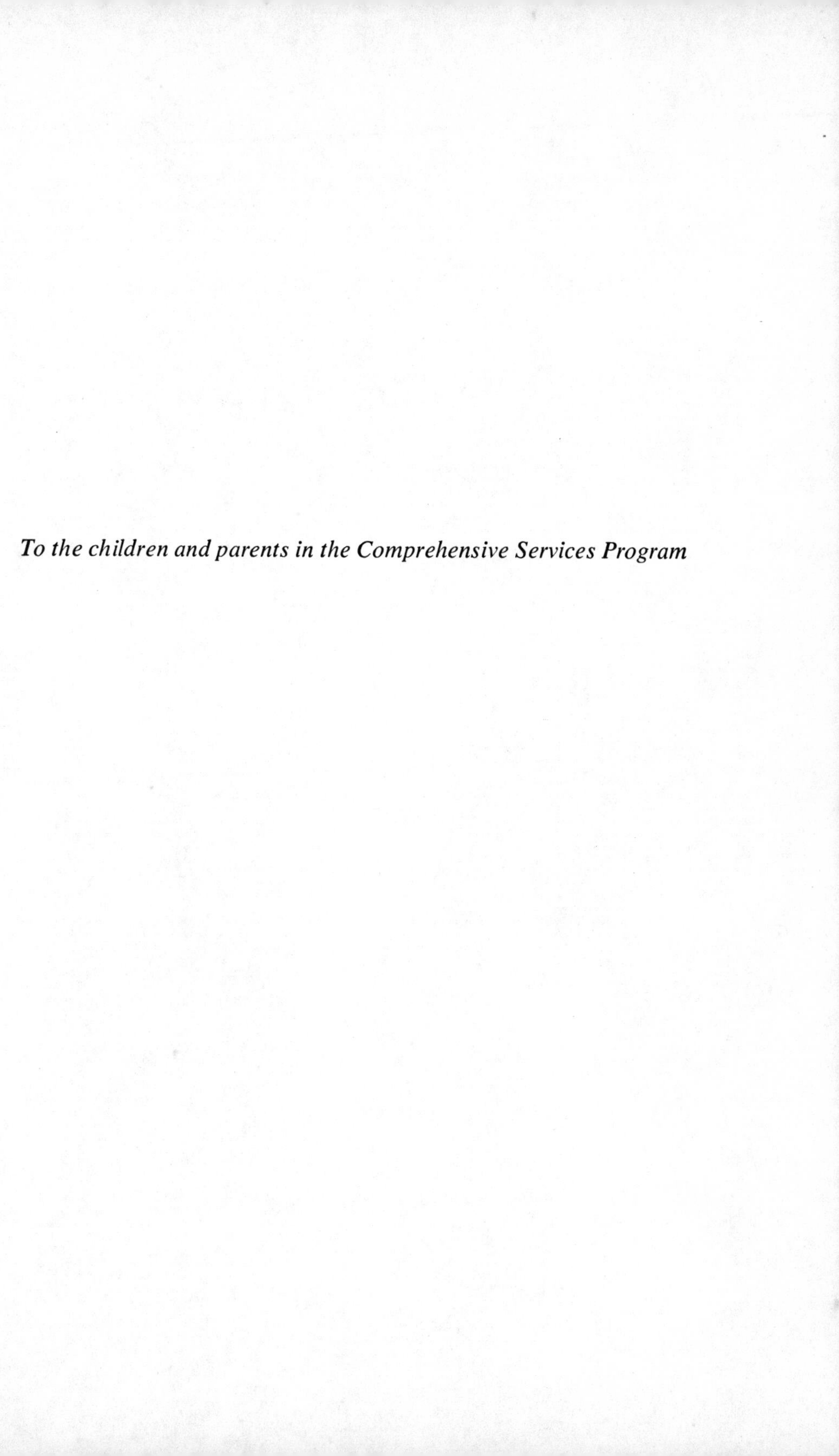

To the children and parents in the Comprehensive Services Program

Table of Contents

Preface

Preschool intervention for children with special needs, although not a new concept, is one that is receiving increasing emphasis. The importance of early diagnosis and programming is no longer a debatable issue. The concern now is with the provision of services and the scope and quality of such service programs. This book addresses specifically two handicapping conditions; hearing impairment and language delay as they relate to children from early infancy to the age of entry into a formal educational system.

Our purpose is to provide information based on the Comprehensive Services Program for Hearing-Impaired and Language-Delayed Infants and Preschool Children currently in operation through the Department of Speech Pathology and Audiology, Speech and Hearing Center, at the University of Virginia. The book presents a "hands-on" collection of information regarding the assessment and educational intervention concerns for hearing-impaired and language-delayed children from early infancy through 6 years of age. Specifically, it illustrates innovative techniques in the auditory evaluation of infants and preschool children, methods of evaluating the overall development and linguistic functioning of young children, and programming considerations from a parent-infant orientation through a preschool group learning environment.

For the purpose of this work, hearing impairment is defined as any auditory disorder that presently interferes, or may potentially interfere, with a child's linguistic or educational development and function. The term therefore includes all degrees of hearing loss and peripheral and auditory processing difficulties. Language delay refers to linguistic functioning other than what is considered normal at specific age levels. The definition includes representations of both delayed and deviant language. Therefore various etiologies are inclusive in this definition.

The Comprehensive Services Program, and therefore this text, is based on the premise that only through intense cooperation between those in the field of audiology, the education of the hearing impaired, and other professions that address hearing and language problems in young children can the needs of such children be adequately met. Further, it is believed that only through early intervention, via appropriate assessment techniques and quality educational programming, is it possible for these children to have the chance to reach optimal functioning potential.

The book is organized around the following topics. In the first part, on assessment, Chapter 1 presents an overview of audiometric assessment techniques used with infants and young children. It also presents the evaluation procedure adopted by the Comprehensive Services Program. Chapter 2 presents both the philosophical and the practical implications of early amplification. Types of amplification and the management of hearing aids are discussed in depth.

In Chapter 3, the issues and concerns related to difficulties in the processing of auditory information are presented. A practical model of auditory processing that may apply to the evaluation and programming needs of young children is illustrated. Chapter 4 examines the purpose, concerns, and instruments in the developmental or psychoeducational evaluation of infants and preschool children and describes the tests and procedures employed in the Comprehensive Services Program.

The first of two chapters devoted to language evaluation, Chapter 5 presents an overview of the purpose, concerns, and available instruments and procedures used in evaluating aspects of linguistic ability in early childhood. Chapter 6 then focuses on the process of language evaluation based on a language sample analysis called Bare Essentials in Assessing Really Little Kids, or BEAR, as developed by Dr. Suzanne Hasenstab. The rationale and procedures in the use of this instrument and the BEAR Concept Analysis Test are described.

In the second part, on intervention programming, Chapter 7 examines parent-infant programming. The focus is on development in infancy, the purpose and scope of parent-infant programs, and the specifics of the parent-infant program as part of Comprehensive Services. In Chapter 8, the development of children from ages 2½ through 4 is examined and related to curriculum and programming. The discussion covers the concerns and needs of parents as integral members of the educational team.

Finally, in Chapter 9, the prekindergarten educational needs of children of ages 4 through 6 are examined, both in their present setting and as related to entry into various alternatives beyond the preschool program. As in Chapter 8, the cooperation of parents is addressed.

It is hoped that the information in this book will be of value to students, professionals, and parents who are engaged in intervention for infants and children with hearing or language problems. The text by no means claims to be inclusive in any of the areas presented. It attempts rather to highlight and illustrate fundamental knowledge and information that will assist in the assessment and educational programming of the children being served.

Acknowledgments

We would like to extend very special thanks to Drs. Zahrl Schoeny and Joan Laughton for their time and effort in coauthoring Chapters 3 and 6 and for their constant behind-the-scenes assistance and support in the realization of this text. An expression of gratitude is also due to graduate students Amanda Connolly, Barbara Summers, and Mary V. Compton for the hours of library time they so generously contributed. Finally, we must add a word of appreciation for the patience and kind words of family and friends throughout this experience.

Part I

Assessment

Federal and state legislation, growing public awareness of handicapped people, and increased positive attitudes on the part of professionals related to the area of education have produced ardent concern regarding the rights of children and the handicapped, as well as educational accountability in these areas. This has resulted in a movement toward the provision of appropriate educational placement and programming for exceptional children.

A crucial component in the provision of appropriate education is assessment. Intelligence tests and achievement tests are combined by teachers, clinicians, and psychologists with various evaluative measures in language, motor growth, and social-emotional development to determine programming needs within the academic milieu. Now there is increased emphasis on early intervention and the education of preschool exceptional children, including children with hearing and language difficulties. Without accurate assessment, programming can become a hit-or-miss ordeal.

DEFINITION

Assessment, as used in the context of this book, refers to the composite of various evaluative measures, both data-based and criterion-referenced, and the observations made by contributing professionals involved with the child and the child's family.

PURPOSE

The primary purpose of assessment is to determine the exact nature and extent of the child's disability so that appropriate intervention and education can commence. Salvia and Ysseldyke (1981) indicate five purposes in assessment or, more specifically, in the administration of tests:

1. screening
2. placement
3. program planning
4. program evaluation
5. assessment of individual progress

All but the first of these five purposes are integral in the overall assessment program presented in this book. Once the educational program is underway, the purpose of assessment expands to provide parents and professionals with continuous new information to aid in expanding and altering the child's program to enhance development. Program planning is ongoing; it is dependent on continuous monitoring of progress and development. This is interrelated with the evaluation of the child's individual progress within the program.

APPROACH

If the purpose of assessment is to be achieved, a multidisciplinary approach is needed. Such an approach will allow for the input of information by various qualified professionals regarding their specialty and the child's functioning in that area. Information from the following areas is considered pertinent:

- The child's physical health—A complete medical history and physical examination report by a family physician or pediatrician, either in private practice or clinic based.
- The child's health as related to the auditory and oral mechanism—A complete medical examination by an otolaryngologist.
- The child's peripheral auditory functioning—A summary of auditory evaluation performed by an audiologist.
- The child's intellectual and developmental functioning—A summary of psychoeducational evaluations administered by a qualified examiner.
- The child's linguistic and speech abilities—A summary of linguistic evaluations conducted by a qualified examiner.
- The child's family—A summary of the child's home and family environment resulting from parent interviews and home visitations by qualified personnel.

In addition, various other specialists may be involved if warranted by a particular case. Fallen (1978) lists eight main specialty areas from which representatives may serve as consultants in determining the presence of handicaps in children. These specialists could, if necessary, also be engaged in the case of a hearing-impaired child. The eight specialty areas are related primarily to the medical field. The first specialist is the geneticist. A referral to a geneticist would be made to determine if a child's hearing loss was due to hereditary factors. The second is the neurologist. The neurologist is consulted quite frequently in cases of multihandicapped hearing-impaired children in order to verify the presence of central nervous system dysfunction. The biochemist is the third specialist who may provide additional information regarding a hearing-impaired child, especially in cases where hyperactivity is evident. The fourth specialist area is concerned with adequate vision. Because the hearing-impaired child is already faced with adjusting to one deficient sensory avenue, it is important that other sensory modes, especially vision, function adequately. Thus, any suggestion of visual problems should be quickly investigated by an ophthalmologist.

In the fifth specialist area, it would be advantageous to enlist the expertise of the orthopedist (or the rheumatologist) in cases where there are obvious or suspected bone or muscle disorders. In the sixth specialist area, dental health may be a factor with hearing-impaired children as well as with hearing children. The dentist and orthodontist can provide services that are not only beneficial to the child's health but also aid in the development of speech. An intact oral peripheral mechanism is an aid to the child in articulation. It is also possible that, in the seventh specialist area, a particular child may demonstrate emotional or social behaviors that would warrant the attention of a child psychologist or psychiatrist. In such cases, appropriate referral should be made. Finally, the eighth specialist cited by Fallen is the otologist or otolaryngologist, who, as indicated earlier, will obviously be involved in the medical evaluation.

AREAS OF CONCERN

The assessment component of the Comprehensive Services Program is concerned with three major categories of functioning, each of which will be discussed in detail in the following chapters:

1. The auditory functioning of the child, which includes the peripheral auditory mechanism and the auditory processing abilities.

2. The overall development of the child, which includes the areas of motor growth, cognitive abilities, social-emotional maturation, and attainment of independence in self-help skills.
3. The specific language and speech abilities of the child, which include receptive and expressive skills within the components of language.

OBJECTIVES

Based on the areas of concern in assessment, objectives may be formulated. The goals in an assessment, very broadly stated, are (1) to determine accurate information regarding the child's performance in all areas of development and (2) to provide a foundation for the development of an educational program for the child.

SUMMARY

Assessment is an integral part of the process of providing adequate and appropriate educational intervention for infants and preschool children with hearing impairment. The actual complexity of the total assessment will depend on the individual child, the extent of the handicap, and the child's particular life situation.

REFERENCES

Fallen, N. *Young children with special needs.* Columbus, Ohio: Charles E. Merrill, 1978.

Salvia, J., & Ysseldyke, J. E. *Assessment in special and remedial education* (2nd ed.). Boston: Houghton Mifflin, 1981.

Chapter 1

Audiological Evaluation

John S. Horner

Although determination of the peripheral auditory abilities of hearing-impaired infants or infants with a language delay constitutes only a part of the habilitation process, this knowledge is pivotal to other testing and the educational plan. Proper utilization of the auditory feedback channel during the earliest habilitation program can determine the relative success or failure of the child to develop effective expressive and receptive oral communication.

This chapter has several purposes: First, it presents a rationale for the earliest identification of hearing loss. Second, it evaluates the auditory responses provided by various test modalities. Third, it describes the tests currently being used in many clinics for audiological evaluation. Finally, it describes the tests and procedures utilized in the Comprehensive Services Program for children in the period between birth and 6 years of age.

EVALUATING NEONATES AND INFANTS

Traditionally, nonverbal children were usually referred to the audiologist for a hearing assessment as a first step in their habilitation. That is, that was the first step if such children were referred at all. Usually the referral was too late (as will be stressed in the next section of this chapter). As a result, irreversible impairment of the potential communication ability of these children was common. An additional effect was the slow development of audiological assessment techniques for children under 3 years of age. It has been only in the past few years that effective hearing measurement techniques for neonates and young infants have proliferated. When pediatricians and other referring agents such as public health nurses realize that quantitative audiological assessment can be performed on infants as young as 4 months, they may begin referring younger infants, which in turn will spawn the development of more effective test batteries (Horner & Horner, 1979).

RATIONALE FOR EARLY IDENTIFICATION OF HEARING LOSS

Most experienced clinicians have followed the speech and language development of a severely hearing-impaired child identified before the age of 12 months and then compared that development with that of a similarly impaired child who was not identified until after the age of 2 years. In such studies, though each child was fitted with amplification and provided with speech and language stimulation, the striking contrast in their eventual ability to communicate could not be overlooked. The late-identified child sounded "deaf," with a "swallowed," hypernasal voice quality and excessive pressure during the articulation of consonant sounds that combined with other "deaf speech" characteristics to make the child almost unintelligible to the untrained ear. The early-identified child, in contrast, sounded almost normal, the residual effects of the hearing impairment on the child's speech suggesting to the untrained ear the possibility that the child had a foreign accent.

When comparing such anecdotal experiences with other professionals, it is tempting for the clinician to hypothesize that early identification and subsequent training are responsible for the surprising communication proficiency developed by the second child. However, the temptation of this hypothesis must be resisted in the absence of confirmed research data. Clearly, early identification by itself does not improve a child's eventual communicative accomplishment. Likewise, early training of a severely hearing-impaired child, without the stimulation of amplified sound, has not been shown to result in a voice quality and speech facility within the normal range. The early-identified child's success is probably due to early stimulation with appropriate amplified sound in combination with the proper training procedures. Yet, to belabor a critical approach one more time, there is no hard evidence to indicate how early is "early," what "appropriate amplified sound" is appropriate, and what "proper training procedures" are proper. In subsequent chapters, appropriate amplified sound and proper training procedures will be addressed.

For many years, professionals associated with habilitation of the hearing impaired have intuitively subscribed to the early discovery and training of their charges. The urgency of their actions has varied with each professional because, although the audiologist and teacher of the hearing impaired knew early intervention was important, it was not uniformly clear that early intervention is *essential*. One had the feeling that, if a child happened to be discovered a little late and if that child was basically intelligent, had an excellent teacher, ideal, motivated parents, and the best amplification, then that child could "catch up" with a less endowed child who had been identified earlier in life. This feeling, however, is not supported by recent data emerging from studies on sound deprivation.

Though most studies involving sound deprivation utilize animals, some human studies report the effects of early chronic otitis media on various aspects of speech and language acquisition.

Data from animal studies suggest a variety of effects of sound deprivation on auditory transmission and processing. Tees (1967) raised hooded rats with earplugs and found that they had significantly poorer tonal pattern discrimination than their normal controls. Rats raised in sound deprivation by Batkin, Groth, Watson, and Ansberry (1970) showed 20 dB less sensitive auditorily evoked potentials than did normal rats. As reported by McGinn, Willot, and Henry (1973), mice raised with earplugs from 17 through 22 days had 12 dB less sensitive auditorily evoked potentials than the controls. Clopton and Winfield (1976) showed that rats having early exposure to patterned sounds demonstrated an increased response selectivity to that particular pattern as compared to similar but unfamiliar patterns when the response was single-unit recordings in the inferior colliculus. Partial to complete loss of binaural interaction was shown in neurons of the inferior colliculus by Silverman and Clopton (1977) when they performed a unilateral ligation of the external auditory meatus of rats. Further studies by Clopton and Silverman using this paradigm demonstrated a critical period of 10 to 60 days for binaural interaction in neurons of the inferior colliculus, with the greatest plasticity shown between 10 and 20 days. Webster and Webster (1977) found incomplete maturation of most brain-stem auditory neurons resulting from both postnatal auditory deprivation and experimentally produced, conductive hearing losses in mice.

All of the above studies concerned themselves with a relatively intact sensorineural system that had been deprived of auditory stimulation by various procedures. Similar deprivation occurs in human infants with early chronic conductive hearing loss due to such things as bilateral congenital atresia or chronic otitis media. Further, although it is difficult to verify without question, there are indications that such infants share the pattern discrimination and other retardation in development demonstrated by animals. Wishik, Kramm, and Koch (1958) found a delay in grade placement in children with chronic otitis media. Ling (1959) reported a significant retardation of arithmetic and reading skills in children with a history of this disease. Holm and Kunze (1969) found that children with a history of recurrent otitis media demonstrated significant difficulty with vocabulary comprehension, use of verbal analogies, grammatic closure, use of visual analogies, and articulation of sounds in isolated words. In a study of infants with a history of early otitis media (between birth and 18 months), Needleman and Menyuk (1977) discovered that such infants showed a significant problem with articulation in isolated words and connected speech and in the reproduction of morphological markers.

Up to this point, the discussion has centered around the development of a normal auditory sensorineural system with early sound deprivation. One might question how the evidence in this area relates to the infant with a typical, severe, sensorineural hearing loss. Without question, this infant does not have a normal auditory sensorineural input. Sound pressures must be increased until those sensorineural units that are still relatively intact can provide the infant with auditory experience. Although sound pressures must also be increased for the infant with conductive impairment to have an auditory experience, there is a major difference in the way in which sensorineural units code the auditory information. Since the conductive lesion attenuates the sound pressure, it effectively reduces the level reaching the cochlea so that all of the coding goes on essentially as in a normal ear. In the ear with a sensorineural impairment, this attenuation does not occur. All of the sound pressure passes into the cochlea to be coded by those neural units that are still functioning. Consequently, at the sound pressure levels of ambient noise and of normal conversational speech, the neural units still functioning in the ear with a severe sensorineural impairment are rarely called upon to code sound.

Therein lies part of the dilemma. When children with a severe sensorineural impairment are discovered and we begin their habilitation with stimulation using amplified sound, for the required task we are essentially calling upon sensorineural units that have had auditory deprivation. Because of their position in the cochlea, these sensory units are usually required to respond only to the high sound pressure levels of loud noises, shouting, and other alerting signals. Now, with amplification, they are called upon to discriminate more subtle speech signals. Whether these units normally have the ability to discriminate subtle cues has not been completely researched. But, since evidence from sensory deprivation studies with conductive hearing losses shows impairment of function and incomplete maturation of most brain-stem auditory neurons, it is unlikely that these units will ever develop subtle discrimination skills without early practice (Webster & Webster, 1977).

It has been suggested that without adequate sound stimulation during a particular critical period of brainstem maturation, the auditory neurons will not develop fully. Whether a critical period during brain maturation exists in mice or in humans is still a matter of controversy. Some researchers believe that the period may not be critical but may be one of more sensitivity (Rubel, 1980). In any case, it is becoming more evident with each reported study that "modifications of 'normal' experience must have differential influence on the ontogeny of neuron structure and function by producing some change, qualitative or quantitative, in the afferent input to the neurons under investigation" (Rubel, Parks, Smith, & Jackson, 1978, p. 2). Certainly, hearing loss is a modification of normal experience and as such will produce some change from normal development and function of brain-stem auditory pathways. The impaired sensory system consequently will never reach its potential for the coding and transmission of complex stimuli in the manner for which it was designed. However, because of the plasticity of the brain during early postnatal development, intensive auditory stimulation of sensory units still functioning in a sensorineurally impaired ear may result in hyperdevelopment of residual pathways and permit the near normal function sometimes found in early-identified, hearing-impaired children. Since it has been shown that the brain stem in the human infant is not mature until after 1 year of age (Salamy & McKean, 1976), surely auditory stimulation early within that first year has the best chance of creating a morphological, and hopefully a functional, change conducive to the better development of speech and language.

Although we are still not sure how early is "early," the evidence suggests that the pediatric audiologist and the educator of the hearing impaired should feel a strong sense of urgency to discover and begin stimulating the hearing-impaired infant as early as possible within the first year.

CONCERNS IN AUDIOLOGICAL ASSESSMENT OF INFANTS

When the audiological assessment of a pediatric population is planned, the first consideration is to decide which aspect of hearing function should be measured. What data from an infant's auditory input and feedback system are most essential to predicting the child's communicative development? We really do not know. Historically, pediatric audiologists have tried to measure the child's hearing sensitivity or the differential frequency response at threshold. These threshold audiograms have had value for medical referrals and for the choice of a hearing aid. This approach had and still has some face validity, since surely one must surpass the hearing threshold with amplified input before the child receives auditory stimulation.

On the other hand, the nature of a hearing-impaired infant's suprathreshold auditory experience cannot be known. Each child probably has a unique "sound" that is experienced as dependent on the frequency response and other processing characteristics of each individual ear. What the child experiences and whether it differs from "normal" or from other hearing-impaired children's experiences really should not concern us. We will probably never know what another's experience is like. What is more disturbing is that we do not know the minimal frequency, intensity, and phase information that an infant must be able to process in order to develop a reasonable receptive auditory function. Furthermore, even if we did have the minimal data necessary to process, we would still have to develop techniques to measure this processing ability before we could begin to predict an infant's potential for the speech hearing function. As a result of these unknowns, the clinician helping to habilitate hearing-impaired infants must measure the possible and guess at the unknowns. This means to measure thresholds and guess at suprathreshold loudness contours, difference limens for frequency and intensity, and other processing parameters.

Evaluating the Auditory Response

The recent proliferation of audiometric techniques utilized with pediatric populations tends to suggest (at least by inference) that we are testing infants' hearing. Perhaps it is time to reexamine just what audiometric tests are measuring. An excellent thought organizer for this purpose is presented by Shepherd (1978). He emphasizes that, following the auditory stimulus, the audiologist looks for an auditory response that is a change in the response system chosen for the production of an auditory response. The response system may be one of the *specific* auditory response systems that responds only to auditory stimulation, such as the cochlea, the auditory nerve, and the brain stem. Or the response system may be one of the *nonspecific* auditory response systems that is not specifically designed to reslond only to auditory stimulation but is influenced by other body systems. These response systems yield such responses as the electrodermal, the electrocardiac, and the behavioral responses. In either case, when the audiologist is observing a change in a specific or a nonspecific response system, the key concept in audiometric procedure is the observation of a response. What that response can tell us about hearing is dependent upon the characteristics of the auditory test protocol. For more specific analysis of the meaning of responses, the test protocols can be grouped into (1) behavioral observation audiometry, (2) electrophysiologic audiometry, and (3) conditioned behavior audiometry.

Behavioral Observation Audiometry

In order to gain knowledge about the performance of the neonate's and young infant's auditory systems, investigators have used observations of behavioral changes following the introduction of an auditory stimulus. The procedure relies upon the hope that the child's poststimulus activity will be distinctive from his prestimulus activity. The change in activity must be evaluated according to previously set response criteria and then scored as a response or a no-response. If no conditioning is involved in this procedure, it is called *behavioral observation audiometry* (BOA), a term introduced by Lloyd and Young (1969). The success of the BOA approach is very dependent upon the prestimulus activity level of the infant and the investigator's observation of the correct response system. The response may be reflexive activity, such as the Moro response or the Auro-Palpebral Reflex, or it may be as subtle as a quieting response. In any case, the BOA procedure yields a simple "yes" or "no" as to the infant's change or behavior in the presence of a stimulus. Consequently, BOA research has shown only those stimuli to which neonates and infants prefer to respond; it has not revealed the capabilities of their auditory processing systems. This is due, in part, to two aspects of the BOA procedure.

First, since the most observable responses are reflexive behaviors elicited by high-intensity signals, sensitivity thresholds are not measured. Even though some investigators choose to observe responses other than reflexes and to reduce stimulus intensities, sensitivity "thresholds" recorded for young infants do not approach normal adult threshold intensities by this method. Thus, BOA procedures must be considered identification audiometry, used to discover auditory systems that are possibly defective.

Second, because the nature of the infant's response is so dependent upon the prestimulus activity level within the response system, the signals chosen as the stimuli, and the age of the infant, it is difficult, if not impossible, to design a BOA procedure to quantify discrete aspects of an infant's auditory capabilities.

Electrophysiologic Audiometry

Other nonspecific auditory response systems besides the behavioral have been utilized in the measurement of infant auditory system capabilities. These are the electrophysiologic response systems in which auditory responses are recorded as changes in the electrical properties of body systems as an indirect result of auditory stimulation. These responses include electrodermal responses, and perhaps the electroencephalic response (although whether the latter response is specific or nonspecific to the auditory system is still under debate).

Other approaches to hearing testing that take advantage of the autonomic nervous system's response to novel stimuli measure changes in respiration, heart rate, and pupillary dilation. These electrophysiological or other autonomic nervous system responses have provided more information regarding auditory threshold sensitivity and also, according to Eisenberg (1979), auditory vigilance in neonates. However, there has been very little success, using the nonspecific autonomic response systems, in establishing infant auditory threshold norms. Nor does it seem likely that a measurement procedure using these systems will yield much definitive information regarding peripheral processing, transmission characteristics of the eighth cranial nerve, integrative functional maturation of the brain stem, or central processing of complex stimuli.

Specific auditory response systems currently being employed to obtain auditory responses are the cochlea, the eighth cranial nerve, and the brain stem. The advantage of specific auditory response systems over nonspecific systems, such as behavioral or autonomic nervous systems, is that the former are relatively inactive in the absence of auditory stimulation, are not under cortical control, and may be only slightly influenced by descending neural impulses from the cortex. The cochlea and the eighth cranial nerve best fit the criteria of specific auditory response systems. It is at the brain stem that we find rich interconnections with other sensory systems and descending cortical connections. However, the methods employed to obtain a response from even the brain stem have not revealed any serious contamination of the auditory response by other sensory or cortical neural impulses. This may be due to the fact that summing and averaging computers are used to enhance the auditory brain-stem response and to reduce the effect of other sensory or cortical responses whose latencies may differ from auditory system responses.

In any case, the response of these specific auditory response systems is only electrical signals. A response, when it occurs, is identified primarily by its time of arrival after stimulus onset and by its voltage amplitude. The presence of a clear response is most helpful since it suggests that the sound is creating a change in the state of the central nervous system. However, absence of a response does not necessarily imply the reverse. Any attempt, therefore, at interpretation of these neuroelectric responses in terms of the functional ability of the organism is a courageous, if not foolish, task—given our present knowledge.

Conditioned Behavior Audiometry

In the past 10 to 15 years, an increasing interest in the application of conditioning to behavior audiometry has led to the development of some exciting techniques for the audiological assessment of the difficult-to-test.

Although dependent on nonspecific auditory response systems, if consistent, repeatable responses are obtained, these measurement techniques have the advantage of quantifying functional abilities of the organism. Most of these techniques can be termed *conditioned behavior audiometry* (CBA) to differentiate them from behavioral observation audiometry (BOA).

BOA requires that the clinician or researcher identify the neonate's or infant's prestimulus activity level in order that a response can be recognized. As defined by Shepherd (1978), the prestimulus activity level is based upon Wilder's law of initial value (LIV) and includes the two interacting conditions of (1) the psychological state and (2) the readiness of a response system to respond only to auditory stimulation. As a consequence of BOA test protocol, many types of responses are acceptable. As reported above, the investigator may observe reflexive activity, quieting, localization, distraction behavior, and so forth.

Conditioned behavior audiometry (CBA), on the other hand, uses the auditory stimulus to signal and condition the child to expect a reward. The neonate's or infant's activity to partake of the reward within a prechosen time interval after the stimulus onset is accepted as the response. This response to the auditory signal must be verified by a number of quiet control intervals. Additionally, the investigator attempts to choose and maintain, if possible, an optimum prestimulus activity level so that the desired response may be observed. This response can be a simple head turn to the reward, increased sucking, button pushing as in tangible reinforcement operant conditioning audiometry (TROCA) or in visual reinforcement operant conditioning audiometry (VROCA), or even putting rings on a post as in play audiometry. In short, BOA observes the prestimulus activity level and accepts various changes of behavior as a response, while CBA tries to choose and maintain a prestimulus activity level for the presentation of the auditory stimulus and to condition a particular behavioral change as the response.

Consequently, the investigator using CBA is not dependent on high-intensity signals to elicit a response. If a stimulus that is truly rewarding to the subject can be devised or discovered and if that subject can be conditioned, then the investigator has only to use imagination and good scientific technique to devise CBA tasks that will permit assessment of the child's auditory capabilities. Since these auditory system talents will be inferred from conditioned behavioral response rather than from neuroelectric changes in portions of the central nervous system, the researcher may feel closer to defining the pragmatic consequences of auditory stimulation. For example, if the CBA technique results in infants consistently responding to pure tones near adult threshold intensities, one feels confident that these infants have hearing that is at least this sensitive. Of course, if the CBA technique results in the absence of an acceptable response, it shares in the dilemma of most other test techniques. Absence of an acceptable response does not necessarily mean that the child cannot function auditorily. An unsuccessful performance on the test may mean that the infant's auditory system is too immature, that performance of the test is not rewarding, or that there are a host of unknown factors involved. On the other hand, the presence of acceptable responses may demonstrate an infant's ability to perform certain auditory tasks. Since the auditory tasks themselves are a part of the tests, successful performance provides information regarding the infant's auditory abilities.

Pediatric audiometric techniques have proliferated as researchers have given increasing attention to the normal characteristics of infant auditory systems. Additional measurement procedures have been developed as the clinician has striven to detect the abnormally functioning auditory system in infants. As the test armamentarium grows, it becomes increasingly important for the researcher and the clinician to evaluate each procedure as to the data each can yield. For example, BOA procedures rarely provide threshold determinations and are subject to infant prestimulus activity levels within the response system. On the other hand, quite often BOA leads to statements that a child's hearing is "probably no worse than. . . ." Electrophysiologic procedures used on the nonspecific auditory response systems may yield information suggestive of auditory threshold, but this information is often contaminated by other activity in the autonomic nervous system. The electrophysiologic tests used on specific auditory response systems are less susceptible to such contamination, but, on the other hand, the responses elicited are potential changes that may or may not be correlated with functional hearing. CBA procedures enable one to have more confidence in thresholds, difference limens, or discrimination abilities because the task is designed to measure the auditory system's abilities by modifying behavior. However, when using these procedures, one must be careful to ensure that the infant is conditioned to respond to the selected stimulus task rather than to specious cues. Whichever test modality is used, we must not mislead ourselves into thinking that we are actually measuring infants' hearing; we must remember that the data we gather by any of the auditory test procedures are just responses. When we interpret these responses as indicative of *hearing*, we are gambling and speculating with probabilities.

Test Selection

Unfortunately, the question of test selection for neonates and young infants in contemporary audiology does not relate to the abilities to be evaluated but rather to which test might yield some information. The younger the infant, the less quantitative and more qualitative the information yielded by present-day tests. Although some researchers have attempted to describe the nature of normal hearing in the very young (Eisenberg, 1976), audiological armamentaria are not definitive of early auditory capabilities. As described previously, BOA procedures show what the neonate and infant *will* respond to, not what they are *able* to respond to. Auditorily evoked response and electrocochleography procedures are quantitative, but they describe the electrophysiologic system and do not necessarily predict behavior. CBA procedures come closest to allowing behavioral predictions, but they have not yet been used routinely on infants younger than 4 months (Horner & Horner, 1979).

Consequently, the audiologist must consider the emotional, physical, social, and mental age of the child and then choose procedures that will maximize the data that could emerge from the tests. Thus, a newborn with a suspected hearing loss would be tested by BOA and/or electrophysiological procedures since we have no existing procedure to quantify a behavioral threshold. On the other hand, if the infant is over 4 months old, CBA techniques could yield auditory thresholds. Variations of a conditioned behavior audiometric technique could easily be devised to demonstrate suprathreshold abilities of young infants. Some variations are being applied to research purposes but have not been incorporated into clinical routines. As norms are developed for input abilities to discriminate auditorily in ways that are less related to the test procedure than they are to the child's actual processing potential, we will be able to increase assessment accuracy. However, these norms have not been developed for children under 3 years of age. Consequently, the hearing threshold is the most definitive auditory system characteristic available to audiologists and educators of the hearing impaired. And of course even this datum is not always obtainable.

Clinician Qualifications and the Child

Not all audiologists are successful in obtaining maximum information regarding the neonates' and infants' auditory capabilities. The well-trained, experienced, "all-around" audiologist brings skills to the pediatric testing situation that are necessary but do not guarantee success. Clearly, audiologists must be so familiar with their equipment that the child can receive their complete attention. An objective attitude must be maintained. The infant's behavior must be understood, and the clinician must be able to interact with a young child.

However, with all of these abilities, pediatric audiologists will fail to obtain accurate, maximum data until they learn the "rhythm" of the infant they are testing. They must develop a feel for the ebb and flow of the infant's changing state. The activity level and attention of an infant will change at a rate dependent on the child's age, physical development and condition, and the social development and social nature of the child. In order to apply either BOA or CBA techniques, one must be tuned in to the rhythm of this change—tuned to introduce the acoustic stimulus at the time appropriate for test modality and at a time when the expected response can be observed. Many audiologists and other clinicians fail to recognize the critical nature of this timing, or they are unable to modify techniques that have been successful with older children and adults to comply with the infant's changing state.

Another important characteristic of pediatric audiologists is that they be observant of the infant's behavior in every situation. Audiologists must observe as they pass the infant and parents in the waiting room, as the parent interacts with child, as a toy drops to the floor, as the door to the sound suite slams, and as they move around the room in preparation for the formal test. Each occurrence can contribute information on how this little person is sampling the auditory/visual environment. Too often audiologists consider the formal test procedure to be the test and are unaware that the test begins when you "lay eyes" (and ears!) on the infant.

The Test Conditions

The pediatric audiologist's primary concern is the testing of the child's hearing. This means assessing how an infant utilizes the auditory sense in interaction with the environment. To obtain a quantifiable measure, one must control the acoustic environment at some point in the test. The early stages of testing may be informal BOA in a quiet waiting room or even while walking to a test suite. To have results expressed in numbers, extraneous sounds must be eliminated in the test environment and the test stimuli parameters must be controlled. Thus, quantifiable test results will be obtained in a sound-isolated room, such as a test suite, and with calibrated instrumentation.

Although the research literature does not report the quantifiable effects of visual distraction on hearing test results with infants, researchers and clinicians always specify that the test environment be free of visual distractions. Perhaps it is more realistic to say that the room should be designed so that visual stimuli may be controlled. A stark, bare room is not necessary with the majority of children and, in fact, may be detrimental to a child's feeling of well-being. On the other hand, visual stimuli need to be controlled because many of the CBA techniques rely on a visual reward. If too many attractive visual stimuli are within sight, they will dilute the effects of the visual reward. The key concept in hearing testing of infants and in the test conditions is *control*. The clinician must control the auditory, visual, and social stimuli so that the infant's behavior may be modified with the test stimuli. Once the child is under stimulus control, the maximum information may be obtained in the time the child will allot. One aid to control of conditions is the use of two clinicians, one to operate the equipment and one to control the test conditions in the patient side of the test suite. This includes social modification of the infant's behavior, if necessary, for CBA.

The time of evaluation is a critical consideration when evaluating infants and young children. A sleepy, hungry, or uncomfortable child will be more concerned with internal stimuli than with those the audiologist uses in testing hearing. Generally, mornings are the best testing times, but not just before feeding or nap time. The parents usually are aware of times when the infant is alert and happy and can aid in scheduling the hearing test.

Since young children will tolerate only a limited amount of control of their behavior, they will terminate the session for the audiologist when they are ready (not necessarily when the audiologist is ready!). This requires that the time of the test be kept short or, perceived a different way, that the audiologist obtain the most important information from the hearing test first. One can think of the infant as a bank account with responses taking the place of money. Unfortunately, audiologists are not permitted to know how many responses are in their account. It behooves the audiologist under these conditions to work quickly, using up responses on only the most meaningful audiometric data and leaving less critical data until last if it is found there are still some responses left in the account.

AUDIOLOGICAL TESTS FOR EVALUATING NEONATES AND INFANTS

Many test procedures have been developed for evaluating the hearing of neonates and infants. Many more will be created as innovative research demonstrates that the very young infant's hearing can be accurately quantified. The purpose of this section is to discuss types of hearing test approaches rather than to describe every variation.

Behavioral Observation Audiometry

Wedenberg Procedure

Wedenberg (1963) developed a BOA procedure for screening babies' hearing with a high-intensity pure tone. This in turn stimulated other early identification programs. Wedenberg's procedure includes two steps. The first step is to stimulate a deep sleeping baby with a 105–115 dB Sound Pressure Level (SPL) pure tone. The normal hearing baby in deep sleep will react to this intense pure tone with an Auro-Palpebral Reflex (APR), according to Wedenberg's findings. As a second step, a baby in deep sleep is stimulated with a tone of 70–75 dB SPL. The neonate with normal hearing will awaken to a state wherein tactile stimulation will evoke an APR. Earlier, Wedenberg (1956) was the first to report screening the hearing of 100 newborn babies. He used pure tones at 100 dB Hearing Level (HL) as the signal, and the APR was the expected response. The reflexive eye blinks are triggered by tactile stimulation and by acoustic stimulation of sufficient loudness. Consequently, interpretation of an APR should be done cautiously. Inadvertent brushing of the neonate's cheek while testing can produce an APR unrelated to hearing. Even APRs obtained solely from acoustic stimulation should not be overinterpreted. Since the sudden loudness of the acoustic stimulation triggers the APR, babies with sensorineural hearing losses demonstrating recruitment can show an APR if their thresholds are surpassed to the point that normal loudness is perceived. This same criticism can be leveled at BOA techniques that use high-intensity signals in an attempt to detect hearing loss. A response may mean normal hearing, or it may mean a cochlear hearing loss 10–15 dB less than the SPL of the stimulus. No response may mean a conductive or retrocochlear hearing loss, or it may mean a severe cochlear hearing loss. It may even mean normal hearing in a baby who is too busy with internal stimuli to respond to an external stimulus.

Eisenberg Procedure

Eisenberg, Griffin, Coursin, and Hunter (1964) described a BOA design typical of those currently used to identify hearing loss among infants in newborn nurseries and neonatal intensive care units. In their procedure, three trained observers positioned themselves at the head and to either side of the infant. They observed and recorded the neonate's prestimulus and poststimulus activity. The examiner at the head of the baby presented four different stimuli 5 times in random order with variable interstimulus intervals. Each of the observers recorded the prestimulus and poststimulus activity according to a coding system. The stimuli were calibrated noise makers consisting of a drum beat, the crumpling of a fresh sheet of onionskin paper, the striking together of a pair of pierced wooden sticks, and the toot of a small plastic whistle. Although procedures similar to this are used for screening infant hearing, Eisenberg (1976) states she was on a "fishing expedition . . . to define certain relations between the physical and functional properties of sound. . . ." (p. 52).

Downs and Sterritt Newborn Screening Procedures

About the same time that Eisenberg was reporting her BOA design for studying infant hearing, Downs and Sterritt (1964) reported the first study of newborn hearing screening in this country. Their study determined that reliability among observers could be high. As a result, a large-scale neonatal hearing screening program was instituted in all Denver hospitals using volunteers from Junior Leagues and hospital auxiliaries. Subsequently, many neonatal hearing screening programs were developed on the Downs format. That is, an intense high-frequency signal between 3 and 6 kHz was presented to the infant while one or more observers recorded prestimulus and poststimulus activity.

Unfortunately, this BOA procedure has all the pitfalls of other techniques that note prestimulus and poststimulus activity when the stimulus is an intense sound. The observer must see and record the prestimulus activity and then watch for one or more changes in activity during the poststimulus time period. Again, these examiners are looking for a stimulus that the infant *will* respond to, not a stimulus an infant is *able* to respond to. Moreover, since the stimulus is intense, little definitive information is gained regarding the intactness of the infant's auditory system.

Consequently, as the Downs screening program progressed, two problems became evident (Northern & Downs, 1978). A number of babies passed at birth were showing up later as having a hearing loss. The second problem was that all but one baby identified as hearing impaired by the screening program fell into a high-risk category for deafness. These findings tended to destroy confidence in this type of mass behavioral screening. On the other hand, the findings added confidence to the use of the high-risk register recommended July, 1972, by the Joint Committee on Infant Screening and amended in 1978:

> The Committee recommends that, since no satisfactory technique is yet established that will permit hearing screening of all newborns, infants AT RISK for hearing impairment should be identified by means of history and physical examination. These children should be tested and followed-up as hereafter described.
>
> The criterion for identifying a newborn AT RISK for hearing impairment is the presence of one or more of the following:
>
> A. History of hereditary childhood hearing impairment.
> B. Rubella or other nonbacterial intrauterine fetal infection (e.g., cytomegalovirus infections, Herpes infection).
> C. Defects of ear, nose, or throat. Malformed low-set or absent pinnae; cleft lip or palate (including sub-mucous cleft); any residual abnormality of the otorhinolaryngeal system.

D. Birthweight less than 1500 grams.
E. Bilirubin level greater than 20 mg/100 ml serum. (Gerber & Mencher, 1978, p. 13)

These criteria for identifying infants at risk for hearing impairment were amended in 1978 to include "significant asphyxia associated with acidosis" (p. 2).

The point of using a high-risk register is, of course, to attempt to reduce the number of infants given a hearing screening without missing infants with a hearing loss. Thus, only 5.5 to 9.4 percent of the total newborn nursery would need a hearing screening test (Mencher, 1978).

Simmons and Russ Cribogram

Ten years after Downs and Sterritt reported a BOA neonatal hearing screening approach for neonates, Simmons and Russ (1974) reported an approach that did not require the presence of observers. This design, called the Cribogram, utilizes a small-motion transducer that is placed on or under the mattress of the infant's crib. The transducer is semiautomated in that a preprogrammed timing device introduces a 2-second, 92-dB SPL narrow band of noise between 2000 and 3000 Hz through a loudspeaker located approximately 10 inches from the neonate's head. At preprogrammed intervals, the instrument turns itself on, records about 10 seconds of baseline activity on a strip chart, introduces a 2-second stimulus while recording, and then records poststimulus activity for 5 seconds. The number of presentations per 24 hours can be programmed according to the test protocol. The strip charts are scored for positive responses by trained judges.

Although this approach lends itself to computer control and analysis and could reduce the manpower necessary for screening, it suffers from some of the same problems as all other BOA test protocols that depend on high-intensity stimuli to elicit a response. Infants with cochlear lesions and recruitment will be passed along with infants with mild to moderate losses of other varieties. The automated approach has many advantages, however. For example, those three early morning tests can be performed by the computer! With further research it is also quite possible that lower stimuli intensities could be used to reduce the number of false negatives.

Ewing and Ewing Hearing Screening with Noisemakers

Sir Alexander and Lady Irene Ewing of Manchester, England, were the first to use noisemakers to test babies' hearing (Ewing & Ewing, 1947). In their exploration of the effectiveness of noisemakers in eliciting hearing responses, they discovered that (1) patterned sounds, especially those in the speech-hearing range, are more effective in eliciting a response than pure tones; (2) stimuli below 4000 Hz tend to produce responses more readily than those above 4000 Hz; (3) soon after the neonatal period, learned responses take precedence over reflexive responses; and (4) localization ability is very evident and becomes increasingly refined after 6 months. Their most reliable response was the orienting response. This was obtained using such noisemakers as tissue paper, a china cup and metal spoon, a rattle, a toy xylophone, and voiced and unvoiced consonant sounds. This form of BOA testing became the standard infant hearing test and has withstood the test of time. When all else fails, the Ewing and Ewing approach becomes the final choice as a hearing test protocol.

Conditioned Behavior Audiometry

Two characteristics of infants formed the basis for the BOA procedure previously described. The first is that an intense sound will cause various reflexive and startle behaviors. The second is that, as the infant matures, reflexive behavior is secondary to localization behavior. And localization behavior can sometimes be elicited with less intense stimuli. Hardy, Dougherty, and Hardy (1959) and DiCarlo and Bradley (1961), in designing identification hearing tests for young babies, took advantage of the infant's tendency to develop localization behavior. Hardy describes placing an infant on the mother's lap facing an assistant who distracts the infant. An examiner presents stimuli from the back and either side of the infant while watching for localization behavior. The stimuli are various noisemakers categorized according to predominant frequency and presented at approximately 40 dB.

DiCarlo and Bradley (1961) designed a two-room system with four loudspeakers in the subject room placed at 90-degree azimuths. The infant, when placed in its mother's lap directly in the center of the room, could be presented with controlled stimuli through any of the loudspeakers. The desired behavioral response was localization to the activated speaker. They did accept other responses, however.

Some researchers have developed test protocols designed to strengthen and increase the frequency of the localization response. These approaches have rewarded localization behavior with a variety of attractive reinforcers.

Conditioned Orientation Reflex Audiometry

Introduced by Suzuki and Ogiba (1961), the conditioned orientation reflex audiometry (CORA) procedure required the pairing of a sound-field pure tone with a visual stimulus (lighted doll) during an initial conditioning period. The pure tones and visual stimuli emanated from various positions around the test suite. As the child became conditioned to turn its head and eyes toward the stimulus speaker, the light/toy no longer accompanied the tone except as an occasional visual reinforcer. Using a population of 250 children, Suzuki and Ogiba investigated the effectiveness of the CORA procedure in conditioning the children to respond. They found that only 44 percent of the children under 1 year of age could be conditioned, while 85 percent of the 1-year-old infants and 87 percent of the 2-year-old infants could be successfully conditioned. Children 3 years and older did not maintain interest in the test, and the conditioning was unsuccessful. However, the major significance of the test was its simplicity of design and the idea that an orientation response could be strengthened by a reward. Many clinicians and researchers were stimulated to develop and refine the technique and the reward. One aspect of the procedure needing refinement was the sound-field mode of stimulus presentation. This technique does not permit measurement of each ear and measures only the better ear unless one ear is plugged. Also, since Suzuki and Ogiba had the speakers at only 45-degree azimuths relative to the subject, the localization responses were poorly defined and the recording of responses was highly subjective.

Horner (1967), unsatisfied with better-ear, sound-field responses, placed the infant on the mother's lap at 90 degrees to an attractive plastic doll that could be illuminated by an enclosed light. Utilizing a bone vibrator that could be activated at tactile intensities, he conditioned the child to make a 90-degree head turn when the stimulus was introduced. The doll was illuminated to reward and reinforce the head turn. Once the head turn was conditioned, bilateral bone-conduction thresholds were obtained. Then individual ear-air conduction thresholds were obtained under earphones. The significance of this study was that the procedure guaranteed a linking of the bone-conduction stimulus with the visual reward in children who might be profoundly hearing impaired. In addition, the procedure permitted threshold testing of individual ears under earphones and the introduction of masking. Horner reported that the procedure was successful in obtaining pure-tone audiograms on infants down to 12 months of age but that above two years of age the number of responses necessary for an audiogram could not be maintained.

Visual Reinforcement Audiometry

In an attempt to measure hearing in individual ears using loudspeakers, Liden and Kankkonen (1969) placed a speaker at 15 centimeters from the head and plugged the nontest ear. They used colorful slide pictures to reinforce a response. Four types of responses were listed: spontaneous responses, reflexive behavior, investigatory responses, and orientation responses. No conditioning protocol was described that would ensure that a profoundly hearing-impaired child could link the test stimulus with a consequent colorful slide. These experimenters compared the results of their procedure—called visual reinforcement audiometry (VRA)—with Suzuki and Ogiba's CORA results. They suggest that the two techniques produce the same results on children between the ages of 1 and 4 years but that after age 4, the VRA is the more successful procedure.

Many refinements in VRA have been contributed by the research group at the Child Development and Mental Retardation Center at the University of Washington. Moore, Thompson, and Thompson (1975) investigated auditory localization behavior as a function of reinforcement using a head-turn response. They had four conditions: (1) no reinforcement, (2) social reinforcement (verbal praise, a smile, a pat on the shoulder), (3) simple visual reinforcement of a blinking light behind a red square of plastic, and (4) complex visual reinforcement (animated toy). A complex noise was presented at 70 dB SPL in the sound field. Each of the four groups corresponding to the reinforcement conditions were given 30 stimulus presentations. Results of this systematic study were significant for VRA testing. The animated toy animal excited many more head-turn responses than the simple visual reinforcement (blinking light), which in turn resulted in more responses than social reinforcement, which, in its favor, stimulated more responses than no reinforcement. These results so clearly indicated the advantage of the animated toy as a reinforcer that a second study was done to examine its effectiveness on infants below 12 months of age.

Moore, Wilson, and Thompson (1977), using the animated toy, investigated the reinforcement of a head-turn response on infants under 12 months of age. They divided their population into three groups. Group 1 contained 4-month-old infants, Group 2 contained 5- and 6-month-old infants, and Group 3 combined 7- through 11-month-old infants. Each group contained 20 subjects (10 control subjects with no reinforcement and 10 experimental subjects). Results clearly demonstrated that the animated-toy visual stimulus strongly reinforced the head-turn response for infants 5 through 11 months of age but did not serve as a reinforcement function for children under 5 months of age. The clinical implications of the findings of these two studies are that a simple, easily seen head-turn response can be used for a variety of audiological measures on infants as young as 5 months of age. The type of assessment (threshold or suprathreshold task) is governed by the test paradigm, since the infant is performing a discriminatory task rather than giving a reflexive or startle response.

Expanding on their excellent contributions to the refinement of the VRA test paradigm, Moore and Wilson (1978) of the University of Washington research group, identified four additional considerations. The first was the use of a vote/logic circuit to govern the response interval. During that interval, the test-room examiner and control-room examiner must vote to permit the animation of the reinforcing toy if each judges the infant has responded. The second was to define the role of the test-room examiner in the management of the infant state and the control of potential sources of bias. The third was to devise a way to reduce the infant's tendency to stare at the visual reinforcer while awaiting a new activation. Infants doing this could not give a head-turn response since their heads were already turned. To combat this tendency, Moore and Wilson enclosed the animated toy in a dark smoked-plexiglass box with two small 40-watt light bulbs. When the animated reinforcer was activated, the light bulbs were illuminated and the toy became visible. The fourth improvement involved testing to see how many responses could be elicited before habituation. The research group stimulated 12 six-month-old infants with 50 presentations of complex noise, reinforcing by using either a clear enclosure or the new smoked-glass enclosure. They found that the rate at which the infants responded deteriorated after approximately 30 signal presentations. Thus, a clinical protocol needs to incorporate this finding in order to maximize data gathering on any one test day.

With its studies on normal-hearing infants, the Washington University research group provided many of the keys to a clinical protocol, but it failed to study (or at least report) a conditioning procedure that would be successful on a pathological hearing population whose thresholds are unknown. In 1978, Horner and Horner reported a protocol that used the VRA head-turn response conditioned via a bone-conducted, pure-tone signal presented at tactile intensities. With this procedure it was not necessary to know the infant's pure-tone threshold for conditioning to take place. Furthermore, they reported that transfer of conditioning from the tactile to the acoustic stimulus was a natural, easy process as the intensity of the bone-conducted tone was reduced during threshold search. In 1979, Horner and Horner reported a study using a bone vibrator and earphones on normal-hearing infants between the ages of 5 and 11 months. They used this procedure in an attempt to document the emergence of adult-like threshold intensities by age. The results showed that the youngest group, the 5-month-old infants, were already demonstrating pure-tone, air- and bone-conduction (AC and BC) thresholds within the normal range for adults at 250, 1000, and 4000 Hz. It was also noted that obtaining the three BC and the six AC thresholds (three on each ear at 250, 1000, and 4000 Hz) was not an impossible time-consuming task. Of the infants tested, 22 took two 20-minute sessions and 3 were conditioned and provided thresholds in one 35-minute session; 5 infants could not be conditioned (1 at 5 months, 2 at 7 months, 1 at 9 months, and 1 at 10 months). The significance of this study is that the procedure used can produce the head-turn response in hearing-impaired infants no matter what their auditory thresholds and can thereby permit conditioning. The conditioning is easily transferred to an acoustic stimulus, and individual ears can be tested under phones rather than by the less useful sound-field procedure reported by most researchers.

The head-turn response used in threshold testing has been applied to suprathreshold, speech discrimination measurement by Eilers, Wilson, and Moore (1977). Their procedure, called the visually reinforced infant speech discrimination (VRISD) paradigm, is designed to study developmental changes in discrimination as a function of age. The VRA paradigm remains the same except that one syllable of a contrasting pair is presented at a suprathreshold level (50 dB). The second contrasting syllable is presented initially at a higher intensity level while maintaining the repetition rate. The infant is reinforced for a head turn that has been elicited either by the increased intensity or by the speech-sound difference. Once the infant demonstrates a consistent response, the intensity difference between the contrasting syllables is reduced until they are equal. The infant demonstrates discrimination of the speech sounds when responding correctly 5 out of 6 times. Eilers, Wilson, and Moore (1978) and Eilers, Wilson, and Gavin (1978) have shown that a high percentage of infants between 6 and 14 months of age can be tested for speech discrimination of subtle contrasts using this method. The implications of this procedure for clinical application are exciting. Not only would it be possible (with further refinement) to assess speech discrimination with amplification but also to develop other suprathreshold tests of the auditory abilities of infants 6 months and older.

Summary

Previous paragraphs have dealt with behavioral measures of hearing. Research from the last 10 years has shown that procedures have been developed that yield behavioral thresholds on infants as young as 5 months of age that are equivalent in sensitivity to adult thresholds. Suprathreshold speech discrimination tests have been done on 6-month-old infants. As Fulton (1978) notes, "behavioral measurement is becoming more and more important. It not only reflects how an organism's biologic system processes an incoming signal but also how that organism interrelates that event with all other impinging events and conditions" (p. 228).

Even though behavioral measures are the procedures of choice, at times it is not possible to obtain audiograms or valid response data from BOA on some children. The failure may be due to psychological factors, nervous system immaturity, debilitation because of a disease of the infant's motor pathways (or even incompetent methodology on the part of the audiologist!). When all behavioral methods fail, one must turn to procedures that require less cooperation from the child being tested.

BRAIN-STEM-EVOKED RESPONSE AUDIOMETRY

One such procedure is brain-stem-evoked response (BSER) audiometry. The brain-stem responses to click or tone-pip stimuli are apparently little affected by sleep, sedation, or state of awareness and thus can be used to measure the difficult-to-test. Consequently, in the period since Sohmer and Feinmesser (1970) and Jewett, Romano, and Williston (1970) reported the recording of responses from the human brain stem, there has been an extremely rapid growth in the number of studies utilizing this procedure. The responses are presumed to be the sum of synchronous discharges of many units in a group of auditory pathway nuclei. They are usually recorded from an electrode placed on the vertex and compared to responses from an electrode placed on either mastoid, with another electrode on the contralateral mastoid serving as ground. Jewett and Williston (1971) demonstrated that the normal human response consists of five to seven characteristic vertex positive peaks that occur in the first 9–10 milliseconds following click or tone-pip stimuli. They showed that of these peaks, labeled with Roman numerals I through VII, Wave V was the most prominent and stable feature of the response across subjects (see Figure 1–1).

The audiological application of BSER measurement in neonates and infants is an attempt to estimate hearing thresholds in a population that cannot be tested behaviorally or that yields unreliable behavioral hearing test results. Although clinicians use this technique to predict the type and degree of hearing loss, it must be realized that the BSER is not a hearing response in the perceptual sense. Rather it is the expression of the responsiveness of neuronal elements in the peripheral and brain-stem auditory tract. As indicated by Thomas Fria (1980), a child who cannot integrate sound at the cortical level may yield "normal" BSER results. Moreover, the failure to elicit a BSER does not always indicate hearing loss. Since the synchronous firing of neurons required for the computer-averaged response is not necessary for a normal behavioral response to pure-tone signals, children with normal audiograms may not yield a recordable BSER (Worthington & Peters, 1979). These limitations on the relationship of a

Figure 1–1 Characteristic Example of the Brain-Stem Response Elicited by High-Intensity Clicks in a Normal Human Subject

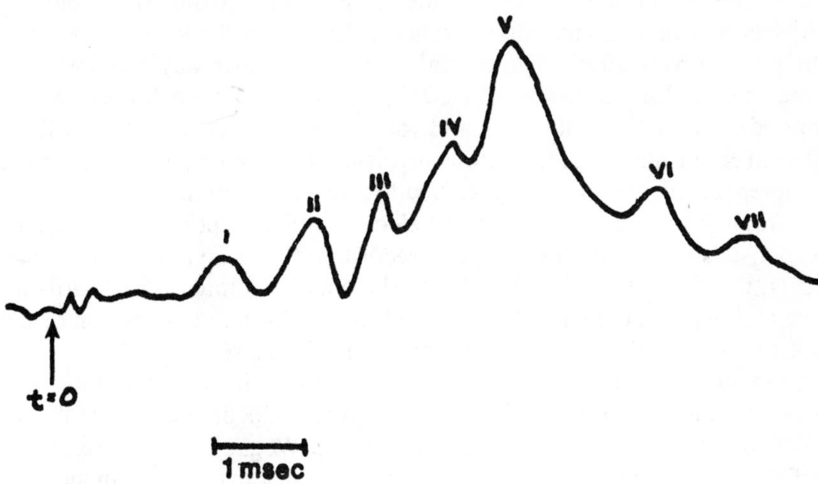

Source: Adapted from Jewett and Williston, 1971.

BSER to hearing thresholds notwithstanding, the technique is still a valuable contribution to the evaluation of a pediatric population's auditory system. When the results are interpreted together with related information, such as case history, physical findings, behavioral audiometric results, and the results of other tests, they permit earlier identification and measurement of hearing loss and consequent intervention.

AUTONOMIC RESPONSE AUDIOMETRY: EDR, EKR, AND RESPIRATION RESPONSE

Through the years, while searching for a hearing test procedure that will permit measurement of hearing thresholds in neonates and young infants, investigators have turned to the changes in the autonomic nervous system that accompany a hearing response. An example of such a change is the electrodermal response (EDR), or the change in skin conductivity as a result of increased sweat-gland activity accompanying an excitation of the nervous system by some stimulus. The EDR is highly sensitive to all sensory stimulation as well as to internal or ideational stimuli. Fear, apprehension, anticipation, or any of the arousal feelings result in an EDR. To enhance the response to auditory stimulation for the purposes of hearing testing, a noxious unconditioned stimulus such as electric shock is associated with the test stimulus in a classical Pavlovian conditioning procedure. This conditioned EDR is quite successful in yielding thresholds on children as young as 4 months (Bordley & Hardy, 1949). However, because the procedure is often unsuccessful when testing mentally retarded children (Irwin, Hind, & Aronson, 1957; Moss, Moss, & Tizard, 1961), brain-injured children (Sortini, 1960), and young nonverbal children (Barr, 1955; Statten & Wishart, 1956), it is not surprising that audiologists have turned to other techniques for young, difficult-to-test populations.

One such procedure measures the electrocardiac response or EKR. This response is frequently measured by recording the interval between heartbeats, the absolute heartbeat rate, or the change in rate of the heartbeat. The technique is dependent on the fact that, prior to a contraction of the heart muscle, a bioelectric impulse passes to the heart and can be detected by sensitive surface (skin) electrodes. A change in the heart rate with presentations of auditory stimuli has been well documented (Schulman, 1970; Schulman & Wade, 1970; Zeamen & Wegner, 1956). Eisenberg (1975) has developed and used the procedure most extensively in measuring the suprathreshold responses of neonates to speech-like stimuli. As one of the most positive advocates of the technique, Eisenberg (1974) states that cardiac measures of audition are potentially important but that the test parameters of the technique still need defining. Schulman, Smith, Weisinger, and Faye (1970) demonstrated a poor correlation of threshold results when they compared the electrocardiac response with averaged electroencephalic responses and behavioral responses of three neonates, five infants, and six young children who had some type of disorder that may have included an auditory disorder. On the other hand, Schulman (1970) found auditory response levels at approximately normal levels in a study of 24 children between 3 weeks and 13 years of age. In this study, Schulman concluded that heart-rate change is a sensitive measure of auditory function and is a feasible technique for clinical application.

It is obvious from the inconsistent research findings that the audiologist who plans to use the electrocardiac response for auditory threshold measurement on a clinical population should first gather normative data on normal-hearing neonates and infants.

Another benign, noninvasive technique with potential for testing auditory sensitivity is respiration audiometry. First described by Rousey, Snyder, and Rousey (1964), this technique has been utilized recently by Bradford (1975) to test neonates' and infants' pure-tone thresholds. The procedure relies upon alterations in the child's respiration pattern following the onset of an acoustic stimulus. These alterations are detected by a sensitive bellows pneumograph that is positioned with the accordion-pleated bellows around the trunk of the infant in such a way that it expands and contracts maximally as respiration takes place. These respiratory changes are recorded on a strip chart along with a marker indicating the onset and duration of the tonal stimuli. Bradford states that a respiratory response will be noticed as one of three characteristic patterns, which he labels as "jamming," "flattening," or "amplitude reduction " and which take place on the inspiration immediately following the onset of the tonal stimulation. These characteristic alterations in respiration are said to be distinguishable from normal respiration patterns. Unfortunately for audiologists, neonates and infants have a tendency toward movement, crying, and verbalizing unless asleep. And, although Bradford reports good results on sleeping infants, most clinic schedules do not have the flexibility to wait for a child to fall asleep before testing. If not asleep, each movement of the child is recorded on the strip chart and masks respiratory alteration responses.

Unfortunately, respiration audiometry suffers from most of the problems associated with any technique that is dependent on a response governed by the autonomic nervous system. The reason is that the response can be elicited by so many other stimuli in addition to the desired acoustic one. External stimuli, internal stimuli, and even ideational stimuli can initiate a change in skin resistance, heart rate, or respiration pattern. Consequently, though conditions may be carefully controlled, many infants will not be testable by these procedures. Unfortunately, the "failures" will probably be those same infants whose responses on other tests are perplexing.

TYMPANOMETRY AND STAPEDIAL REFLEX TESTING

Although tympanometry and stapedial reflex tests are not tests of hearing, any text dealing with measurement of auditory systems would be incomplete if these tests were not mentioned. It is beyond the scope of this chapter to repeat the excellent descriptions of these techniques in detail when full chapters, and even whole books, have been published on them (Feldman & Wilbur, 1976; Jerger, 1975; Northern & Downs, 1978). However, a brief description is included to illustrate the principles of these valuable techniques.

Both tympanometry and stapedial reflex testing rely upon an instrument that, through a probe sealed in a person's ear canal, can introduce a known quantity of sound. The amount of sound remaining in the sealed canal and not passing beyond the tympanic membrane into the middle ear can also be measured via a microphone and bridge circuit attached to the probe.

Tympanometry is a procedure by which we can determine how much energy the middle ear and tympanic membrane transmit to the inner ear, or how resistive they are to this transmission, when the air pressure in the closed cavity of the canal is modified from about 200–400 mm H_2O. The sound level within the closed canal is continuously plotted as the air pressure is changed. This procedure results in a graph representing the compliance of the middle-ear system to the passage of acoustic energy when it is stressed by positive pressure, then gradually stressed less and less under diminishing air pressure, and then increasingly stressed by a negative pressure (or a vacuum). The resultant graph in the normal ear looks like a pointed mountain peak with the peak appearing at ambient air pressure while the slopes fall away at both sides as the tympanic membrane is stressed by increasing positive or negative canal air pressure. The peak represents the point of maximum compliance and of maximum acoustic energy flowing through the middle ear. Figure 1–2 is a schematic representation, demonstrating a normal tympanogram.

Figure 1–2 A Schematic Representation Demonstrating a Normal Tympanogram *

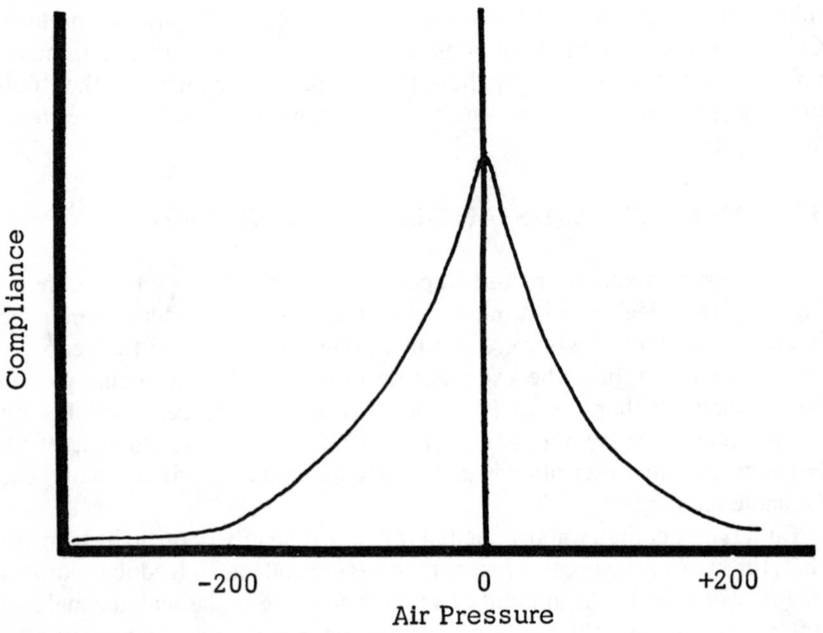

*Maximum compliance falls at ambient air pressure.

Tympanograms of pathological middle ears also have relatively typical configurations whose shapes reflect the changes in the physical transmission characteristics of the system. For example, a middle ear whose pathology is negative air pressure resulting from a nonfunctioning Eustachian tube might have a normal-appearing compliance peak, but it would be displaced on the tympanograph so that the peak would appear at the negative pressure point identical to the negative pressure in the middle ear. Thus the tympanogram demonstrates that compliance in this example is normal when the pressure is equalized on both sides of the tympanic membrane. Figure 1–3 illustrates the tympanogram of an ear with significant negative middle-ear air pressure without effusion.

With the increased use of tympanometry for diagnostic purposes, audiologists have come to recognize many other tympanographic patterns indicative of the changes in transmission characteristics caused by various pathologies of the middle ear. Thus, interpretations of tympanograms have

Figure 1–3 A Schematic Representation of a Tympanogram of an Ear with Significant Negative Middle-Ear Pressure without Effusion *

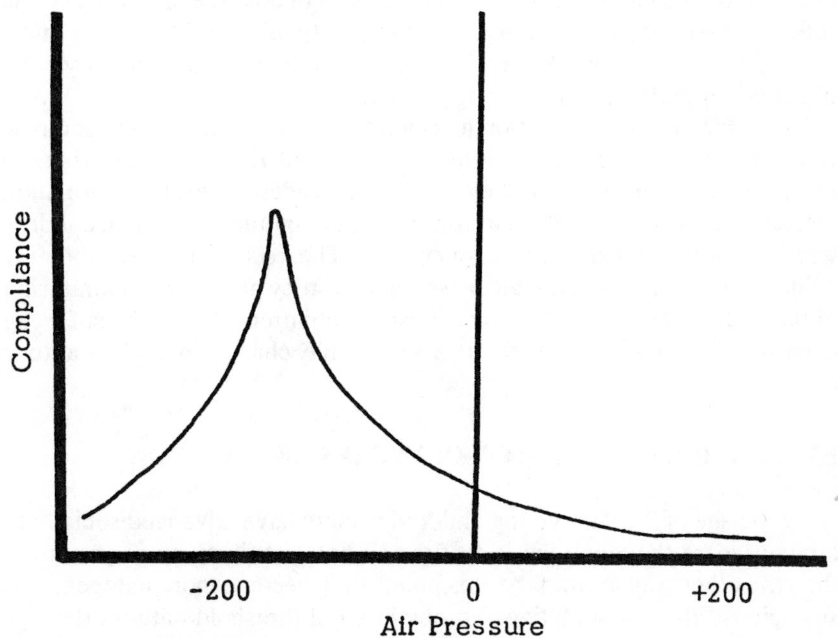

*Maximum compliance falls at – 150 mm H_2O.

added considerable accuracy to evaluations of the auditory systems of nonresponsive or difficult-to-test infants and children.

Utilizing the same probe tube sealed in a person's external canal with a low-frequency probe tone transmitted into this closed cavity, a person's stapedial reflex can be measured. This reflex of the middle-ear stapedius muscle is elicited by introducing an intense acoustic stimulation to either ear, puffs of air about the eyes, tactile stimulation about the face, or galvanic shock to the ear canal. Introduction of a 70–100 dB HL pure tone between 500–4000 Hz in normal ears results in a bilateral change in compliance as a result of this stapedius muscle contraction, which stiffens the middle-ear transmission system. This contraction and resultant stiffening may also be measured at lower intensities for various broad- and narrow-band noises. The benefits to the audiologist of observing a stapedial reflex to acoustic stimulation are considerably greater than if a reflex is absent. Its presence indicates the relative intactness of the complex network of auditory-tract and facial-nerve-tract synapses in the brain stem; of the facial nerve itself, at least down to the sprig innervating the stapedius muscle; of the attachments of the stapedius muscle; and of the middle-ear vibratory system itself. Since the entire system is complex, the absence of an observable reflex is a much less definitive sign and could be the result of a variety of factors. Nevertheless, presence or absence of an observable reflex in response to the above-mentioned stimuli provides much information when used in conjunction with audiological data, history, and observation of the individual being tested.

Even from a brief description it is clear that tympanometry and acoustic reflex testing are valuable additions to clinical test batteries. Using a physical monitoring system, they can yield considerable useful information concerning the status of the auditory system of infants and young children without requiring extensive cooperation. The techniques are not only valuable for original audiological assessment, they also permit monitoring of the middle-ear status of hearing-impaired children who can be suffering from middle-ear disease without a noticeable change in their auditory responsiveness.

EVALUATING CHILDREN OVER 2 YEARS OF AGE

By the age of 2 years, young children usually have advanced socially to a point where they may try to test the audiologist (in many ways) rather than the other way around. At this point, they become more independent, suspicious, and manipulative. To obtain valid threshold data on this age group requires all the skill and "clinicianship" an audiologist can muster. The children are now mobile and often will be up out of their chairs quickly while the audiologist is in midair in the process of sitting down. This may happen several times until the audiologist finds a way to keep the children in place until the audiologist is seated. While it was a purposeful and desirable technique to keep infants younger than 2 years of age in a semibored state so that the test stimuli and the associated rewards would be welcomed, children of 2 years and older usually cannot tolerate boredom. If bored, these children will reject the test situation. Consequently, test protocols like visual reinforcement audiometry will work for only a short period of time before these children give the impression that they are saying, "Okay, what else is new?" Since their attention span is short and they are generally very active and inquisitive, tests for this age group should permit some active physical participation beyond the head turn as a response. Reinforcements of the response may have to be changed frequently. If the reinforcement/reward is animation of a toy, the toy may have to be exchanged frequently. If the reinforcement/reward is a game where tokens, toys, light pegs, or similar things are accumulated or passed through a child's possession, these may have to be varied. But it is important that the response itself remains the same regardless of changes in reinforcement/rewards. A hand-raising or a manipulandum button-pushing response should be continued no matter what the change in reinforcement/reward.

Concerns in Audiological Assessment of Children 2 to 5 Years of Age

The concern for infants below 2 years is to obtain any information regarding their audiologic processing system which it is possible to get. This usually results in learning something about their hearing sensitivity. For many of these infants, one can only make statements like, "Hearing thresholds are no worse than. . . .", and, "Hearing loss does (or does not) contribute to this child's lack of speech and language development." For infants and children 5 months of age and older, a pure-tone audiogram can often be obtained. When this is possible, planning for medical intervention or educational management becomes much more precise. Children over 2 years of age, more often than not, yield such threshold data but also provide the opportunity for speech discrimination and other central processing tests. These suprathreshold tasks become more feasible as children grow more mature and develop more speech and language.

Audiological Tests for Evaluating Children 2 to 5 Years of Age: Conditioned Behavior Audiometry

By the time children are 2 years of age or older, the relatively unrewarding BOA technique will rarely have to be utilized and most children are able to be tested by some form of CBA. By this age, the VRA technique has also become boring for most children, and another form of conditioned behavior should be used. Children throughout this age range still enjoy the appearance of the animated toy in the plexiglass box but need to participate in the test more than by giving a head turn. One test protocol that permits this participation was introduced by Wilson and Decker (1976). This technique, called visually reinforced operant conditioning audiometry (VROCA), is essentially like the tangible reinforcement operant conditioning audiometry (TROCA) design of Lloyd (1966), with a visual reward such as an animated toy substituted for the tangible reward of edibles or tokens. Both techniques are button-pushing designs in which the child is conditioned to respond to the test stimulus by pressing a manipulandum within a specified time span after stimulus onset. If the response occurs within the time span, the child's response is reinforced by the visual or tangible reward. Although the procedure is initially more time-consuming than VRA, once the child is under stimulus control, conditioning is maintained quite well.

Stimuli used in the above procedures can be varied to yield information regarding the child's auditory processing abilities. Pure-tone threshold tests by air conduction can demonstrate the child's sensitivity for various frequencies and allow predictions of function. With pure-tone thresholds by bone conduction (or with results of impedance tests), the frequency response characteristics of the child's ear provide information regarding the status of the middle ear as well as the inner ear. With speech stimuli, tests of central function are more and more feasible as the child develops speech and language.

Another form of CBA that has been around for many years is the technique called play audiometry. In this procedure, the child is permitted to engage in some play activity as a response to each stimulus presentation. The activity is usually some repetitive procedure, such as putting rings on a peg, building block towers, putting pegs in holes, or the like. Although good audiometric data can be obtained with the procedure of play audiometry, the value of the information is quite often in direct proportion to the clinical ability of the audiologist and the cooperativeness of the child. The dilemma of play audiometry is perhaps best stated by Fulton (1978):

> Play audiometry is probably often used because children who are initially shy and withdrawn can more easily be engaged in play activity. Most clinicians, however, assume this display of extraverted behavior to be a resolution of the problem. It is not uncommon for clinicians to obtain the play behavior, then find themselves unable to control random playing. Thus the clinician must

> resort to a subjective judgment that "this play" is related to the signal presented but "that play" is not related. This procedure fosters a paradoxical state—a child is instructed to engage in a behavior he finds enjoyable, but then, because he enjoys it and begins playing when the clinician does not want him to, he is punished. (p. 217)

Many clinicians have found themselves in the situation Fulton describes, and yet the success rate for the play procedure has been respectable. More often than not, however, the success was due to a good clinician rather than to a good procedure.

As the child in the age group under discussion becomes more mature, play audiometry can be discarded for a more conventional hand-raising or button-pushing response and audiometry. This procedure simply requires the child to indicate hearing the stimulus by raising a hand, pushing a response button, or merely stating, "I hear it." When a child is mature enough to cooperate with this procedure, social reward in the form of praise can often maintain the response. However, it behooves the clinician to work rapidly, or the child will terminate the test session. If the child does refuse to go on, every effort should be made to obtain one more response of some sort so that the clinician can be the one to terminate the session, if at all possible. Hopefully, the final response can be followed by praise, perhaps a tangible reward, and a feeling in the child of positive accomplishment. If this can be managed, the test session on the next clinic visit will have a better chance of success.

Many variations of conditioned behavior audiometry have been developed and used successfully. The advantage of this protocol is that the good clinician can design a procedure that is tailor-made for an individual child and still adhere to an adequate psychophysical technique.

AUDIOLOGICAL TESTS AND PROCEDURES USED IN THE COMPREHENSIVE SERVICES PROGRAM

For infants newborn to 4 months of age, the Comprehensive Services Program relies heavily on the case history, developmental signs, and the various BOA hearing test procedures. It is not that brain-stem-evoked response tests and autonomic nervous system tests are not used if necessary. It is just that behavioral results are believed to provide information more relevant to the prediction of behavioral function than do electrical potential changes or modifications of heart rate, respiration, or skin resistance. Of course, in difficult-to-measure infants, every test in our armamentarium could be utilized.

The purpose of the audiological test results is threefold: first, to determine if there is a medically reversible hearing loss or pathology present; second, to determine whether a hearing aid is necessary for speech and language development; and, third, to determine the need for educational intervention. Many infants can be saved from hearing loss and a life of special education if their reversible condition is detected early enough (in the first few months of life) and medical and/or educational intervention is begun. Consequently it behooves every professional specialty associated with a pediatric population to be aware of the consequences of "waiting until the child is a little older" and to realize that persons of virtually *any* age can be given a hearing test.

At the age of 4 to 5 months, an infant seen in the Comprehensive Services Program will be given a pure-tone hearing test by air conduction and bone conduction, using the VRA approach. The audiogram thus generated will be put together with results from tympanometry, acoustic reflex testing, and the case history. In most instances, this will provide all the necessary audiological data, but, if it does not, BSER testing will be performed as the next test of choice.

Since the VRA protocol of the Comprehensive Services Program has not yet appeared in print in specific detail, it is described in the following paragraphs.

Instrumentation

A clinical pure-tone audiometer used to produce the pure-tone stimuli is located in one room of a two-room, double-walled audiometric test suite. An electrically animated toy reward is located in the subject's room of the test suite. When the lights are off in its chamber, the toy is obscured from view by a thick, dark plexiglass box. When the lights in the plexiglass box are turned on, the toy suddenly appears and becomes animated. This visual reinforcer is located at eye level and 90 degrees to the right of the infant's line-of-sight so that the child has to turn both head and eyes for a response. Several toys are available, so the reward can be changed to renew interest.

Procedure

In a test booth the infant is held on the parent's lap (or the clinical aide's lap if necessary), faced at right angles to the reinforcement stimulus. A few enticing, colorful toys are placed on a table separating the clinician from the parent and child. As soon as possible, without restraining the child unduly, a bone vibrator is placed on one mastoid of the child, with instructions to the parent not to permit the infant to remove it. The parent is asked not to speak to the infant or to react to any sounds that might be heard. The clinician attempts to distract the infant immediately so that the bone vibrator is forgotten. A relatively calm unhurried atmosphere is generated by the clinician, keeping the child in a mildly bored, but not uphappy, emotional state if possible.

Then the child is conditioned with a bone-conducted tone at 250 Hz at a tactile level of at least 25–40 dB HTL. A 7-second tone is presented. After 4 seconds, the animated toy reward is activated for approximately 3 seconds, with simultaneous termination of tone and toy. This procedure is continued until the child gives two consecutive head- and eye-turn responses to the tone before onset of the toy. After conditioning, a threshold search for best bone-conduction responses begins at −10 dB HTL at 250 Hz, ascending in 5-dB steps until a response occurs. After each response, the signal level is attenuated 10 dB and another ascent begun. This procedure is continued until the lowest three responses on the ascent are obtained. The same three frequencies are tested under phones for each ear. Silent control periods are interspersed among the tonal presentations to ensure the validity of the responses and to assess the number of random head and eye turns.

In a study reported by Horner and Horner (1979), this protocol yielded thresholds within normal adult ranges for 22 infants 5 to 11 months of age in two 20-minute sessions. Three infants were able to complete the tests in one 35-minute session.

The VRA procedure described above is generally successful on most children up to and sometimes exceeding 2 years of age. However, when a child's interest in the VRA procedure fades or if the child is too active, it is an easy transition to switch to the VROCA procedure. In this procedure, the details of conditioning using the bone vibrator at tactile intensities are essentially the same except that the child is conditioned to respond by pushing the button of the manipulandum instead of making a head turn. This is accomplished by illuminating a light under the manipulandum striking surface when the test tone is initiated. An assistant leads the child's hand to press the button that activates the animated toy. Thus rewarded for a response, the child must then learn that button pushing is rewarded only when the manipulandum light and the test tone are present. Once the child is conditioned to this combination, the light within the manipulandum is dimmed until the test tone is the only signal that a reward is available. After this is accomplished, the ascending threshold search is begun and the protocol that was established for the VRA procedure is followed.

Quite often the VROCA procedure will be sufficient for any age group up to and including those children who are usually tested by play audiometry or conventional hand-raising audiometry. Naturally, if the child is extremely difficult to test, other behavioral tests such as TROCA will be used. The TROCA protocol is the same as the VROCA procedure but substitutes a tangible reward for the animated toy visual reward. The TROCA procedure is generally kept as a last resort in the behavioral battery of tests because it is often quite time-consuming. When results from behavioral procedures are not forthcoming, BSER is the test of choice.

SUMMARY

In the past 10 years great strides have been taken in the development of behavioral and electrophysiologic procedures to measure auditory function. Whereas 10 years ago we felt fortunate to obtain a pure-tone audiogram on a child 2 years of age, today we succeed in this task with many infants only 5 months of age. Indeed, much information regarding auditory system function can be gained on infants even younger than 5 months of age. The next few years should see us obtaining equivalent data on infants as young as newborn. As professionals dealing with pediatric populations realize that infants can yield precise information regarding their auditory systems, they can begin referring infants at earlier and earlier ages. This can only result in more effective intervention as we learn more about infant audition, language, and speech development.

REFERENCES

Barr, B. Pure-tone audiometry for preschool children. *Acta-Oto-Laryngologica,* 1955, *121,* 89–94. (Supplement)

Batkin, S., Groth, H., Watson, J. R., & Ansberry, M. Effects of auditory deprivation on the development of auditory sensitivity in albino rats. *Electroencephalography and Clinical Neurophysiology,* 1970, *28,* 351–359.

Bordley, J. E., & Hardy, W. G. A study in objective audiometry with the use of a psychogalvanic response. *Annals of Otology, Rhinology and Laryngology,* 1949, *58,* 751–759.

Bradford, L. J. Respiration audiometry. In L. J. Bradford (Ed.), *Physiological measures of the audio-vestibular system.* New York/San Francisco/London: Academic Press, 1975.

Clopton, B. M., & Winfield, J. A. Effect of early to patterned sound on unit activity in rat inferior colliculus. *Journal of Neurophysiology,* 1976, *39,* 1081–1089.

DiCarlo, L. M., & Bradley, W. H. A simplified auditory test for infants and young children. *Laryngoscope,* 1961, *71,* 628–646.

Downs, M. P., & Sterritt, G. M. Identification audiometry for neonates: A preliminary report. *Journal of Auditory Research,* 1964, *4,* 69–80.

Eilers, R. E., Wilson, W. R., & Gavin, W. *Linguistic experience and phonemic perception in infancy: A cross-linguistic study.* Manuscript submitted for publication, 1978.

Eilers, R. E., Wilson, W. R., & Moore, J. M. Developmental changes in speech discrimination in infants. *Journal of Speech and Hearing Research,* 1977, *20,* 766–780.

Eilers, R. E., Wilson, W. R., & Moore, J. M. Speech discrimination in the language-innocent and the language-wise: A study in the perception of voice-onset-time. *J. Child Language,* 1978, *20,* 766–780.

Eisenberg, R. Auditory vigilance in neonates. Unpublished presentation at a symposium at the University of Virginia, 1979.

Eisenberg, R. B. Measurement of sensory capabilities. In R. E. Stark (Ed.), *Sensory capabilities of hearing-impaired children.* Baltimore: University Park Press, 1974.

Eisenberg, R. B. Cardiotachometry. In L. Bradford (Ed.), *Physiological measures of the audio-vestibular system.* New York: Academic Press, 1975.

Eisenberg, R. B. *Auditory competence in early life.* Baltimore/London/Tokyo: University Park Press, 1976.

Eisenberg, R. B., Griffin, E. J., Coursin, D. B., & Hunter, M. A. Auditory behavior in the human neonate: A preliminary report. *Journal of Speech and Hearing Research,* 1964, *7,* 245–269.

Ewing, I. R., & Ewing, A. G. *Opportunity and the deaf child.* London: University of London Press, 1947.

Feldman, A. S., & Wilbur, L. A. (Eds.). *Acoustic impedance and admittance—the measurement of middle ear function.* Baltimore: Williams and Wilkins, 1976.

Fria, T. J. The auditory brain stem response: Background and clinical applications. *Monographs in Contemporary Audiology,* 1980, *2,* 2.

Fulton, R. T. Pure-tone tests of hearing-age one year through five years. In F. N. Martin (Ed.), *Pediatric audiology.* Englewood Cliffs, N.J.: Prentice-Hall, 1978.

Gerber, S., & Mencher, G. Supplementary statement of Joint Committee on Infant Screening. In S. Gerber and G. Mencher (Eds.), *Proceedings of the Saskatoon Conference on Early Diagnosis of Hearing Loss.* New York/San Francisco/London: Grune and Stratton, 1978.

Hardy, J. B., Dougherty, A., & Hardy, W. G. Hearing responses and audiologic screening in infants. *Journal of Pediatrics,* 1959, *55,* 382–390.

Holm, V., & Kunze, L. Effects of chronic otitis media on language and speech development. *Pediatrics,* 1969, *43,* 833–839.

Horner, J. P., & Horner, J. S. (Producers). *A pure-tone threshold protocol for infants ages 4½–11½ months.* Videotape presented at ASHA convention, San Francisco, 1978.

Horner, J. S. *Modifications of COR audiometry in pure-tone threshold testing of infants.* Paper presented at SHAV convention, Charlottesville, Va., 1967.

Horner, J. S., & Horner, J. P. *Pure-tone earphone and BC thresholds on 5–11 month infants.* Paper presented at ASHA convention, Atlanta, Ga., 1979.

Irwin, J. V., Hind, J. E., & Aronson, A. E. Experience with conditioned GSR audiometry in a group of mentally deficient individuals. *Training School Bulletin,* 1957, *54,* 26–31.

Jerger, J. (Ed.). *Handbook of clinical impedance audiometry.* New York: American Electromedics Corp, 1975.

Jewett, D. L., Romano, M. N., & Williston, J. S. Human auditory evoked potentials; Possible brain stem components detected on the scalp. *Science,* 1970, *167,* 1517–1518.

Jewett, D. L., & Williston, J. S. Auditory-evoked far fields averaged from the scalp of humans. *Brain,* 1971, *94,* 681–696.

Keating, L. W., & Olsen, W. O. Practical considerations and applications of middle-ear impedance measurements. In D. Rose (Ed.), *Audiological assessment* (2nd ed.). Englewood Cliffs, N.J.: Prentice-Hall, 1978.

Liden, G., & Kankkonen, A. Visual reinforcement audiometry. *Acta Otolaryngologica* (Stockholm), 1969, *67,* 281–292.

Ling, D. *The educational and general background of children with defective hearing.* Thesis, Cambridge University Institute of Education, Cambridge, Mass., 1959.

Lloyd, L. L. Behavioral and audiometry viewed as an operant procedure. *Journal of Speech and Hearing Disorders,* 1966, *31,* 128–136.

Lloyd, L. L., & Young, C. E. Pure-tone audiometry. In R. Fulton & L. Lloyd (Eds.), *Audiometry for the retarded with implications for the difficult-to-test.* Baltimore: Williams and Wilkins, 1969.

McGinn, M. D., Willot, J. F., & Henry, K. R. Effects of conductive hearing loss on auditory evoked potentials and audiogenic seizures in mice. *New Biology,* 1973, *244,* 255–256.

Mencher, G. Prologue, the Saskatoon conference: A perspective. In S. Gerber & G. Mencher (Eds.), *Proceedings of the Saskatoon Conference on Early Diagnosis of Hearing Loss.* New York/San Francisco/London: Grune and Stratton, 1978.

Moore, J. M., Thompson, G., & Thompson, M. Auditory localization of infants as a function of reinforcement conditions. *Journal of Speech and Hearing Disorders,* 1975, *40,* 29–34.

Moore, J. M., & Wilson, W. R. Visual reinforcement audiometry (VRA) with infants. In S. Gerber and G. Mencher (Eds.), *Proceedings of the Saskatoon Conference on Early Diagnosis of Hearing Loss.* New York/San Francisco/London: Grune and Stratton, 1978.

Moore, J. M., Wilson, W. R., & Thompson, G. Visual reinforcement of head-turn responses in infants under 12 months of age. *Journal of Speech and Hearing Disorders,* 1977, *42,* 328–334.

Moss, J. W., Moss, M., & Tizard, J. Electrodermal response audiometry with mentally defective children. *Journal of Speech and Hearing Research,* 1961, *4,* 41.

Needleman, H., & Menyuk, P. Effects of hearing loss from recurrent otitis media on speech and language development. In B. Jaffe (Ed.), *Hearing loss in children.* Baltimore: University Park Press, 1977.

Northern, J. L., & Downs, M. A. *Hearing in children* (2nd ed.). Baltimore: Williams and Wilkins, 1978.

Rousey, C. L., Snyder, C., & Rousey, C. Changes in respiration as a function of auditory stimuli. *Journal of Auditory Research,* 1964, *4,* 107–114.

Rubel, E. Personal communication, 1980.

Rubel, E. W., Parks, T. N., Smith, D. V., & Jackson, H. Experiential afferent influences and development in the avian N. Magnocellularis and N. Laminaris. Paper presented at the 17th International Congress of Ornithology, 1978.

Schulman, C. A. Heart rate response habituation in high-risk premature infants. *Psychophysiology,* 1970, *6,* 690–694.

Schulman, C. A., Smith, C. R., Weisinger, M., & Faye, T. H. The use of heart rate in audiological evaluation of nonverbal children. *Neuropaediatric,* 1970, *2,* 187–196.

Schulman, C. A., & Wade, G. The use of heart rate in the audiological evaluation of nonverbal children: II. Clinical trials on an infant population. *Neuropaediatric,* 1970, *2,* 197–205.

Shepherd, D. C. Pediatric audiology. In D. Rose (Ed.), *Audiological assessment*. Englewood Cliffs, N.J.: Prentice-Hall, 1978.

Silverman, M. S., & Clopton, B. M. Plasticity of binaural interaction: I. Effect of early auditory deprivation. *Journal of Neurophysiology*, 1977, *40*, 1266–1274.

Simmons, F. B., & Russ, F. N. Automated newborn hearing screening, the Crib-o-gram. *Archives of Otolaryngology*, 1974, *100*, 107.

Sohmer, H., & Feinmesser, M. Cochlear and cortical audiometry conveniently recorded in the same subject. *Israeli Journal of Medical Science*, 1970, *6*, 219–223.

Sortini, A. J. Hearing evaluations of brain damaged children. *Volta Review*, 1960, *62*, 536–540.

Statten, P., & Wishart, D. E. S. Pure-tone audiometry in young children: Psychogalvanic skin-resistance and peep show. *Annals of Otology, Rhinology and Laryngology*, 1956, *65*, 511.

Suzuki, T., & Ogiba, T. Conditioned orientation reflex audiometry. *Archives of Otolaryngology*, 1961, *78*, 84–150.

Tees, R. C. Effects of early auditory restriction in rats on adult pattern discrimination. *Journal of Comparative and Physiological Psychology*, 1967, *63*, 389–393.

Webster, D. B., & Webster, M. Neonatal sound deprivation affects brain stem auditory nuclei. *Archives of Otolaryngology*, 1977, *103*, 392–396.

Wedenberg, E. Auditory test on newborn infants. *Acta Otolaryngologica* (Stockholm), 1956, *45*, 5.

Wedenberg, E. Objective audiometric tests on noncooperative children. *Acta Otolaryngologica*, 1963, *175*, 32. (Supplement)

Wishik, S., Kramm, E., & Koch, E. Audiometric testing of school children. *Public Health Report*, 1958, *73*, 265–278.

Worthington, D., & Peters, J. *Quantifiable hearing and no BER: Paradox or error?* Paper presented at ASHA convention, Atlanta, Ga., November 1979.

Zeamen, D., & Wegner, H. Cardiac reflex to tones of threshold intensity. *Journal of Speech and Hearing Disorders*, 1956, *21*, 71–75.

Chapter 2

Hearing Aid Considerations for Preverbal Hearing-Impaired Children

John S. Horner

INTRODUCTION

Amplification systems like hearing aids are a pain in the neck for parents and teachers of hearing-impaired children. How often have we heard these pleas: "How do I know when they are working and when they are not?" "The children change the settings when I am not looking." "They drop them, lose them, break them, spill juice and cereal on them, put 'silly putty' in every orifice, and throw them in the toilet." Unique modes of hearing-aid destruction are being invented each day, yet the serious teacher or parent picks up the hearing aid, wipes it off, drys it out, and starts over. Why do we bother? Perhaps it is because amplification and the use of residual hearing is the single most important avenue to learning for the hearing-impaired infant. This is true even though the hearing aid was chosen for the child under optimal acoustic conditions, using controlled levels of test stimuli, under low levels of distortion and reverberation, and using excellent signal-to-noise ratios. The hearing aid, it has been demonstrated, does not handle transient signal mixtures such as speech and noise with even reasonable fidelity. The classroom, the home, the supermarket, and other "real" situations provide meaningful signals immersed in a sea of clicks, bangs, and roars that are much less than optimal for cognitive processing through the distorting amplifying device. Furthermore, the hearing-impaired child is expected to process low-redundancy, meaningful signals buried in noise using an auditory sensory system that is restricted severely in frequency bandwidth and threshold sensitivity. Consequently, the redundancy of processing elements utilized by the normal-hearing person to function with low-redundancy signals in noise is not available to the hearing-impaired child. Additionally, if the hearing impairment was prelinguistic, the child cannot even make a good guess regarding the meaning of a signal based on past cognition.

Again, why do we even bother to fit a hearing aid on a hearing-impaired youngster if optimum acoustic conditions are critical to truly effective use of this inadequate amplification? Obviously, such a question, given the bleak conditions we have described, cannot have a completely satisfying answer. Yet, simply put, amplification—optimal or less than optimal—is still the best tool we have for neurological development of the auditory nervous system. It is still the best educational route to normal communicative function for most hearing-impaired children, if started in the first 6 months of life.

The main problem of prelinguistic, hearing-impaired children is that their hearing loss restricts the input of the major sensory channel used for reception and expression of oral communication. Although the ideal solution to this problem would be to prevent hearing loss, such a solution may take many more generations of research. Consequently, the underlying premise of this chapter and the Comprehensive Services Program is that early identification and the currently most appropriate fitting of amplification are the most important habilitative aids for prelinguistic, hearing-impaired infants. Since most of these children have considerable residual hearing, proper amplification can permit potential-reaching speech and language development.

Although early identification of hearing loss in infants has become more a reality in the last few years, the provision of a "currently most appropriate" fitting of amplification on a preverbal infant is another matter. With verbal adults, many tests of fitting effectiveness can be performed, and the adult can express satisfaction or concern with a chosen hearing aid. Since the infant cannot provide verbal feedback, however, the audiologist must use other information in the choice of amplification parameters. The successful decisions that have been made on adults can be applied to fittings on children. Such decisions, appropriate for an adult auditory mechanism that in many cases has been normal during language and speech learning periods, can be used to fit infants with immature auditory pathways and little-known processing abilities. In such a situation, the clinical audiologist either can attempt to utilize the best information derived from research literature and to make consistent fitting decisions, improving them as more is learned, or can use a minimal criterion for fitting and essentially "give up." Unfortunately, there are advocates with "proofs" of the effectiveness of both philosophies. Hopefully, as ways are developed to measure the frequency response and sound pressure of the amplified signal reaching of the individual infant's eardrum and as ways are improved to measure the infant's suprathreshold loudness experience, the fitting of personal amplification can be consistent. With this consistency, research can show the way to maximize the effectiveness of amplification in the development of speech and language.

Several steps are basic to the fitting of a hearing aid on a preverbal child. First, it is necessary to quantify the child's hearing sensitivity (preferably for each ear). This information needs to be supplemented, if possible, with other types of hearing measures, such as loudness discomfort levels. The more we are able to quantify the infant's hearing, the more appropriate will be the hearing aid we choose.

Second, we need to define the acoustic properties of the speech signal that will optimize the speech and language learning of a child with the hearing characteristics we have quantified. For example, if the child has hearing out to 4000 Hz, the amplified sould should include that acoustic information, since it has been shown to contribute to speech discrimination (Pascoe, Niemoeller, & Miller, 1973). On the other hand, if an infant has hearing sensitivity restricted to 2000 Hz and below, the acoustic information contained in those frequencies above 2000 Hz should not be sacrificed by choosing an aid with a limited bandwidth. The premise, "if a child cannot hear frequencies above 2000 Hz, why bother to send this acoustic information into the ear?" has reasonable face validity. However, there is little question that the band from 2000 to 6000 Hz contributes greatly to perception. If we choose an aid (such as a transposer aid) that faithfully reproduces the information from the band of 2000 to 6000 Hz by transposing it into a frequency range that can be heard by the child, our chances of ultimately improving the child's communicative function are enhanced.

In the United States, failures of this type of amplification have resulted in its rejection in recent years. However, these failures may well be due to fitting the infant too late rather than to a faulty concept or inadequate instrumentation. With the advent of techniques for early identification of hearing loss and pure-tone threshold quantification in infants as young as 4½ months (Horner & Horner, 1978), a transposer hearing aid can be fitted in the first 6 months of life. Thus, all or most of the acoustic information necessary for the development of speech discrimination can be present in the infant's receptive system during the period when the brain stem is maturing and neural elements are proliferating and refining their function. Even if this hypothesis does not stand the tests of trial, using amplification with a restricted bandwidth that does not reproduce in any way the frequencies above 2000 Hz is "throwing away" meaningful discrimination data. To optimize the speech and language learning of the child whose hearing we have quantified, we must continue to search for an input to the child's sensory system that does not consciously restrict the meaningful information necessary for the eventual development of normal communication.

Third, it is important (in view of the foregoing rationale) to define amplification with the electroacoustic properties that will provide infants with maximal information for the physiologic and discriminatory development of their acoustic sensory systems. Fourth, the adequacy of the criteria for selecting the hearing aid must be evaluated. Finally, the electroacoustic system must be modified and adjusted as we monitor the performance and growth of the infant's use of amplified sound. Aided-sound-field measurements on a monthly basis (at first) will ensure the proper functioning of the amplification when compared to regular electroacoustic analysis of the aid. The child's progress with amplification, however, will be demonstrated or substantiated by the parents and teachers who observe behavioral manifestations in real-life situations, such as in the home, in the preschool, and in outside play. It is only as speech and language develop that we can expect the formal sound-field tests to provide data sufficiently specific to allow dramatic changes in type of amplification. Consequently, those early critical months as the infant is in a rapid growth period must have very careful monitoring by regular specific questionnaires filled out by the child's managing adults. The clinic tests can monitor the hearing aid's electroacoustic function and the infant's otologic stability, but parental and teacher feedback are necessary to assess the effectiveness of the amplification on emerging communicative behavior.

Obviously, such close monitoring of an infant's amplification and communicative development is difficult in many clinical settings. Yet the "I shot an arrow in air, it fell I knew not where" philosophy of hearing aid fitting has been eminently unsuccessful in the past. If we are to achieve an optimum communicative result, we can no longer afford to fit a child with a hearing aid, give the parent some orientation, and send both home until recheck time. It is only within a complete habilitative atmosphere, such as that in the Comprehensive Services Program, that the child has a chance to develop communicative potential. There are too many unknowns, too many advances coming rapidly from research, too many necessary program modifications to permit a child to go home with a lay parent for training, never to be seen again until recheck time. The infant develops rapidly, and since experience apparently has a differential influence on the ontogeny of neuron structure and function (Rubel, Parks, Smith, & Jackson, 1978), the quality of that experience must be regularly monitored and kept optimal. This is not to say that an informed cooperative parent is not essential to successful habilitation. Rather it means that no one of the managing adults—whether it be a professional audiologist, a hearing aid dispenser, a teacher of the hearing impaired, or a parent—is sufficient to manage all the aspects of communicative habilitation if we expect hearing-impaired children to reach their potential.

DEFINING A CHILD'S HEARING

It was not many years ago that audiologists were starting "audiological impressions" on a hearing-impaired youngster with the statements, "Hearing is no worse than __dB. . . " or "Hearing loss is the most probable cause for the lack of speech." These statements reflect the gross definition of the various parameters of hearing resulting from the behavioral observation audiometry (BOA) techniques used to measure hearing on children unable to cooperate with play audiometry. The results of this mode of testing did not permit electroacoustic selection procedures for hearing aids with any semblance of precision. Behavioral selection of a hearing aid also suffered from the lack of precision of BOA procedures. Consequently, the fitting of a hearing aid on a preverbal child became an art practiced by professionals whose success was related to their knowledge, intuition, and "talent." Woe to the infant whose communicative future was entrusted to a "budding artist" or to one of little talent.

Today, fitting of a hearing aid to a preverbal child is still an art. However, a much more accurate definition of the child's hearing is now possible due to the evolution of visual reinforcement audiometry (VRA) and brainstem-evoked response audiometry (BSER). Now, artistry takes over at a much more refined stage of the modification of the fitting rather than at the hearing-measurement stage. Consequently, a refinement of hearing aid fitting that took months (or years) to accomplish 10 or 15 years ago is where many children of today start. The reason for this advance, of course, is that we can now obtain pure-tone thresholds on infants as young as 4½ months of age (Horner & Horner, 1978). For infants younger than 4½ months, BSER data can be correlated with behavioral observations to supply almost equivalent information for the electroacoustic setting of a hearing aid. When acoustic reflex thresholds are available for a child, we can then define the upper power limits of the aid, using a physiologic response correlated with the child's tolerance thresholds.

Whatever the age of the infant and whatever the measurement procedure, it is necessary to define the hearing in several ways. Obviously, the first step is to determine the degree of hearing loss so that we may decide whether amplification will be needed.

Second, is the loss conductive, sensorineural, or mixed? If the child may benefit from medical intervention, there may be no need for a hearing aid. In any case, it is at this step that otologic evaluation and clearance and/or treatment of the child's ears should be arranged. This will contribute to good comprehensive medical care of the hearing impaired and prevent unnecessary fitting of hearing aids to those children whose hearing can be restored medically.

A necessary qualification of the term "medical clearance" should be noted. Too often, when giving medical clearance to wear a hearing aid, physicians feel responsible for making a decision of whether a child needs, or should wear, a hearing aid. This decision is well within the responsibility of the physician if an active or chronic pathology would be aggravated by the use of a hearing aid. However, if the ears are otologically sound, and if the physician is basing the decision and opinion on whether the child needs amplification, the physician is wrong to voice that opinion to the patient or the patient's managing adults. Too many children have had irreparable delays in obtaining amplification because the physician did not fully comprehend the continuing consequences of sensory deprivation during critical physiologic and behavioral development periods. The medical clearance the physician provides should be confined strictly to matters of physical health.

Third, some measurement or estimate of dynamic range is necessary. Thus, in those children in whom the acoustic reflex is present, a physiologic response correlating with tolerance thresholds is measured. In children whose reflex thresholds are absent at the limits of the audiometer, some estimate of tolerance threshold should be obtained by watching for Auro-Palpebral responses, signs of discomfort, and any behavioral indication that tolerance levels are being approached as pure-tone or noise stimuli are increased in intensity. These stimuli should be relatively frequency specific so that the maximum power output (MPO) can be set by prescription.

HEARING-AID SELECTION PROCEDURES

Physical Characteristics of the Hearing Aid

Before considering the electroacoustic characteristics of a hearing aid, one must be concerned with the physical aspects of this wearable electronic box. An aid that is too small, falls off, and emits a whistling, squealing feedback because it drags the earmold loose, is just as useless as a large heavy box of an aid that encumbers the small baby during normal physical play behavior. Whichever aid is chosen, it must have consistent operating characteristics despite the child's conscious or accidental attempts at its destruction. All this strength and stability must be packaged in a container that has physical dimensions appropriate for the size and type of the child's daily activity.

If the aid has a cord, it should be available in a heavy-duty model that resists breaking as a result of flexing. Although cords are dispensable as are batteries, one does not want to replace either one any more often than necessary.

External controls, such as the volume control, tone control, mike/telecoil control, and on/off control, should be sturdy, usable by the child, and clearly labeled. How often has a hearing control been so poorly labeled that you could not tell whether the aid was on or off without listening to it or without making it produce feedback. Internal controls for versatility of gain and MPO adjustment should be available for dispenser or clinic modification of the output. As the child's needs change or as more definitive measurements of the child's auditory system are possible, optimum fitting of amplification becomes more likely, and the aid should have the capability of being modified. Hearing aids and earmolds will have to be replaced often enough as the child's physical size changes without having the additional expense of buying a new hearing aid when an electroacoustic modification is necessary.

Another consideration when selecting a hearing aid for a preverbal child is whether to recommend an in-the-ear, postauricular, or body-type fitting. In the Comprehensive Services Program, an in-the-ear fitting is never used, for some obvious reasons. This type of fitting has severe limitations in control flexibility. Infants go through rapid growth periods requiring regular earmold revision, and this type of fitting cannot be enlarged easily. Such a fitting necessitates a commitment to a particular hearing aid that restricts the possibility of switching hearing aids on a trial basis.

Postauricular fittings would be the ideal choice if it were not for the size of the infant and the infant's life style. These aids, when fitted binaurally, restore the head-shadow effect (Tillman, Kasten, & Horner, 1963), remove the body-baffle effect, and provide the child's developing sensory system with more "normal" cues for speech discrimination in most acoustic environments. Unfortunately, for several reasons, the postauricular aids cannot reasonably be recommended for infants and children below 3 or 4 years of age. As mentioned earlier, the infant's size and life style affect the choice of an optimum hearing aid. Although modern postauricular aids are now sufficiently powerful and have the electroacoustic control flexibility to meet the needs of most hearing-impaired children, the child's short neck and small pinna restrict the use of such a fitting. On really small infants a postauricular aid may even lay on the children's shoulders! Since infants spend much of their time (at first) in the crib, this aid is often rubbing against the mattress or blanket. Consequently, "clothing noise" is a constant reduction of the signal-to-noise ratio.

Another major problem is in the control of feedback. Since the microphone and earphone on a postauricular aid are close together, effective control of acoustic feedback is maintained by proper seating of a tightly fitting earmold in the canal of the user. The infant lying in a crib often displaces the earmold by mattress pressure on the hearing aid. In addition, the infant's ear canal grows quickly in the first few years of life, requiring new earmolds more often when the control of feedback is so critically dependent on a tight earmold-canal seal.

Consequently, for the initial fitting in the Comprehensive Services Program, a body-type fitting is the one of choice. This provides the child and the parent with a durable, flexible aid that can be made to give them their money's worth while learning on an instrument that is easier to adjust and manage.

The final factor to be considered regarding the physical characteristics of the hearing aid is whether a monaural or binaural fitting should be chosen as the initial aid. In the Comprehensive Services Program, a binaural fitting is almost always recommended. Although when using body-type hearing aid fittings, we cannot expect all the binaural advantages that accrue when they are head-borne, we feel we cannot afford to lose the brain-stem interactions from binaural stimulation during physiological development. Consequently, the policy of the Comprehensive Services Program is to make an initial fitting with two separate amplification systems—one for each ear. Although there is no head-shadow effect, these aids are separated on the infant's small body as far as possible so that differential information can reach each ear. When the child reaches 3 to 4 years of age, these body-type instruments are exchanged for postauricular aids to provide more natural binaural conditions. At this time, both the parents and the child are more sophisticated in caring for the hearing aid; the child's pinna and canal are larger, making earmold impressions more accurate; and the child can provide more definitive behavioral responses during fitting procedures. These instruments offer the option of microphone placement near the pinna and reestablish the head-shadow effect for more truly binaural listening.

Naturally, the philosophy of fitting outlined above cannot be adhered to for all children. Yet, the habilitation benefits are hypothesized to be so great for eventual communicative proficiency for the early-identified, hearing-impaired infant that few are managed in any other way. Results of this hearing-aid-fitting philosophy and of others that deviate only slightly (Ross, 1980) should be measurable in the next few years.

Choosing Electroacoustic Parameters of the Hearing Aid

Most audiologists would say that the least enjoyable procedure required by their profession is choosing the electroacoustic parameters of a hearing aid—particularly for a preverbal infant. This attitude is understandable. How many years can a person feel inadequate? How long can you live with frustrating failures because the task you are called upon to perform has what looks like an infinite number of variables? Let us look at the past history of hearing and fitting procedures and determine whether we are showing progress toward the goal of making excellent fittings routine.

Before looking at the history, however, we must consider some relatively self-evident odds and ends that influence hearing-aid fitting. First, few people would argue with the concept that amplified sound must surpass the hearing-impaired child's threshold before it can be perceived. How can you perceive meaningful acoustic information if you cannot hear it? This concept is not as sophomoric as it sounds when you consider that the meaningful acoustic information we are most concerned with is speech—a combination of sounds with constantly changing spectral characteristics covering a range of frequencies from 250 to above 4000 Hz. Consequently, when we say that amplified sound must surpass the hearing-impaired child's threshold before it can be perceived, we are saying that the information used as phonemic or morphemic markers in speech must surpass threshold as well as the peak energies in the speech. Obviously, then, a single gain figure chosen for a hearing aid will not describe whether speech will surpass the hearing impaired's threshold.

Second, the amplified sound should not reach the loudness discomfort level (LDL) for the child. This concept is not so self-evident. It is really not known if sounds at LDLs impair the development of perception of speech in hearing-impaired youngsters. On the other hand, many children reject amplification when it surpasses their LDL; thus, "a hearing aid that is worn is better than one that is not."

Third, all of the acoustic information contained in the speech signal should be presented within the hearing-impaired child's dynamic range—between the sensitivity threshold and the LDL. This concept is also not completely self-evident, although it has great face validity. We know that adults, who know the language, can function quite well with a reduction in the redundancy of the speech signal. Whether acoustic information could be subtracted from the speech signal and still not compromise the learning of a congenitally hearing-impaired child is not known. Research suggests, however, that we cannot afford to eliminate any of the acoustic energy contained in speech. The hearing-impaired child is listening with a damaged auditory system through a low-fidelity electroacoustic instrument, both of which reduce transmission of high frequencies. With regard to the importance of high frequencies, Ross (1980) suggests that the information provided by frequencies of 4000 to 8000 Hz is likely not to be redundant at all but rather minimal cues necessary for developing speech and language skills. This stance is supported by studies performed by Watson (1960), Olson (1971), Pascoe et al. (1973), and Triantos and McCandless (1974).

Fourth, a hearing aid's bandwidth, amplification (gain) at each frequency and maximum power output (MPO), or saturation sound pressure level (SSPL) can be measured with great accuracy in a 2-cc coupler with present-day electroacoustic instrumentation. Since many hearing aids have flexible adjustments of gain, bandwidth, and SSPL, one would think our fitting problems would be solved. We can set the hearing aid gain so that normal speech intensities surpass the hearing-impaired child's thresholds. We can choose a bandwidth to include all important speech frequencies. We can set the SSPL so that the LDL is not surpassed. These adjustments can be accomplished. But, lo and behold, when the hearing aid is coupled to the child's small canal with a space-occupying earmold, the frequency response of the amplification measured at the child's eardrum bears little resemblance to the "ideal" settings derived in the coupler of the hearing-aid test chamber (Niemoeller, McCormick, & Miller, 1974). Furthermore, once a satisfactory fitting has been accomplished, before long the child will need a new earmold. This new mold will usually change the acoustics so much that the hearing aid seems to be a different model.

Finally, as we will see from examining the history of hearing-aid-fitting procedures, little is known about the contribution of various speech frequencies to better perception of speech in the hearing-impaired child's auditory system. To explain, let us first consider the speech signal in a normal unoccluded ear. If we electronically mix the voices of men and women reading from different texts, we find that this long-term average spectrum of speech is remarkably constant (Niemoeller et al., 1974). However, when this spectrum is put into an open ear canal, the perceived frequency response of the averaged speech signal changes so that, instead of perceiving the frequencies as they are present in the impinging speech signal, subjects report the areas of frequency emphasis. These areas lie at about 630 and 2500 Hz (Pascoe, 1978). Furthermore, Pascoe notes that one hearing-impaired subject (reported typical of a group of eight) demonstrated this same perceived two-humped configuration when the listener was tested unaided with an unoccluded ear canal. However, when this listener was tested through a hearing aid, whether the canal was closed with an earmold or fitted without an earmold, the speech spectrum was perceived without the two-humped configuration in a formation typical of hearing-aid frequency responses. The importance of these findings is that this hearing-impaired listener had good unaided speech discrimination but poor aided discrimination (with or without an earmold).

Several questions arise as a result of these findings. Will a two-humped perceived spectrum of speech centering at 630 and 2500 Hz provide an ideal stimuli configuration for optimum perception for all degrees and shapes of hearing impairment? If so, how can we test the preverbal infant's perception to see if the desired spectral result has been obtained? Is long-term, averaged, speech-spectrum "noise" sufficiently typical of conversational speech so that it can be used to set hearing aids? And, will this single test stimulus be appropriate for all varieties of hearing loss configurations? Obviously, some of these questions can be answered immediately from past experience and by recalling the hearing-loss configurations of many congenital hearing-impaired children who apparently can hear no frequencies above 1000 Hz. On the other hand, if the above research can help achieve optimum fittings for some, it needs to be confirmed by more extensive study.

The above concepts that affect hearing-aid-fitting procedures have appeared in one form or another throughout the history of our discipline. In 1940, Watson and Knudsen noted that great claims had been made for selective amplification although little was known about its application to hearing aids. They point out that the claims for this procedure are supported by meager quantitative data. By definition, the term *selective amplification* means that the frequency response of the hearing aid is modified to meet the hearing-impaired subject's presumed needs. Unfortunately, the key phrase here is "subject's presumed needs." As Watson and Knudsen are quick to point out, the fundamental principles of fitting with selective amplification have not been researched. And, although professionals who fit hearing aids intuitively lean toward selective amplification as a rational approach in meeting the hearing-impaired's needs, little agreement has been reached on specifying those needs.

Hearing Aid Gain and Frequency Response

As we have noted, one of the first considerations in providing optimal amplification for the preverbal hearing-impaired child is deciding how much gain the hearing aid should have. *Gain* is defined as the increase in intensity of the signal provided by the hearing aid. For example, if a 50-dB pure tone strikes the microphone of a hearing aid and a 100-dB pure tone is emitted from the earphone, then the hearing aid is said to produce 50-dB gain at that frequency (output minus input equals gain). On the other hand, if a 50-dB speech signal, which consists of many simultaneous frequencies, strikes the microphone of a hearing aid and a 100-dB speech signal is emitted from the earphone, what is the hearing aid's gain? Again the gain is 50 dB, but because of the frequency response of the hearing aid you do not know how the energy is distributed across the various speech frequencies. The 50-dB gain could be "peak gain" representing energy at one frequency, or it could be "average gain" representing the average energy at several frequencies.

The intelligibility of the speech signal will obviously be affected by the distribution of energy. This distribution of energy, or gain at each frequency, is called *frequency response*. Since the goal of even the early hearing aid fitters was to provide energy at all frequencies in the speech range above the hearing-impaired person's thresholds, the concept of using a single gain figure in choosing gain became less attractive than selective amplification. As noted earlier, selective amplification modifies the frequency response or the relative gain at each frequency to meet the hearing-impaired's needs. When we look at the hearing-impaired's audiometric threshold losses, those needs would appear to be obvious. If the hearing-impaired's pure-tone threshold at 1000 Hz is 70 dB worse than normal, it stands to reason that the hearing aid gain should be set to compensate by 70 dB at 1000 Hz. The modification of gain at each of the other frequencies could be based on the same reasoning, and the resulting hearing-aid frequency response would be a perfect mirror image of the person's hearing loss, thus theoretically bringing the person's hearing back to normal by prescription.

Although advocated by some researchers before 1940, and by others even more recently (Reddell & Calvert, 1966), this procedure ignores the fact that the hearing-impaired person's threshold configuration does not describe suprathreshold listening experience. This fact was most dramatically demonstrated by the findings of the research group that produced the well-known Harvard Report (Davis, Steven, Nichols, Hudgins, Marguis, Peterson, & Ross, 1947). These researchers showed that, despite widely disparate threshold configurations, their hearing-impaired subjects demonstrated amazingly similar loudness contours at about 100 dB SPL. Despite the fact that some subjects had flat hearing losses and others had sharply falling hearing losses, the loudness experienced by the subjects, when measured with 1000 Hz at 100 dB SPL as a reference, was apparently alike.

Taking to task the mirroring philosophy of hearing aid fitting, the Harvard research group recommended two concepts that, because they were accepted by many audiologists, set back hearing aid research 10 to 15 years. The first idea was that "the fitting of hearing aids should be based primarily on the maximum acoustic gain required by, and the maximum acoustic output acceptable to, the wearer'' (p. 8). The second, and more devastating idea in terms of research was the Harvard group's recommendation regarding the frequency response of hearing aids. The group's conclusion was that a hearing aid with either a flat or a 6-dB-per-octave rising response was appropriate for the majority of hearing aid users. As an apparent result of this conclusion, little appeared in the professional literature on the subject of selective amplification until the middle 1960s.

Since the mid-1960s, however, there has been increasing interest in at least some form of selective amplification. This has been evidenced by articles, book chapters, and convention reports by such authors as Lybarger (1963), Gengel, Pascoe, and Shore (1971), Berger (1976), Wallenfels (1967), Byrne and Tonnison (1976), Shapiro (1976), and Ross (1980). Although these authors differ somewhat in their approach to hearing aid fitting by selective amplification, several common ideas are present in their rationale in one form or another.

First, each of these researchers, and many other clinicians not cited, have apparently decided that differential emphasis of frequencies within the speech range is most beneficial to the hearing-impaired communicative performance. Second, they appear to have concluded that differential amplification should place speech within the hearing-impaired person's dynamic range somewhere close to the most comfortable listening level (MCL). Some, such as Pascoe (1978), feel that the perceived intensity configuration should have a particular shape. For Pascoe, this is a two-humped configuration with emphasis at approximately 630 and 2500 Hz, which he feels provides better speech discrimination.

Various clinical procedures have been used to adjust the amplification so that it is within the listener's dynamic range. One increasingly popular method is to adjust the hearing aid gain by formula (Berger, 1976; Byrne & Tonnison, 1976; Gengel, et al., 1971; Lybarger, 1963; Shapiro, 1976; Wallenfels, 1967). Some clinicians use a single gain figure to represent the average increase in signal intensity necessary to insert the signal into the hearing-aid user's dynamic range. Others feel that a single gain figure is not precise enough to provide optimum comfort and discrimination. They attempt to adjust the gain at each frequency within the hearing aid's bandwidth. Berger (1976), for example, bases his gain-frequency response formula on the following and other postulates: (1) most speech is in the 55 to 75 dB SPL range, (2) the amplified signal reaching the impaired ear should improve speech intelligibility over that unaided for typical conversational levels, (3) the desired gain will have an average magnitude slightly greater than one-half of the client's pure-tone hearing level, (4) amplification of low-frequency ambient noise is detrimental, (5) less intensity is required at 500 Hz and below than at the frequencies more important to the understanding of speech, and (6) speech sounds above 4000 Hz are extremely weak and relatively unimportant to intelligibility. Thus, it can be seen that, although he includes some generalities regarding the speech spectrum within his formulation, Berger adheres more strongly to the one-half rule for hearing-aid gain fitting. This one-half rule relates to the finding that hearing aid users consistently set their gain control so that they receive 1-dB gain for every 2 dB of their hearing loss (Brooks, 1973). Berger, however, uses his modification of the one-half rule for specific frequencies (500, 1000, 2000, 3000, and 4000 Hz) rather than for an average gain figure, as do some clinicians (Lybarger, 1963).

Trying to relate their gain settings more specifically to the speech spectrum, Pascoe (1978) and Ross (1980) amplify the speech signal to deliver to the hearing aid user the frequencies of speech in proportions of intensity that relate to the long-term spectral characteristics of that speech. Unfortunately for the student of hearing aid fitting, their descriptions of these characteristics differ substantially. Ross describes the following frequency response average at normal conversational intensities (Ross, 1980, p. 224):

250	500	1000	2000	3000	4000
60	60	55	45	40	40

with a range of +12 dB to −18 dB. Pascoe (1978, p. 16), on the other hand, reports the average spectrum at the same normal conversational intensity of 65 dB as:

Frequency:	250	500	1000	1500	2000	3000	4000	6000 Hz
Maximum:	68	71	60	61	62	55	54	50 dB SPL
Mean:	58	61	50	51	52	45	44	40 (third-octave)
Minimum:	48	51	40	41	42	35	34	30 (band levels)

The principle Ross and Pascoe set forth has great face validity; must we not provide all the frequencies of speech in the proper intensity relations to achieve good development of speech discrimination? In his formula, however, Ross still relies on the threshold configuration of the hearing impaired to determine the amount of gain necessary to provide these speech frequencies in the appropriate intensity relations. He starts by using a modification of the one-half rule for his gain estimation, adds this to his version of the long-term spectral characteristics of speech, and determines whether the resulting signal will lie between the child's hearing threshold and the maximum permissible output determined by acoustic reflex thresholds (or estimations, if these thresholds cannot be elicited).

Maybe this is the best we can do? Ross, like most clinicians, determines the "boundaries" of hearing and tosses the amplified sound in the proper intensity proportions within those boundaries so that the "edges" of the stimuli do not touch any of the boundaries. Unfortunately, the boundaries of hearing do not describe a person's experience at suprathreshold sensation levels. Those carefully controlled intensity proportions of the frequency relations in speech may well be lost completely to those unknown loudness functions of a pathological ear. In fact, they probably are, as evidenced by some original research with adults (Davis et al., 1947).

Pascoe (1978) uses a testing procedure that helps to describe the suprathreshold experience of the hearing impaired. He states that "we will have, in fact, all the basic information we need to select a hearing aid" (Pascoe, 1978, p. 16). His procedure is to present monaurally, in field conditions, pulsed third-octave bands of noise. The untested ear is plugged and muffed. The listener is given a five-point scale from which to describe each signal presentation. This scale allows these decisions: (1) very soft; (2) soft, but clear; (3) just right; (4) a little loud, but OK; and (5) too loud, uncomfortable. Intensity levels are repeated often enough during the test to establish consistency. Using the information regarding suprathreshold experience thus derived, Pascoe determines the gain necessary to raise the speech spectrum signal into a comfortable listening level for the hearing-impaired person and maintains the relative intensities of the signal except for the two-humped characteristic at 630 and 2500 Hz, which he feels provides better speech discrimination.

This procedure provides an excellent starting point for adults. Unfortunately, with present audiological techniques, the preverbal infant cannot provide the clinician with judgments of "very soft, soft but clear, just right, and so on. On the other hand, the procedure demonstrates a recognition of the need for measuring and including an individual suprathreshold experience in a hearing-aid gain prescription. And, although it is not a practical procedure with preverbal infants at this time, if Pascoe's protocol results in optimum hearing aid fittings, it may generate research leading to the development of an infant procedure.

Another aspect of hearing-aid gain setting not yet discussed is the post-fitting evaluation of the appropriateness of the electroacoustic system. The need for such an evaluation stems from some facts previously mentioned. As we noted earlier, hearing aid gain, SSPL, and bandwidth can be measured quite accurately and consistently with present-day 2-cc couplers and associated hearing-aid test chambers. This procedure would appear to define the electroacoustic characteristics of the hearing aid for purposes of fitting. However, it has been demonstrated that, when coupled to the ear via an earmold, the carefully chosen electroacoustic characteristics are changed all out of proportion from what one would expect. The obvious solution practiced by many clinicians is to measure the gain,

SSPL, and bandwidth characteristics with the aid coupled to the ear canal by using a tiny miniature microphone inserted into the ear canal close to the eardrum. In this way, the effects of sending the test signals into the confined space of a small ear canal are measured so that modifications necessary to provide the desired signal can be made.

One would think that electroacoustic fitting problems are now solved! With this procedure we know the precise characteristics of the amplified signal reaching the auditory system of the hearing impaired as measured right at the eardrum. Is that not enough? Unfortunately not.

This solution suffers from the same misleading ills inherent in all scientific procedures that attempt to solve the problems of a defective multicomponent system with many unknowns. The traditional approach is to solve the problems of each component, couple it to the next component, check the function of the two together, and so forth. The ultimate test of effectiveness of the solutions, however, is to test the whole system for the signal processing. In this case, it is to test the hearing-impaired listener's function. When this is done, we find that the insertion gain, or the gain of the hearing aid measured at the eardrum, differs from the functional gain, the increase in the listener's threshold sensitivity when using the hearing aid. Rumoshosky and Preves (1977) and Preves and Orton (1978) demonstrated that insertion gain is greater than functional gain at all frequencies between 250 and 6000 Hz. Since these researchers were using subjects with "normal" middle-ear measurement, they felt the answer to the discrepancy could be found in a hypothesis of Wever and Lawrence. In 1954, Wever and Lawrence suggested that the sensitivity of the ear changes when it is occluded due to an alteration in its acoustic impedance.

Fortunately, as noted earlier, the procedure for the measurement of a whole-signal processing system that includes the hearing-aid listener already exists. The procedure is to generate an aided-sound-field audiogram that can be compared with an unaided-sound-field audiogram to determine the functional gain produced by the amplifying hearing aid. Although this procedure will not describe the hearing-aid user's suprathreshold experience, it permits control of the signal as it enters the final stage of signal processing, that is, as it reaches the user's threshold. As stated before, Pascoe's (1978) procedure will carry the signal one step further for adults. A comparable step for preverbal infants must still await research.

Saturation Sound Pressure Level

The hearing aid's maximum output is one of the most important electroacoustic parameters in fitting an aid on children (Ross, 1980). In fact, most clinicians feel that the SSPL may be the most critical of the factors involved in the electroacoustic part of fitting by prescription (Berger, 1976; Martin, 1971; McCandless & Miller, 1972). The two reasons usually cited for this conclusion are, first, that sounds that are uncomfortably loud or painful will elicit dissatisfaction in adults and fear and rejection in the child who is not accustomed to amplified sound, and, second, that excessive amplification of background noise tends to be uncomfortable for the user and to reduce speech intelligibility through an upward spread of masking (Berger, 1976).

Current practices for setting maximum permissible SSPL of hearing aids for adults are usually based on discomfort levels. Sometimes called threshold of discomfort (TD), sometimes uncomfortable loudness level (UCL), and sometimes loudness discomfort level (LDL), they are all measured in much the same way. The adult is asked to report when a pulsed warble tone, a narrow band of noise or speech, reaches an intensity level that would be uncomfortable to listen to for a specified length of time. These intensities are converted to sound pressure levels that are used in the prescription to limit the maximum output of the hearing aid. Although this is a rational approach for fitting aids on adults, it fails to solve the problem of the preverbal infant who cannot report levels of discomfort.

With the increasing use of tympanometry and acoustic reflex testing, a possible solution to setting the SSPL on hearing aids for infants shows promise in some cases. McCandless and Miller (1972) reported a study that showed that the sound pressure for the acoustic reflex thresholds (ART) and the level at which the sound first becomes uncomfortable at five frequencies were about equal (95–100 dB SPL) for 15 normal listeners as well as for 20 subjects with cochlear hearing loss. In the same study, they noted that the ART for speech was 89 dB and the LDL was 95 dB SPL. The pure-tone findings were essentially confirmed by Horning (1975), Rainville (1976), Woodford and Holmes (1977), and Preves and Orton (1978).

However, as noted by Rappaport and Tait (1976), Keith (1976), and Dennenberg and Altshuler (1976), there is disagreement over the concurrence of the ART and LDL for speech. These researchers suggest that the ART is more closely associated with the most comfortable level than it is with the LDL. These disagreements would not appear to be serious, however, since all of the findings agree that, for speech, LDLs are higher than the ARTs. Consequently, if ARTs can be elicited and used with a conservative correction factor to set the hearing aid's maximum SSPL, one could feel some confidence that the amplified sound was not surpassing the LDL. This conclusion is, of course, based on the premise that preverbal infants exhibit the same ART/LDL relationships as the adults in the cited studies.

BSER Use in Fitting Hearing Aids

It is unfortunate for clinicians who attempt to develop precision in controlling electroacoustic parameters for optimum hearing-aid fitting that many hearing-impaired adults and children do not demonstrate acoustic reflexes. This is particularly unfortunate in the case of preverbal infants who do not provide us with discrete quantitative behavioral responses. This most difficult clinical population, however, may eventually be aided by a promising technique that utilizes brain-stem-evoked response audiometry (BSER) or, as it is also called, auditory brain-stem-evoked response (ABER).

First reported by Mokotoff and Krebs (1976), the BSER procedure has recently been explored to determine whether it would reveal hearing-aid frequency-response settings that provide the best speech discrimination and whether it would show clear-cut identification of the optimum gain settings chosen by the subjects (Cox & Metz, 1980). Using adult subjects divided into groups demonstrating flat, sloping, or precipitous audiometric configurations, Cox and Metz were able to devise a task that allowed them to compare ABER latencies of Wave V (with various stimuli clicks, 1000, 2000, and 4000 Hz tone pips) with speech discrimination scores obtained with three frequency-response settings. They also checked (among other things) Wave V latencies at 10 dB above and below optimum gain of the hearing aid. The significant results of their study were that ABER Wave V latencies were shortest with 75-dB stimuli through hearing-aid frequency-response settings producing the best speech discrimination scores. Furthermore, these latencies were longer at 10 dB below the chosen optimum hearing aid gain and were shortened as gain was increased to the optimum setting. No further decreases in latency were noted as gain increased beyond the optimum setting.

These test results provide considerable confidence that a method can be devised using the ABER that will permit accurate, consistent electroacoustic setting of a hearing aid on preverbal hearing-impaired youngsters. As Cox and Metz point out, however, the results of their tests are by no means conclusive. In the first place, adults were used as subjects for the study, and the results would have to be extrapolated for infants. Also, their study utilized only eight subjects, and more data are necessary to confirm the results.

At least one more recent attempt to use ABERs as indicators of hearing aid performance has been reported (Kileny & Desrochers, 1980). These clinicians describe a case report of an 18-month-old infant who, when tested unaided with ABER, demonstrated questionable responses bilaterally to 85- and 90-dB clicks. With amplification of a hearing aid in the sound field, however, she showed well-defined, typical brain-stem response patterns from one ear down to 30 and 40 dB. Subsequent behavioral observations confirm that the child is progressing in the use of her amplified hearing.

Although it is difficult to evaluate the details of the procedure in this case study because of the meager information provided in the report, two salient points are suggested. First, some success in fitting amplification to nonverbal hearing-impaired infants can be obtained using ABERs. Second, further research on an ABER test stimulus must be performed to discover the stimulus that is least distorted by present hearing aids and that provides optimum frequency-specific fitting information.

HEARING-AID SELECTION AND MANAGEMENT PROCEDURES IN THE COMPREHENSIVE SERVICES PROGRAM

Defining the Hearing Problem

For infants newborn to 4 months of age, the Comprehensive Services Program uses the combined behavioral and BSER audiometry approach described in Chapter 1 to define the infant's hearing and need for a hearing aid. Infants at any age will of course be given this combined approach if they fail to respond to behavioral procedures. Definition of hearing problems in older infants and young children is usually accomplished using pure-tone audiometry with the VRA/VROCA approach. Obviously, when possible, speech-awareness and speech-reception thresholds are tested. As noted in Chapter 1, tympanometry, acoustic reflex testing, and the case history are essential parts of the evaluation.

Electroacoustic Selection Procedures

For Preverbal Children without Behavioral Pure-Tone Thresholds

Children on whom we are unable to measure behavioral pure-tone thresholds constitute the most difficult group to fit with optimal hearing-aid electroacoustic characteristics. Many in this group are less than 6 months old and therefore present additional mechanical problems of coupling an electroacoustic "box" to a small body and even tinier ear canal. These problems can be worked out, however, and appropriate use habits can be incorporated into the family's life style.

Electroacoustic choices are another matter. Because no verified optimum procedures have been devised, the Comprehensive Services Program utilizes an approach that may go down either of two paths. The first path is the "standard" procedure that starts by defining the infant's hearing in ways previously outlined. Using the thresholds obtained by BSER, a hearing aid is chosen that is highly flexible in its gain, SSPL, and frequency-response settings. The gain is set using the 50 percent rule as applied to the best estimate of hearing found when using BSER audiometry. The SSPL of the aid is set between 105 and 125 dB SPL, depending on the severity of the hearing loss. Of course, behavioral observation of ARTs might influence whether a gain or SSPL is modified upward or downward. In the first month of hearing-aid use, the children are monitored weekly by BOA and parental conferences. They are then monitored monthly until they have matured sufficiently to be tested quantitatively with pure-tone audiometry. At this stage, they are reevaluated by a more refined procedure used with more mature children.

The second path an infant without behaviorally determined, pure-tone thresholds might take starts after BSER thresholds have been measured. This path leads to an experimental fitting procedure that utilizes aided BSER audiometry. Again, aids are chosen that are flexible in the control of their electroacoustic characteristics. The aids are taken from a pool of amplifiers whose transient response characteristics have been measured and whose effects on brain-stem response latency are known. In the Comprehensive Services Program, it is felt that each aid will contribute its own effect on latency and will modify in individual ways the time and frequency parameters of the brain-stem audiometer's tone-pip and click stimuli. These hypotheses are presently being researched.

In the meantime, in accord with an urgency stemming from a firm philosophy of fitting the amplification as early as possible during the infant's physiological development, one of the aids is fitted to the infant's custom earmold. The gain of the aid is set according to the 50 percent rule, using the child's unaided BSER thresholds. If no thresholds can be obtained by BSER, they are presumed to be at 100 dB HL. Aided BSER thresholds are then measured in the sound field with stimuli at 70 dB SPL at the face of the hearing aid microphone. Hearing-aid gain settings are thought to be adequate when the shortest aided BSER latencies are achieved with the 70-dB SPL stimulus. As noted before, this experimental procedure is utilized with a select group of infants whose pure-tone behavioral thresholds could not be elicited.

For Preverbal Children with Behavioral Pure-Tone Thresholds

Children who respond to VRA conditioning or other behavioral tests and reveal their pure-tone thresholds (usually those 4 to 5 months of age and older) are fitted with the 50 percent rule applied to the thresholds to set the hearing-aid gain in a prescription similar to the one reported by Ross (1980) and Berger (1976). Both of these clinicians incorporate some version of the long-interval spectrum of speech into the choice of gain values at speech frequencies. They differ, in quite rational ways, in the specific values at each frequency. As reported earlier, Pascoe (1978) uses a procedure and rationale that provide a further contrasting view in the hearing-aid gain-setting protocol dilemma.

In the Comprehensive Services Program, the goal is to provide an aided pure-tone threshold configuration that approximates the two-humped frequency emphasis advocated by Pascoe. In many cases of congenital hearing impairment, however, this is not possible. Berger and others caution that "if the unaided hearing level at 2000Hz is 110dB or worse, or at 3000Hz is 90dB or worse, or at 4000Hz is 75dB or worse, the gain furnished may not assist in the reception of speech sounds in these frequency ranges at one meter or more distant, even if the speech is loud" (Berger, Hagberg, & Rane, 1977, p. 13). In the case of children with pure-tone thresholds, as much as possible of the two-humped configuration is achieved as an interim measure while the case for transposing hearing aids and signal processing is reexplored.

The setting of the SSPL for infants who can supply aided pure-tone thresholds is accomplished in the Comprehensive Services Program by using acoustic reflex thresholds when available. It is believed that SSPL can be set 6 dB above the ART and still not surpass loudness discomfort levels (Dennenberg & Altshuler, 1976; Horning, 1975; Keith, 1976; Preves & Orton, 1978; Rainville, 1976; Rappaport & Tait, 1976; Woodford & Holmes, 1977). If the infant does not exhibit aided ARTs, the aid is again set between 105 and 125 dB SPL, depending on the severity of the hearing loss. It is the philosophy in the Comprehensive Services Program to underfit until positive behavioral observations suggest the need for increases in either the gain or the SSPL.

Hearing Aid Management

Essential to adequate hearing-aid management in the Comprehensive Services Program is the realization that hearing-impaired infants and young children need what Ross reports as a "a very heavy 'hands-on' approach" (Ross, 1980, p. 231). As reported earlier, those children whose only thresholds are those estimated by BSER audiometry and who are fitted with a hearing aid are monitored weekly in the first month of hearing-aid use via BOA procedures in the clinic, the nursery school, and parental conferences. In these conferences a questionnaire is filled out covering the infant's responses to amplification (see Exhibit 2–1). Attention is paid to specific areas dealing with the child's changes: in response to environmental sounds; in response to voice; in crying behavior; in communicative

Exhibit 2–1 Weekly Questionnaire for Parental and Nursery School Teacher Feedback on the Infant's Adjustment to the Trial Hearing-Aid Fitting

Name ______________________________
Age______ Date ______________________________
Hearing Aid Brand ______________________________
Model____________ Ear______________________________
1st Week Gain__________ SSPL______________________________

1. *Environmental sounds.* Does the child seem more aware of sounds in the home, such as doors slamming, pots and pans, motors (vacuum cleaner, food processor, etc.), doorbell, telephone, or other sounds?
2. *Voice.* Does the child react to voices more frequently?
3. *Crying behavior.* Does the child cry more or less with hearing-aid amplification? Has the cry changed in any way? Does the child cry when the aid is turned on? When it is turned off?
4. *Communication landmark behavior.* Any change in babbling, cooing, lalling, etc.?
5. *Tolerance.* Does the child show any signs of distress in the presence of loud sounds? Is there any sign of physical irritation of the ear canal (redness, a lesion)?
6. *Visual behavior.* With the aid in place and adjusted, is the child more, or less, alert when others make rapid movement, like walking into the room (especially when accompanied with sounds of the movement)?
7. *Acceptance of amplification.* Does the child seem to accept the aid being put on? Does the child seem to accept the amplified sound?
8. *Special problems.* Are there any special problems not covered by the above questions? These may be related to the manipulation or physical management of the hearing aid.

Note significant answers to the above.

Recommendations:

landmark behavior such as babbling, cooing, lalling, and so on; in visual reactions (alertness); in tolerance reactions to loud sounds; and in acceptance of amplification. At this point, any special problems are noted and dealt with.

Children with multiple handicaps may require weekly monitoring beyond the first month. Most of the others will go on a monthly monitoring schedule at the discretion of the clinician. This monthly schedule is maintained until the child matures sufficiently to yield behavioral pure-tone thresholds or until the clinician is confident that such close monitoring is not necessary.

Older children, or children who have been fitted according to their behavioral pure-tone thresholds have their aided thresholds monitored with VRA/VROCA, play audiometry, and the questionnaire on a monthly basis for about 3 months. After this period, at the clinician's and teacher's discretion, the monitoring schedule usually changes to once every 2 months. Naturally, as the child develops, more formalized procedures—such as performance scales and language, speech, cognitive development, and social-emotional measures—are used to monitor progress.

Many hearing-aid management suggestions are well documented. Some valuable day-to-day recommendations on how to help a child adjust to the hearing aid are specified by Northern and Downs (1978). Parent hearing-aid orientation and troubleshooting information can be found in Ross (1980).

SUMMARY

It is clear from the cited literature that hearing-aid fitting-procedure problems of adults are gradually yielding to basic and applied research. Not that any clinician is satisfied with the progress—but when is a clinician satisfied with less than perfect remediation of a handicap?

As might be expected, however, the progress achieved with adults has not been realized with preverbal children. Electroacoustic adjustment of a hearing aid for preverbal children is still as much as 90 percent art. This is not to say that objective progress has not been made. With the improvements in conditioned behavior audiometry and the development of BSER audiometry, measurable, repeatable hearing-aid-gain and SSPL settings can be evaluated as to their contribution to optimum speech reception in the hearing-impaired infant. As art is translated into science, we should see an acceleration in the curve depicting successful hearing aid prescription versus time.

REFERENCES

Berger, K. Prescription of hearing aids: A rationale. *Journal of the Auditory Society of America,* 1976, *2,* 71–78.

Berger, K., Hagberg, E., & Rane, R. *Prescription of hearing aids: Rationale, procedures and results.* Unpublished monograph, Kent State University, 1977.

Brooks, D. Gain requirements of hearing aid users. *Scandinavian Audiology,* 1973, *2,* 199–205.

Byrne, D., & Tonnison, W. Selecting the gain of hearing aids for persons with sensorineural hearing impairments. *Scandinavian Audiology,* 1976, *5,* 51–59.

Cox, L., & Metz, D. ABER in the prescription of hearing aids. *Hearing Instruments,* 1980, *31*(9), 12–15.

Davis, H., Steven, S., Nichols, R., Jr., Hudgins, C., Marquis, R., Peterson, G., & Ross, D. An experimental study of design objectives. *Hearing aids.* Cambridge, Mass.: Harvard University Press, 1947.

Dennenberg, L., & Altshuler, M. The clinical relationship between acoustic reflexes and loudness perception. *Journal of the American Auditory Society,* 1976, *2*(3), 79–82.

Gengel, R., Pascoe, D., & Shore, I. A frequency response procedure for evaluating and selecting hearing aids for severely hearing impaired children. *Journal of Speech and Hearing Disorders,* 1971, *36,* 341–353.

Horner, J. P., & Horner, J. S. (Producers). *A pure-tone threshold protocol for infants ages 4½–11½ months.* A videotape presented at ASHA Convention, San Francisco, 1978.

Horning, J. Tympanometry and hearing aid selection. *Hearing Aid Journal,* 1975, *28*(6), 8.

Keith, R. *An acoustic reflex technique of establishing hearing aid settings.* Paper presented at ASHA Convention, Houston, Tex., 1976.

Kileny, P., & Desrochers, C. *Auditory brain stem responses as indicators of hearing performance.* Paper presented at ASHA Convention, Detroit, 1980.

Lybarger, S. Simplified fitting system for hearing aids. In *Radioear specifications and fitting information manual.* Radioear Corp, October 1963.

Martin, M. Electroacoustic characteristics of hearing aids and sensorineural hearing loss. *Scandinavian Audiology,* 1971, *1,* 99–108. (Supplement)

McCandless, G., & Miller, D. Loudness discomfort and hearing aids. *Hearing Aid Journal,* 1972, *25*(6), 28, 32.

Mokotoff, B., & Krebs, D. *Brainstem auditory-evoked responses with amplification.* Paper presented at meeting of the Acoustic Society of America, Miami, Fla., 1976.

Niemoeller, A., McCormick, L., & Miller, J. On the spectra of spoken English. *Journal of the Acoustic Society of America,* 1974, *55,* 461.

Northern, J., & Downs, M. *Hearing in children* (2nd ed.). Baltimore: Williams and Wilkins, 1978.

Olson, W. O. The influence of harmonic and intermodulation distortion on speech intelligibility. *Scandinavian Audiology Supplement,* 1971, *1,* 109–125.

Pascoe, D. An approach to hearing aid selection. *Hearing Instruments,* June, 1978, *29*(12), 6.

Pascoe, D., Niemoeller, A., & Miller, J. *Hearing aid design and evaluation for a presbyeusic patient.* Paper presented at meeting of the Acoustic Society of America, Detroit, Mich., 1973.

Preves, D., & Orton, J. Use of acoustic impedance measures in hearing aid fitting. *Hearing Instruments*, 1978, *29*(6), 22–34.

Rainville, M. Impedance measurements in evaluation of hearing aid performance. *Hearing Instruments*, 1976, *27*(11), 39.

Rappaport, B., & Tait, C. Acoustic reflex threshold measurement in hearing aid selection. *Archives of Otolaryngology*, March, 1976, *102*, 129–132.

Reddell, R., & Calvert, D. Selecting a hearing aid by interpreting audiometric data. *Journal of Auditory Research*, 1966, *6*, 445–452.

Ross, M. Hearing aid selection for preverbal hearing-impaired children. In M. Pollock (Ed.), *Amplification for the hearing-impaired* (2nd ed.). New York: Grune & Stratton, 1980.

Rubel, E. W., Parks, T. N., Smith, D. J., & Jackson, H. *Experiential afferent influences and development in the avian N. Magnocellularis and N. Laminaris*. Paper presented at the 17th International Congress of Ornithology, 1978.

Rumoshosky, J., & Preves, D. Hearing aid evaluations using custom in-the-ear and stock behind-the-ear aids. *Hearing Aid Journal*, 1977, *30*(10), 11, 46–49.

Shapiro, I. Hearing aid fitting by prescription. *Audiology*, 1976, *15*, 163–173.

Tillman, T., Kasten, R., & Horner, J. *Effect of head shadow on reception of speech*. Paper presented at ASHA Convention, Chicago, 1963.

Triantos, T., & McCandless, G. High frequency distortion. *Hearing Aid Journal*, 1974, *27* (9), 38.

Wallenfels, H. *Hearing aids on prescription*. Springfield, Ill.: Charles C Thomas, 1967.

Watson, N., & Knudsen, V. Selective amplification in hearing aids. *Journal of the Acoustic Society of America*, 1940, *11*, 406–419.

Watson, T. J. Some factors affecting the successful use of hearing aids by deaf children. In S. A. Ewing (Ed.), *The modern educational treatment of deafness*. Manchester, Eng.: Manchester University Press, 1960.

Wever, E., & Lawrence, M. *Physiological acoustics*. Princeton: Princeton University Press, 1954.

Woodford, C., & Holmes, D. Relationship between loudness discomfort level and acoustic reflex threshold in a clinical population. *Audiology Hearing Education*, 1977, *3*(6), 12.

Chapter 3

Auditory Processing

M. Suzanne Hasenstab and Zahrl G. Schoeny

For the purpose of this chapter, auditory processing is defined as the reception, categorization, and utilization of information received primarily through the auditory channel. In order to bring a consistent viewpoint to bear when dealing with auditory stimuli in general, we have chosen to identify problems in the utilization of auditory stimuli as *auditory deficits*. The steps or mechanisms associated with the utilization of auditory stimuli we refer to as *auditory processing*. The value of this orientation is twofold: (1) the conceptual base does not require identification of a specific auditory processing deficit, such as auditory memory disorder, for classification and (2) the identification of types of pathology becomes implicit. In turn, this alleviates the problem of identifying whether the auditory disorder is peripheral, central, or a general cognitive processing problem unrelated to specific sensory input, such as mental retardation. The decision to place the pathology in one of the above categories cannot at present be made with confidence and requires more extensive knowledge of the entire auditory processing system and its function and purpose before such categories can be meaningfully applied in a practical context. Meanwhile, the definitions presented here will help provide practitioners with a functional framework and will avoid the necessity of overspecification when in fact, the present knowledge base is insufficient for such application.

DEFINITIONS FROM THE LITERATURE

In addressing auditory processing, or problems related to the function of the auditory system, it is first necessary to establish a general working orientation. Myklebust (1954), for example, defines auditory disorders as "incapacities relating to the reception or interpretation of sound whether they be physical or pyschological" (p. 4). From this definition it may be inferred that problems in auditory processing are a subcategory within the area of auditory disorders. The definition of auditory processing presented by Witkin, Butler, and Whalen (1977) focuses on the mechanisms of auditory processing, specifically the immediate short-term processing of auditory information. They further elaborate that auditory processing is positioned medially between the physical reception of an auditory signal (peripheral hearing) and the process of cognition. Piavio (1971) describes auditory processing as a system that is specialized to handle auditory stimulus patterns that are serially organized in time.

A superficial examination of these definitions and others presented in the literature indicates a wide discrepancy in the reference and understanding of the conceptual framework associated with auditory processing. In light of the critical nature of the auditory system in all learning and interactive situations, individuals in many specialties and disciplines have been forced to conceptualize the role of the auditory system as related to their particular orientation. The result has quite naturally led to many definitions reflecting the various specialty areas concerned with auditory processing.

An adequate working definition of auditory processing must be broad enough in scope to encompass the wide range of definitions presented in the literature. It must refrain from specificities that are not supported by the current data base regarding auditory function. Further, it must be sufficiently flexible to address, in a systematic fashion, the present demand for the clinical management of individuals with disorders identified with auditory processing deficit. For these reasons, a general definition of auditory processing, as presented above, has been adopted. Once again, any difficulty in the utilization of auditory stimuli is identified as an auditory deficit.

PERSPECTIVES IN AUDITORY PROCESSING

The basics of information that are used in communication behaviors are derived from experimental interaction with the surrounding environment. However, there must be "avenues" through which such experiences can reach the linguistic and/or cognitive areas of the brain for identification, interpretation, and comprehension or memory of events to occur. These avenues are our processing systems of vision, audition, touch, taste, and smell, as well as the kinesthetic and vestibular mechanisms. It is important to note that many concerns and characteristics of auditory processing are common to other sensory processing systems. It should also be remembered that the processing of incoming information in the normal individual results from the balance of unique information from each perceptual system provided to the "central processing station." Furthermore, when one sense, such as hearing, is affected, the total perceptual balance of the individual is altered. Thus, not only will the change in the value of each dimension in audition occur, but an overall change in the coordination of sensory input will result.

As a result of external stimulation, the auditory processing system converts the information with a message or electrochemical code that is compatible with neural function. Researchers have yet to answer all of the questions regarding this transfer of information and how it is actually interpreted by the brain. However, as Garwood (1979) points out, there are some general points that can be made. He presents three that may be applied to any of the input systems. First, external stimulation is coded as increased or decreased neural activity. Second, each system relays stimulation via respective exclusive neural pathways. Third, specialized areas of the brain utilize incoming information for specific input systems. Although this specificity exists, it is usually the integration of several input systems that provides the most comprehensive information. At the present time, there is incomplete understanding as to how the brain accomplishes this task of integration as well as interpretation.

COMPONENTS OF AUDITORY PROCESSING

When auditory processing is viewed as a unitary ability, it is seen as related to a larger area, such as language or reading (Rees, 1972). But, in itself, auditory processing is also comprised of subcomponents (Witkin et al., 1977). The nature and number of these subcomponents are subject to variation, due to the same reasons noted for diversity in labels and definitions. Auditory processing has been dissected so as to include auditory discrimination, auditory memory, adaptation to novel speech-sound tasks, interpretation of sound without orthography, resistance to distortion, masking and distraction, auditory closure, matching auditory stimuli, judging order of auditory sequential stimuli, auditory figure-ground orientation, and other such auditory "skills" (Bever, 1970; Hanley, 1956; Hirsh, 1967; Solomon, Webster, & Curtis, 1960; Witkin, 1971a). These skills or mechanisms have been perceived as hierarchical and as part of a continuum. Furthermore, whatever specific aspects or subcomponents might exist as part of auditory processing, the central focus is that the auditory system must analyze and relay the internal representation of the dimensions of acoustic information.

An overview of the subcomponents of auditory processing can be gained by examining the aspects of auditory processing in terms of increased complexity along a continuum of analyses and decisions imposed by the auditory system. The aspects summarized and presented by Sanders (1977) as related to speech perception actually can be applied to auditory processing, based on the definition proposed in this chapter, and serve as a most comprehensive summary listing.

Awareness of the Acoustic Signal

The first aspect or level of auditory processing signals the beginning step in the processing of an auditory stimulus. It is concerned with the awareness of sound as opposed to no sound. This fundamental ability to distinguish sound from no sound is imperative for linguistic, cognitive, and psychological development (Ramsdell, 1970). Sanders emphasizes that psychological implications stem from the fact that the auditory system, by virtue of its function as a monitoring system, creates a bridging between self and environment. Much more obvious is the relationship of awareness of an auditory signal to both linguistic and cognitive development. Unless a child is aware that a sound, whether linguistic or environmental, has occurred, ceased, or changed, higher levels of auditory processing cannot occur. For example, if children are not aware of a sound, they will not demonstrate localization behavior.

Localization

The aspect of localization relates the listener with the source of the sound, whether that be a person, object, or event. Sound localization is also termed *search behavior*. Once children are aware of a sound, if it is salient to them, motivation to determine from where the sound originates will occur. Sound localization forms the basis for the awareness of figure-ground relationships between a particular sound set against a background of all other sounds occurring within the environment at the same time. This is also referred to as *signal-to-noise preception*. Localization to a sound is crucial to all attending behavior as part of the perceptual process. Localizing behavior presents the necessary condition for intensive concentration on the source of the stimulus.

Attention to the Acoustic Signal

Closely related to acoustic awareness and localization, and actually dependent upon those aspects, auditory attention involves the listener in following the growing pattern of auditory information over a time period. This attention, based on localization of sound, also separates the auditory stimulus from other sounds within the surrounding context. Garwood (1979) describes two attentional functions that serve as a basis for effective utilization of cognitive and linguistic activity. The first, the *attention-sustaining* function, establishes the needed optimal condition of elimination of interfering stimuli in order that the system can be devoted to the target information. Time is the essential component in the sustained-attention function. The duration of sustained attention is referred to as the *attention span,* which is vital in the sequencing of increasingly relevant information.

The second attentional function is *selective attention.* The auditory system is constantly presented with various auditory stimuli; but, in order to process acoustic information effectively, some priority must be established in attending behavior. It is at this point that listening occurs. The importance of attention, both selective and sustained, lies in the reality that if information is unattended it cannot be identified, comprehended, interpreted, remembered, or applied (Garwood, 1979).

Differentiation between Environmental Sounds and People Sounds

The differentiation between environmental and people sounds is vital and must be made early in the processing of auditory information. This is critical to other processing aspects and resulting processing decisions. Within this component, levels of finer differentiation are made. First, the listener determines if the sound is an environmental sound or a people sound. Second, if it is a people sound, is it speech or one of the other various sounds that people produce (cough, laugh, belch, etc.)? At this level of differentiation, aspects such as meaningful versus nonmeaningful, speech versus nonspeech, and linguistic versus nonlinguistic are initially determined. This processing component is the foundation for those later discrimination levels that assist in the interpretation of incoming acoustic information. There presently exists a substantial amount of evidence from various studies indicating that speech-linguistic sounds are perceived and interpreted in the left hemisphere of the brain cortex (Gazzanega, 1967; Geschwind, 1972; Kimura, 1961; Lenneberg, 1967). Other sounds, such as music, are processed and interpreted in the right hemisphere (Molfese, 1972, 1973). Thus, this aspect of auditory processing has been determined to be crucial to the mastery of developing communication behaviors in young children.

Auditory Discrimination

Auditory discrimination has received much attention; because it is necessary in the resynthesizing of the auditory pattern, it is generally included in all listings of subcomponents of auditory processing. Differentiating between auditory patterns is based on certain perceptual variables, such as length, complexity, nature (such as linguistic or nonlinguistic), structure, temporal relationships of frequency, and intensity. Once the differentiation of a speech-linguistic sound as opposed to a nonspeech-linguistic sound is made, further discrimination can be effected with respect to perceptual variables. The characteristics of one auditory form can be distinguished from another within the larger category of speech-linguistic sounds or nonspeech-linguistic sounds. Sanders (1977) emphasizes that auditory discrimination is complex and interdependent with the other components of auditory processing. Actual discrimination can take place only when the auditory pattern is "compared with the internal model and categorized" (p. 207). It should be noted that auditory discrimination is commonly referred to as the ability to distinguish between phonemes. In reality, however, it constitutes the distinction between all forms of auditory patterns.

Suprasegmental Discrimination

Dependent on auditory discrimination, suprasegmental discrimination or prosodical distinction involves the analysis of pattern variation in spoken language, such as the intonation contours of sentences or the emotive cues carried by pitch and stress variations. It is generally believed that a close developmental relationship exists between this ability and the acquisition of phonology and syntax (Ling, 1976). The suprasegmental feature discriminations in English are based on stress (including word and syllable stress), tone or pitch variation, intonation contour or the pattern of rhythmic stress across an utterance, and timing factors such as pauses indicating word boundaries.

Segmental Discrimination

While suprasegmental discrimination is concerned with those features that provide "quality" to speech or vocalizations (such as babbling), segmental discrimination focuses on the differentiation and identification of phonemes and, most important, on phoneme patterns. Language components or morphology and phonology are highly dependent on this form of discrimination. However, it is the mutual interaction of suprasegmental features and phonemic order that signals the linguistic rules that make speech meaningful to a listener. This involves discrimination for both aspects. Although as mentioned previously, phonemes have served as the basis for determining auditory discrimination abilities in children, this component also includes distinctions among larger linguistic patterns in semantics and syntax. Indeed, this is an even more important function when auditory processing is examined in connection with communication behavior.

Auditory Memory

Another subcomponent of auditory processing that has received much attention is auditory memory. An auditory stimulus occurs over a time period. Therefore, the acoustic information must be held or stored as it is resynthesized. The stimulus pattern is organized into units or "chunks" of information that can then be processed cognitively. The function of "chunking" information into units allows restructuring into larger and larger meaningful units within the capacity of the system, thereby increasing the capacity of memory. The retention capacity of memory is approximately seven units or chunks of information for adults. The way in which information can be chunked depends on previous experiences and requires recognition of recurrent patterns, regulations, and associations of stimuli that can be redefined into more and more complex units of information. Through the chunking process, phonemes can be grouped into morphemes, morphemes into words, and words into sentences or sentence components. Memory in this context includes immediate and short-term memory. Long-term memory is not addressed here, lest we begin to digress from our point of focus.

Auditory Sequencing

Sequencing is related to auditory memory but specifies the order of components in addition to specific parts or patterns. It is felt that this aspect is an important factor in determining meaning and is closely related to structural rules of sentence formation. Developmentally, shifts or reversals may be seen in word pronunciation or word orders in sentences, however persistence of these language restrictions in school-age children indicates language processing problems (Aten, 1974). Sequencing problems, it should be remembered, can also be noted for nonspeech-linguistic auditory stimuli.

Auditory Synthesis

As the bits of auditory information are received, blending must occur in order for identification of the pattern to take place. This blending is called auditory synthesis. In order for the acoustic event to be relevant, the information must be synthesized. This goes back to the chunking process described under auditory memory. Synthesis is the merging of the information chunks that allows total pattern identification and further cognitive activity in order that interpretation, application, comprehension, and long-term memory storage can occur. It is intimately dependent on all the other processing components.

Whatever the actual number of analyses involved in auditory processing and no matter what we choose to label them, it must be emphasized that they are mutually interdependent; all are necessary for accurate cognitive utilization of auditory information. As Sanders (1977) points out, it is impossible to regard these aspects as discrete skills, yet, in evaluation and intervention programming the processing aspects are often treated as such. The concept of the development or remediation of individual auditory "skills," however inappropriate, serves as the usual basis for assessment and programming.

A MODEL OF AUDITORY PROCESSING

Research in the areas of psychoacoustics and psycholinguistics casts more and more doubt on the skills concept. In an attempt to provide a functional reference for information processing, we propose a synthesized model for information analysis based on a perceptual-behavioral orientation (see Figure 3–1). The foundation of this model emerges from physiological research and draws heavily on concepts from the field of memory and attention. The purpose and value of the model is to provide an integrated structural framework for the viewing of input processing behaviors of an individual. Although it is not an exact specification of perceptual behavior action, the model permits structured observation of behavior and processing that can be used to assist in organizing our evaluation of an individual, based on the impact of incoming information about the individual rather than skills alone. It can also be used to develop an organized understanding of processing behavior and can serve to focus inquiries regarding the validity of the generalizations based on current understanding of auditory processing.

Since we view auditory processing as a function of an integrated system, the Figure 3–1 model is essentially basic to all sensoriperceptual modalities. Sanders classifies theories of auditory processing into two main categories: passive and active. A passive theory presents a "direct relationship between the acoustic pattern and neural representation of that pattern" (Sanders, 1977, p. 5). An active theory includes an "intermediary process to recode information . . . prior to perception" (Sanders, 1977, p. 5). The Figure 3–1 model is based on an active theory. Specifically, it is based on the formulations of Broadbent (1958), Loftus and Loftus (1976), Barlow

Figure 3–1 A Schematic Model for Auditory Processing

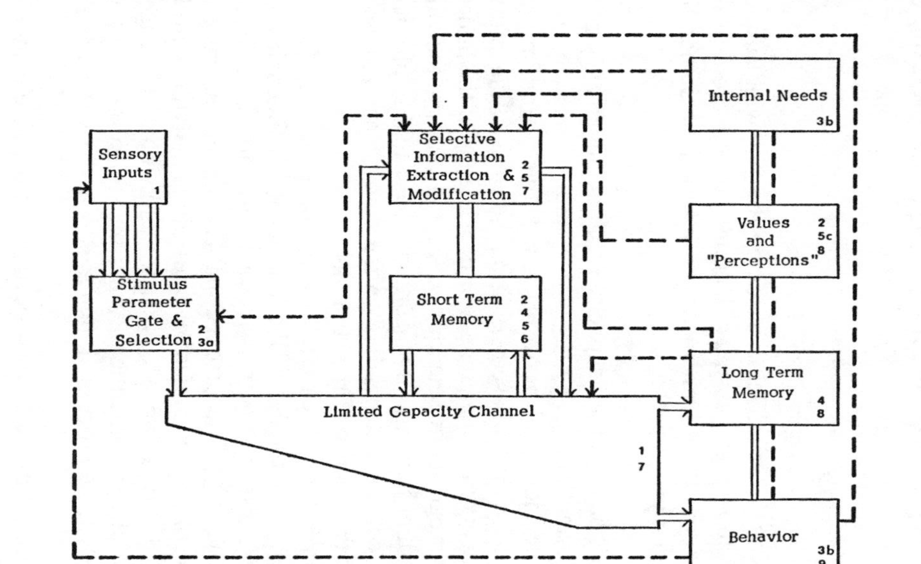

Note: The above model shows the interrelationships between input shaping, processing alternatives, and processing determinants. The numbers in the elements of the model designate location within the model related to the underlying assumptions presented in the text. Solid lines indicate potential flow patterns for the incoming information. Dashed lines indicate controls that can affect processing. The central core of the model is the limited capacity channel that spans input shaping, processing alternatives, and processing determinants. Information is routed through the limited capacity channel to various levels within processing alternatives, then to long-term memory and/or behavior. Information may also proceed directly to these final stages (long-term memory and/or behavior) through the limited capacity channel.

(1961), Norman (1973), Warrington and Weiskrantz (1973), Iversen (1973), and Gallistell (1973). It represents an extraction from the findings in research dealing with attention, memory, and learning. However, numerous simplifications have been made in order to increase the utility of the model for practical application. Of necessity these simplifications introduce certain biases that may be untestable at the present time. However, it is felt that the practical use of our formulation justifies the taking of such liberties.

Assumptions of the Model

Our auditory processing model is based on the following assumptions regarding the individual's processing of incoming information. Its focus is on what an individual does with incoming information rather than on physiology or anatomy:

1. The individual has a limited capacity for attending to and processing incoming information.
2. Therefore, the individual performs a selective operation upon the input information that is based either on the value of the information to the individual or the uniqueness or consistency of the information itself. Another part of the selection process is to attend to features of the stimulus that have an organizational base that is physically or perceptively constant, depending on the developmental level of the individual or the quality of the stimulus.
3. The selection process is ordered by the properties of the sensory events and by certain states of the individual: (1) Examples of properties of the sensory events that are known to be important are intensity, frequency of occurrence, pattern, change in sense modality, and so forth. (2) Examples of states of the individual are behaviors related to drives and needs. If the individual is engaged in a certain mode of behavior, then events that reinforce that behavior are more likely to be processed than events that do not contribute to that behavior.
4. Information that is associated by occurrence or value is more likely to be "learned" or stored in long-term memory than information that is fragmented. Furthermore, information that is related to an ordered series of stimuli (the base of the order is established by the individual's capacity to attend and process incoming information) has the highest likelihood of being processed effectively.
5. Incoming information may be temporarily stored to establish processing by allowing the accumulation of information; however, this

accumulation process will only last a few seconds. When sufficient accumulation of information has taken place, the extracted information will be passed on to the central processor for action. Barlow (1961) presents three principles that underlie the transmission of sensory information: (1) The processing system functions as a detector, selecting key information from the incoming stimulus that has special saliency to the individual. (2) Components of the processing system modify the incoming information to fit the requirements of other parts of the nervous system. (3) the processing system functions in a manner that selects significant or salient information from a highly redundant stimulus such as speech.

6. The limitations of short-term storage are overcome by allowing return of information to the limited capacity input stage. This permits a longer storage or access time by recycling information; however, this also reduces the capacity of the individual to attend to new incoming information.
7. Attention can be shifted very rapidly from one type of stimulus or information to another. However, processing of one type of stimulus or information requires a minimum time and therefore controls the number of events or stimuli that an individual can both attend to and process at any given time.
8. Successfully processed information, based on the individual's perceptive system, leads to an increased probability that further information of similar content will be both successfully processed and rewarding to the individual.
9. Information processing is done in such a way as to permit optimization of the individual's behavior related to the internal needs of the individual and the individual's perception of social organization.

The Figure 3–1 model illustrates these points graphically.

Application of the Model

The construct and underlying assumptions of the model permit the practitioner to evaluate any auditory task expected of a child in terms of the steps that the child would follow in processing auditory information. The value of this approach is that it allows an integrated evaluation of a task while, at the same time, it permits the practitioner to assess the specific elements of the task in light of the child's present capabilities.

Although this model may be applied to the processing of any sense modality singly or in combination with other modalities, it can also be used as an overview in the understanding of auditory processing function.

Current models based on the concept of discrete auditory skills necessitate understanding and identification of specific auditory processing skills or abilities. Present identification of "skills" is not adequate, as evidenced by a cursory review of the literature and by the lack of consistency in the identification of specific skills. The advantage of our model is that, because it does not view the steps of auditory processing as isolated events but rather as a continuum, it permits the integrated assessment and understanding of auditory function. This understanding, in turn, makes possible the effective evaluation and programming related to auditory processing when combined with audiological and linguistic evaluation information that is not achieved by a skill orientation or approach.

EVALUATION OF THE AUDITORY PROCESSING FUNCTION

The assessment of an auditory processing deficit in a child is an area that is still open to considerable debate. The how and what of evaluation in relation to auditory processing is again a variable question, often based on the orientation of specific points of view. In Chapters 1 and 2, an overview of the assessment of auditory function and abilities was presented. It will be recalled that, from the definition of auditory processing presented earlier in this chapter, auditory function is an integral part of the auditory processing system. Therefore, evaluation of that functioning is inherent in the evaluation of auditory processing, and vice versa. In this chapter, considerations of evaluation will be restricted to those aspects of auditory processing that are viewed from specializations other than audiology.

Earlier definitions in the study of auditory processing disorders included only those children who manifested a gross neurological involvement. This criterion is, however, no longer of prime importance. The definition is thus now expanded so that the population of children with auditory processing problems is seen as one that has a general competence or ability but that appears to be unable to benefit from auditory experiences as "normal" children might. Though a deficiency in auditory learning exists, this should not be mistaken for an incapacity for such learning.

Attempts to design tests to identify auditory processing problems based on this expanded definition have been clouded by the uncertainty and disagreement as to what should be and what actually is measured. If one adheres to the premise that auditory processing problems stem from a dysfunction of skills or abilities, emphasis on perception of sound (most often speech) as related to various skills is usually central to diagnosis.

Describing an Auditory Processing Problem

In general, evaluation of the hearing-impaired child has been primarily concerned with measures of sensitivity and discrimination. However, recent evidence indicates that many children with peripheral hearing loss may also exhibit auditory processing problems. Furthermore, children with apparently normal hearing have also been found to have auditory processing disorders. These problems may be associated with a minimal central lesion or may be associated with developmental factors related to early deficiency in the peripheral or central mechanism, such as a long history of recurrent otitis media.

Usually children with an auditory processing problem have difficulty with the processing of auditory information, linguistic, nonlinguistic, or both. The results are manifested in areas that require the processing of auditory nonverbal information, listening skills related to language and speech acquisition and function, and the auditory abilities related to the academic areas of reading, writing, and mathematics. School-aged children with such disorders, but with intact hearing, are most often found in special education classes for students with learning disabilities (Wallace & Kauffman, 1978) or in language therapy programs (Northern & Downs, 1978).

Terminology

Labels such as learning disorder, language dysfunction, symbolic language dysfunction, auditory perceptual disorder, minimal brain dysfunction, receptive aphasia, psychoneurological learning disorder, psychosensory learning disorder, and central auditory processing disorder have been applied as descriptions for children displaying auditory processing deficits (Garwood, 1979). Although there is extensive variation in terminology in these descriptions, there is a central focus. The great commonality in this group of children—despite which label is applied, and whether or not peripheral hearing loss exists—is the failure to achieve academically and/or linguistically and a displayed deficiency in certain auditory abilities.

The auditory inability to make processing decisions may be manifested in various ways. For example, difficulty in auditory discrimination results in the inability to distinguish differences between sounds, linguistic, nonlinguistic, or both; or the child who is unable to derive meaning from spoken language or acoustic environmental events may be said to be demonstrating difficulty in auditory comprehension.

The Use of Standardized Tests in Evaluating Auditory Processing

One approach, indeed a popular one, is to undertake the evaluation of a child's ability to process auditory information through the use of standardized assessment instruments. The use of standardized measurements or techniques establishes a reference point or focus for what is deemed "normal" behavior, function, or performance. In theory at least, if the area to be evaluated is totally understood and represented by observable, measurable behaviors, including factors such as developmental levels and sequence, a standardized approach may yield accurate results. However, in the application of standardized tests without a clearly outlined awareness and knowledge of the problem under study, or when the specifics of behavior are not readily defined or measured, limitations are imposed by the current state of the art. This state of affairs may be said to apply to the area of auditory processing. Thus, unique components associated with an individual case can be overlooked because the standardized methodology regiments consistent application of the test procedure in order to permit generalization. It is therefore imperative that beyond the use of standardized measurements, equal weight be given to the unique behaviors of the individual in a particular setting.

In the majority of cases involving an auditory deficit, the child exhibits a related language and/or speech delay. For whatever reason, the child does not fully benefit from receiving linguistically related auditory information. A standardized test may reveal that the child cannot discriminate between vowels in isolation, or even syllables or words out of context; or a test of auditory memory, such as digit span, may indicate that the child can only sequence in order up to four digits. What this approach does not reveal, but yet what is central to this particular child's auditory deficit problems, is how these results are related to the child's communication handicap.

Educational Evaluation

In the area of psychoeducational and related evaluation, the assessment of auditory processing ability is accomplished primarily through the use of standardized, normed tests. Often auditory processing is addressed as a subcomponent of an instrument in which various auditory skills are measured, as related, for example, to reading.

Various reading tests, both those designed as diagnostic in nature so as to ascertain a reading disability and those that are achievement or progress tests in nature, contain items that are intended to measure auditory processing "skills." In many of the tests used to evaluate auditory processing, the main emphasis is on the child's ability to *discriminate*, usually between phonemes individually or in various combinations. In other words, processing proficiency is measured by how well a subject "hears" the difference between speech sounds. The value of identification of isolated sounds is questionable. Berry (1969), for example, emphasizes that auditory processing of language in regard to discrimination is based on sets of phonemes occurring in prescribed context, not in isolation. Because language as spoken is received in patterns governed by rules of the various linguistics components, measurement of fragmented aspects of the pattern in relation to discrimination cannot be generalized to the pattern or continuum itself. In other words, because a child cannot distinguish the difference between /*i*/ and /I/ or even b*i*d and bId does not mean the child cannot gain meaning from those phonemes or words in context.

Evaluation of auditory processing, if focused on speech, must involve the suprasegmental features and respect the fact that phonemes do not occur in isolation or in nonsense syllables in communication, whether verbal or written. An important additional point is that in many instances auditory processing is treated as being synonymous with speech perception. This, however, is only one condition, albeit an important one, of auditory processing. As mentioned previously, auditory deficits may also include difficulty with environmental information.

Educationally, auditory processing problems as related to skills have been classified as problems in auditory discrimination, wherein the child is unable to distinguish between sounds; auditory comprehension, or the inability to determine meaning from environmental sounds and/or speech; auditory memory, which is the inability to remember or sequence auditory stimuli; auditory figure-ground, or the inability to prioritize auditory stimuli; and auditory closure, in which partial words or information are perceived. Again, in most cases the emphasis has been primarily on speech or, in the case of written language, the recoding of the visual representation to the auditory counterpart.

Since successful programming for children depends on accurate and complete assessment of the child, whether school-aged or younger, it is imperative that interventionists and teachers recognize that standardized test measures, although valuable in many instances, are not the sole means of determining how and where the child operates. Chapters 1 and 2 have already focused on auditory evaluation; Chapters 5 and 6 will address specifically the evaluation of language. If these two areas of evaluation are adequately understood and appropriately applied, evaluation of auditory processing or auditory deficit may be accomplished, based on the definition proposed in this chapter.

Informal Evaluation

We do not wish to infer that formalized testing, whether based on standardized measures or criterion performance, is the only form of evaluation. Informal evaluation carried out by parents or teachers within the program format is also important. This type of evaluation takes the form of task-oriented activities designed by the interventionist or teacher to determine progress and mastery by the child. With the young child, activities involving direct experience can provide a wealth of information to augment more formalized testing results.

As in formalized testing, caution must be exercised, and the evaluator must be cognizant of what is being evaluated and how that behavior is related to the child's auditory and language problem. Evoking or attempting to obtain imitative responses from a 30-month-old child for consonant clusters is inappropriate because of developmental reasons and has little to do with auditory function. However, the 30-month-old child who produces imitatively and spontaneously a variation pattern in intonation contour is presently performing appropriately. The performance information indicates that pitch variation of that pattern is being processed auditorily.

Ongoing Evaluation

In addition, as Meyen (1972) points out, initial evaluation should be viewed only as a starting point in gaining information regarding a specific child. The process of continuous assessment is in reality the basis of ongoing teaching (Wallace & Larsen, 1978). This ongoing evaluation includes not only formal and informal evaluation but also the day-to-day observations by teachers, parents, and support personnel who interact with the child. Ultimately, the true evaluation of ability is how the child functions auditorily and linguistically within the social context of the child's environment. It is the combination of formal evaluation, although not necessarily standardized tests, informal teacher evaluation, and observation of the child within the home and school that provides the needed information to maintain programming consistent with the child's growth and progress.

INTERVENTION STRATEGIES

The foundation for the majority of programs or strategies designed for use with children designated as demonstrating difficulty in auditory processing is, as mentioned previously, comprised of individual skills that must be treated or remediated. However, because each aspect is inseparable from and interactive with all the others, as has been emphasized, auditory processing cannot feasibly be viewed as a matter of individual skills. If auditory processing is to relate to language and communication, which indeed it must, the idea of discrete skills is not plausible (Sanders, 1977; Williamson & Alexander, 1975).

As we have noted, a dysfunction of auditory processing is generally manifested in a language and/or speech delay. Later in school, this manifestation may also become evident in reading, which is also a linguistic function. Emphasis in intervention should be on the auditory function as related to language along a developmental continuum, because it is this interference along the developmental continuum that results in the difficulty of learning in linguistically related areas.

If a developmental view of auditory processing as part of the overall language system is accepted (Rees, 1973), then the tests of auditory learning skills and consequent intervention and educational strategies that presently exist are inadequate. It is debatable whether the specific auditory problems cause the language problem or whether the difficulty in auditory processing is a result of the language disorder (Northern & Downs, 1978). Either way, communication limitation is a central issue.

Researchers have made attempts to determine the differences, in both normal and "learning disabled" children, in the auditory processing of stimuli defined as linguistic and nonlinguistic and meaningful and nonmeaningful (Aten & Davis, 1968; Carrow & Maudin, 1973; Liberman, Cooper, Harris, MacNeilage, & Studdert-Kennedy, 1967; Rosenthal & Eisenson, 1971; Sabatino, 1969; Zigmond, 1969). The variables in these efforts have included linguistic stimuli, such as words, sentences, nonsense syllables, synthetic phonemes, pure tones, filtered noise, and environmental sounds.

A study by Laskey, Jay, and Hanz-Ehrman (1975) contrasted four dimensions of auditory stimuli interactively with both normal and learning-disabled children. The four dimensions were nonlinguistic-nonmeaningful sounds (pure tones), linguistic-meaningful information (words), linguistic-nonmeaningful stimuli (nonsense words), and nonlinguistic-meaningful auditory information (environmental sounds). Laskey observed that, for both populations, auditory processing was easier for the nonlinguistic-nonmeaningful pure tones and the linguistic-meaningful words than for either the linguistic-nonmeaningful nonsense syllables or the nonlinguistic-meaningful environmental sounds. If the evidence of this and similar studies is sound, there is a need to question the advantage of using nonsense words or syllables to aid in developing auditory learning or of assuming that teaching a child to attend to environmental sounds is any easier than teaching speech information or that such teaching can be thought to generalize to the auditory processing of spoken language. Northern and Downs (1978) have determined that, if a developmental theory is accepted, based on a linguistically oriented model, then language facilitation becomes the viable and appropriate intervention approach.

This factor is crucial in developing a program for the infant or preschool child with an auditory deficit, whether classified as hearing impairment or an auditory processing disorder. For the young child who demonstrates an auditory deficit, awareness and understanding of environmental sounds is indeed important. But it must be remembered that linguistic sounds and environmental sounds (speech and nonspeech) are processed at different locations of the brain. Thus, the traditional approach to developing listening skills initially as related to "gross environmental sounds" does not ensure transfer to auditory reception, comprehension, and the application of linguistic signals represented in speech. Because there is indeed a recognized relationship between audition and language acquisition and usage, it is somewhat questionable for intervention to consider one without the other. Language development can be facilitated by emphasizing functional, or residual, hearing in the case of hearing impairment (Ling, 1976), and intervention of auditory deficit problems must include attention to linguistic stimuli. In children with auditory deficits, differences between acoustic and nonacoustic processing cannot be compared to those of normal-hearing children because the auditory deficits necessitate verbal labeling or referent association with even the simplest acoustic stimuli. We are not dealing with a dichotomy because all acoustic events for auditory impairment must be learned by definition. The use of residual hearing, Ling (1976) maintains, is the "potentially most important [sense] because it is the only sense directly capable of appreciating the primary characteristics of communicative speech, which are acoustic" (p. 22). Sanders (1977) underscores the view that auditory processing involves how the child processes acoustic information or the "raw material" of sound stimuli. Because the obvious display of an auditory deficit is observable through language behavior, programming goals must concern the manner in which the child employs the systematic rules of language.

Intervention and Speech Perception

After much debate regarding the minimal unit of speech pérception (Foder, Bever, & Garrett, 1974; Massaro, 1975), there is now general agreement that it is at least a syllable and, in actuality, even an increased amount of information, for example, a morpheme or a word. Individual phoneme perception is not necessary for a listener to identify a word. Indeed, each phoneme, when combined with other phonemes, is altered within each context. Attention to phoneme elements via an analytic approach to recognition or discrimination of speech violates current linguistic theory. A child's mastery of auditory processing of discrete phonemes of even nonmeaningful syllables will not guarantee success in the processing of connected language. This aspect of programming must include syntax, semantics, and pragmatics, as well as phonetic intervention.

Discrete Skills Versus Interdependent Components

Intervention strategies and programming that relate to auditory deficit within the processing domain must address the problem by going beyond attention to a discrete auditory skill or skills and by relating the problem to the resulting language and speech behaviors of the young child. As we have noted, components of auditory processing are indeed highly interactive and mutually dependent on one another. A problem in one area will reflect on other areas as well. It is therefore illogical to assume that one aspect can be isolated for study or remediation (Witkin, 1971b). McGrady and Olsen (1970) point out that addressing auditory skills alone cannot provide a successful intervention program. However, this is the general approach that is still employed in many intervention systems.

SUMMARY

The area of auditory processing still presents many unanswered questions. Increased knowledge in the areas related to sensory and cognitive processing and the physiology of the neurological system will undoubtedly contribute vastly to our current understanding. In the meantime, the lack of agreement as to definition, aspects, and so on, necessitates the development of a view of assessment and intervention that emphasizes audiological functioning as a process that is highly interrelated with language. Furthermore, auditory processing must be viewed not as discrete or isolated skills but as a complex continuum of interrelated analyses and decisions concerning acoustic information made by the auditory system.

REFERENCES

Aten, J. L. Auditory memory and auditory sequencing. *Acta Symbolica*, 1974, *5*, 37–65.

Aten, J. L., & Davis, J. Disturbances in the perception of auditory sequence in children with minimal cerebral dysfunction. *Journal of Speech and Hearing Research*, 1968, *2*, 236.

Barlow, H. B. Possible principles underlying the transformations of sensory messages. In W. A. Rosenblith (Ed.), *Sensory communication*. Cambridge, Mass.: MIT Press, 1961.

Berry, M. F. *Language disorders in children*. New York: Appleton-Century-Crofts, 1969.

Bever, T. G. The cognitive basis for linguistic structures. In J. R. Hays (Ed.), *Cognition and the development of language*. New York: John Wiley and Sons, 1970.

Broadbent, D. *Perception and communication*. New York: Pergamon Press, 1958.

Carrow, E., & Maudin, M. Children's recall of approximations to English. *Journal of Speech and Hearing Disorders*, 1973, *16*, 201–212.

Foder, J. A., Bever, T. G., & Garrett, M. F. *The psychology of language*. New York: McGraw Hill, 1974.

Gallistell, C. R. Self stimulation: The neurophysiology of reward and motivation. In J. A. Deutsch (Ed.), *The physiological basis of memory*. New York: Academic Press, 1973.

Garwood, S. G. *Educating young handicapped children, a developmental approach*. Germantown, Md.: Aspen Systems Corporation, 1979.

Gazzanega, M. S. The split brain in man. *Scientific American*, 1967, *217*, 24–29.

Geschwind, N. The organization of language and the brain. *Science*, 1972, *170*, 940–944.

Hanley, C. N. Factorial analysis of speech perception. *Journal of Speech and Hearing Disorders*, 1956, *21*, 76–87.

Hirsh, I. J. Information processing in input channels for speech and language: The significance of the serial order of stimuli. In C. H. Millikan & F. L. Darley (Eds.), *Brain mechanisms underlying speech and language*. New York: Grune and Stratton, 1967.

Iversen, S. B. Lesion and memory in animals. In J. A. Deutsch (Ed.), *The physiological basis of memory*. New York: Academic Press, 1973.

Kimura, D. Cerebral dominance and the perception of verbal stimuli. *Canadian Journal of Psychology*, 1961, *15*, 166–171.

Laskey, E., Jay, B., & Hanz-Ehrman, M. Meaningful and linguistic variables in auditory processing. *Journal of Learning Disabilities*, 1975, *8*, 570–577.

Lenneberg, E. H. *Biological foundations of language*. New York: John Wiley and Sons, 1967.

Liberman, A. M., Cooper, F. S., Harris, K. S., MacNeilage, P. F., & Studdert-Kennedy, M. Some observations on a model for speech perception. In W. Wathen-Dunn (Ed.), *Models for the perception of speech and visual form*. Cambridge, Mass.: MIT Press, 1967.

Ling, D. *Speech and the hearing impaired*. Washington, D.C.: A.G. Bell, Association for the Deaf, 1976.

Loftus, G., & Loftus, E. *Human memory, the processing of information*. Hillsdale, N.J.: Lawrence Erlbaum Associates, 1976.

Massaro, D. W. (Ed.). *Understanding language*. New York: Academic Press, 1975.

McGrady, H. J., & Olsen, D. A. Visual and auditory learning processes in normal children and children with specific learning disabilities. *Exceptional Children*, 1970, *37*, 581–588.

Meyen, E. L. *Developing units of instruction: For the mentally retarded and other children with learning problems*. Dubuque, Iowa: William C. Brown, 1972.

Molfese, D. L. *Cerebral asymmetry in infants, children and adults: Auditory evoked responses to speech and noise stimuli*. Unpublished doctoral dissertation, Pennsylvania State University, 1972.

Molfese, D. L. Cerebral asymmetry in infants, children and adults: Auditory evoked responses to speech and music stimuli. *Journal of the Acoustic Society of America*, 1973, *53*, 363.

Myklebust, H. R. *Auditory disorders in children*. New York: Grune and Stratton, 1954.

Myklebust, H. R. *Progress in learning disabilities* (Vol. 2). New York: Grune and Stratton, 1971.

Norman, D. A. What have the animal experiments taught us about human memory? In J. A. Deutsch (Ed.), *The physiological basis of memory*. New York: Academic Press, 1973.

Northern, J., & Downs, M. *Hearing in children* (2nd ed.). Baltimore, Md.: Williams and Wilkins, 1978.

Piavio, A. *Imaginary and verbal processes*. New York: Holt, Rinehart, and Winston, Inc., 1971.

Ramsdell, D. A. The psychology of the hard of hearing and deafened adult. In H. Davis & R. S. Silverman (Eds.), *Hearing and deafness* (3rd ed.). New York: Holt, Rinehart, and Winston, Inc. 1970.

Rees, N. S. A talent for language. *Journal of Communication Disorders*, 1972, *5*, 132–141.

Rees, N. S. Auditory processing factors in language disorders: The view from procruste's bed. *Journal of Speech and Hearing Disorders*, 1973, *38*, 304–315.

Rosenthal, W., & Eisenson, J. *Auditory temporal order in aphasic children as a function of selected stimulus features*. Paper presented at meeting of the American Speech and Hearing Association, Chicago, 1971.

Sabatino, D. The construction and assessment of an experimental test of auditory comprehension. *Exceptional Children*, 1969, *35*, 729–737.

Sanders, D. *Auditory perception of speech*. Englewood Cliffs, N.J.: Prentice Hall, 1977.

Solomon, L. N., Webster, J. C., & Curtis, J. F. A factorial study of speech perception. *Journal of Speech and Hearing Research*, 1960, *3*, 101–107.

Wallace, G., & Kauffman, J. M. *Teaching children with learning problems*. Columbus, Ohio: Charles E. Merrill, 1978.

Wallace, G., & Larsen, S. C. *Educational assessment of learning problems: Tests for teaching*. Boston: Allyn & Bacon, 1978.

Warrington, E. K., & Weiskrantz, L. Analysis of short-term and long-term memory defects in man. In J. A. Deutsch (Ed.), *Physiological basis of memory*. New York: Academic Press, 1973.

Williamson, D. G., & Alexander, R. Central auditory abilities. *Maico Audiological Library Series*, 1975, *13*.

Witkin, B. R. Auditory perception—implications for language development. In S. Duker (Ed.), *Listening: Readings* (Vol. 2). Metuchen, N.J.: Scarecrow, 1971. (a)

Witkin, B. R. Auditory perception—implications for language development. *Speech and Hearing Service in Schools*, 1971, *4*, 31–52. (b)

Witkin, B. R., Butler, K. G., & Whalen, T. E. Auditory processing in children: Two studies of component features. *Language, Speech and Hearing Services in Schools*, 1977, *8*, 140–154.

Zigmond, N. Auditory processes in children with learning disabilities. In L. Tornopoe (Ed.), *Learning disabilities: Introduction to educational and medical management*. Springfield, Ill.: Charles C Thomas, 1969.

Chapter 4

Psychoeducational/ Developmental Evaluation

M. Suzanne Hasenstab

In any service or facility that provides a comprehensive offering or program to infants and preschool children with hearing impairment or language delay, knowledge of the child's functioning in all areas of development is imperative. Since appropriate educational or intervention programming is a prime objective, a clear and accurate profile of the child must be ascertained. This is accomplished through evaluation beyond the determination of peripheral auditory abilities, specifically in the growth areas of motor development, cognitive ability, social-emotional maturity, and self-help skills (the area of language will be treated separately). The purpose of this chapter is to present the information pertaining to evaluation of preschool children and the assessment procedures utilized in the Comprehensive Services Program for children between the ages of birth and 6 years.

EVALUATING INFANTS

Perhaps the most difficult age range to address in the evaluation of preschool children is that of infancy, that is, ages under 30 months. Historically, we have evaluated the child in this age range in relation to various milestones of development (Cattell, 1940b; Doll, 1966; Gesell, 1940). However, today the focal point in observing or ascertaining growth in a child is the realization that development is an ongoing process in the perfection of skills. The ability to walk, for example, is one aspect of a continuous growth pattern in the area of motor development. Certain coordination and muscle control must precede actual stepping, and afterward the child continues to perfect leg and body movement through walking, running, and other leg-coordinated motor activities.

This shift in the view of child growth from isolated milestones to a continuum of developmental change has affected the approach in the evaluation of children via psychoeducational means. This type of evaluation is no longer a "checklist" approach in determining child accomplishment in various areas; it is now an awareness and discernment of interactive behaviors in all areas of development. For example, in analyzing a child's verbal production of language, the concern is much deeper than the mere utterance of "mama" or "no" or "all gone." To be at the stage of one-word utterances is a representation of ongoing development in auditory, visual, cognitive, linguistic, experiential, and motoric growth. Each growth area is affected by the others. Thus, the developmental view is the central focus in the evaluation and consequential programming of infants.

Concerns in the Evaluation of Infants

In the psychoeducational evaluation of a child, a primary component is that of determining a measure of intelligence. However, with infants, accuracy in assessing or predicting intelligence is tenuous. A major concern requires a shift in emphasis to the determining of a child's developmental functioning level. Fallen (1978) indicates that the measure is sensorimotor development rather than intelligence. Therefore, caution must be exercised in selecting, administering, and interpreting evaluation instruments. Performance indicates where a particular child is functioning at the time of evaluation; it does not predict the success or failure of a child over a period of years in the future. This fact demands care on the part of the examiner in several areas.

Test Selection

The selection of the test must be based on a thorough knowledge of what a particular instrument is designed to evaluate and on that instrument's reliability and validity regarding this end. Standardized tests have been criticized in recent years concerning the value of their use, especially with preschool children. The issue of "culture free" testing, priority behaviors, and interpretation of infant behavior have been addressed in the literature.

The question of test selection relates to the abilities to be evaluated. What do we want to know about the child that psychoeducational testing can reveal? Salvia and Ysseldyke (1981) indicate two types of information that can be obtained from evaluation instruments: Quantitative information is the actual test score, while qualitative information refers to observations that provide information as to how the child achieved the score. Both types of information are valuable and must be applied to areas of evaluation.

Salvia and Ysseldyke (1981) also state that no educational or psychological evaluation is totally free from error. Therefore, measurement error must be dealt with by the examiner. Nunnally (1967) indicates two main types of error. The first is systematic error or bias that occurs systematically across all results. In systematic error, if a measurement device is biased, for example, it may inflate scores by 10; then all results using that measurement will be inflated by 10 points. The second type, random error, may occur as a result of inconsistent measures or inconsistent results.

Reliability involves the presence of random error. It refers to the absence of error in measurement (Salvia & Ysseldyke, 1981). It is concerned with the consistency or stability within an evaluation instrument. Kerlinger (1973) indicates that reliability is synonymous with terms such as predictability, dependability, accuracy, and stability. Obviously, in psychoeducational evaluation we desire reliable instruments, not ones in which an individual's score will randomly fluctuate. The freer an evaluation instrument is of random error, the more reliable it is.

Another issue in test selection is validity, which is concerned with what a testing instrument measures and the extent to which it measures what it purports to measure. Usually, three interrelated types of validity are considered in tests: content validity, criterion-related validity, and construct validity.

Content validity, according to Salvia and Ysseldyke (1981), involves three factors. The first is the appropriateness of the items included in the test as to the purpose of the test, the age of the individual to be tested, and that individual's particular background and makeup. The second is the completeness of the item sample. The test must include enough items to represent adequately what it is designed to measure. The third factor relates to how the items assess the test content. Several alternatives are available. Depending on content, multiple choice, supplying a correct answer, applying a process related to the content, and imitating the behavior of the examiner are but a few of the alternatives. How content is assessed should fit the nature of the content and the population addressed.

Criterion-related validity involves two factors. The first is concurrent criterion-related validity; this refers to performance at the time of testing and to how accurately the examiner can determine an individual's performance on a criterion measure based on the test score. For example, does a score on a reading test provide an accurate indication of how well a child reads? The second factor is predictive criterion-related validity, which refers to the accuracy in determining future performance on a criterion measure. For example, how well does the reading test administered in Grade 1 estimate the child's reading performance in Grade 6?

The third type of validity is construct validity. The term *construct,* in this instance, means the theory or idea that explains what is to be measured, such as cognition, language, or motor ability. In order to determine the construct validity of the measurement device, the test must prove that it evaluates the foundation idea or construct on which it is based.

One other issue pertaining to test selection should be addressed. If standardized testing instruments are to be employed, it is wise to examine the normative data involved in the test. The purpose of norms is to assist in interpreting individual test scores by allowing a comparison of performance between the child and others tested with the same instrument. However, the child being evaluated may not conform to the population used to procure the normative data. In each case, therefore, test manuals containing information on the normed population as well as on test validity and reliability should be thoroughly studied by the examiner to determine if the child to be tested is comparable to the normative group.

In tests designed for infants or preschool children, there are usually age norms, percentile norms, and standard score norms. Age norms represent an average age at which normed children received a particular score. These norms are usually expressed by the age in years and months. For example, a child may have a motor age equivalent of 6 months or of 2 years, 4 months. Performance is compared across age groups. A percentile norm is expressed as a percentile rank, denoting the position of a child's performance along a continuum, relative to others scoring higher or lower on the test. Raw scores are converted to percentile ranks from tables included in testing manuals; this allows the examiner to view performance in relation to the normed group. Standard score norms also show the relation of the child's performance to the group picture. The standard score indicates the child's score in relation to the mean or average of the normative group performance. The child's score is compared to standard deviation units within a normal spread or curve. The examiner can determine if the child's performance is above or below the average for the test used. Standard scores are usually expressed as either T-scores or Z-scores.

The abilities selected for evaluation in the Comprehensive Services Program are based on the interactive areas in child development of cognition, language, audition, motor abilities, social-emotional maturity, and self-help skills. These areas also form the basis for program and curriculum design. Therefore, test selection must center on appropriate evaluation of these areas.

Qualifications of the Examiner

Related to the appropriateness of the evaluation instrument is the qualification of the examiner to administer a particular test. In the school situation, this task has been left primarily to the school psychologist. However, in most centers that offer infant or preschool intervention services, such a staff member is nonexistent. Testing then becomes the responsibility of the teacher or clinician. Wallace and Larsen (1978) note an important consideration regarding this issue, based on P.L. 94–142, the Education for All Handicapped Children Act (1975). P.L. 94–142 requires that teachers participate in the decision of placement and programming of the exceptional child.

Whether the examiner is the psychologist, teacher, or clinician, some specific rules should be followed. It is of the utmost importance that the examiner be intimately familiar with the instrument regarding purpose, limitations, administrative procedures, scoring, and interpretation. Of equal importance is the ability to interact with a young child. The best designed testing instrument will be ineffective if the examiner fails to establish a relaxed, interactive setting with the child. A combination of knowledge of the evaluation measure and test administration skill together with knowledge of young children and their particular behaviors will enable the examiner to evaluate children successfully in the infancy stage.

The Individual Child

The understanding of child/infant behavior in general must be supported by some basic familiarity with the individual child to be evaluated. This leads to an additional area of concern, that of the child's particular life circumstances. Salvia and Ysseldyke (1981) emphasize that awareness of the individual's current life circumstances permits understanding of what the child brings to the evaluation task. Each infant or preschool child enters into the evaluation session from a particular set of experiences, the quality and quantity of which varies from child to child. A child's age, sex, and handicap; the geographical location of the child's home; the socioeconomic status and educational level of the parents; the family structure and level of acculturation—all can affect what experiences an individual child brings to the evaluation session. The history of the child, the parent interview, and visits into the home environment will provide helpful information regarding the child's particular life circumstances. If the child has been seen by other professionals, summaries of the relevant reports will also provide information helpful in evaluation of the child. This familiarization relates closely to the question of norms; that is, the child and the population normed for the test must be comparable. It also calls for a reasonable amount of sensitivity and awareness on the part of the examiner regarding individual differences among children.

Testing Conditions

The actual setting of the examination session is the area most neglected in listing testing considerations. Cazden (1970) points out that the child must be made to feel secure and comfortable during evaluation if a natural and realistic approximation of the child's daily behavior is to be achieved. In addition, the test environment must be free from distraction so that the child's full attention can be directed to the presented tasks. Generally, two alternatives are available in regard to the place of evaluation: the infant can be evaluated either in his home or at the site of services. Very often, we have found that by evaluating the child in the home we can obtain a much more accurate set of results than we can by transporting the child to the center. The feasibility of using the home as the evaluation environment should be discussed with the parents. A desirable testing environment in the home should be physically comfortable for both the examiner and the child and should be free from distraction by other family members, pets, or other household interruptions.

Variation of place may also be exercised within the clinic. For example, the nursery school may be ideal for a three-year-old child but inappropriate for a 12-month-old infant. As with testing in the home, the examiner should select a place that is physically comfortable and free of distraction. The time of evaluation is another critical consideration in testing infants and young children. A fussy, sleepy, or hungry baby is an untestable baby. Generally, early mornings after a good sleep and adequate breakfast are opportune times for evaluating the very young child. Times near meals and naps should be avoided. Parents should be consulted regarding a schedule of the child's daily sleeping, eating, and awake times.

Also related to time is the length of the testing session. Young children tire easily and will become bored if a situation does not particularly appeal to them. Unlike adults, they will not tolerate boredom and will attempt to terminate the session by rather direct verbal or physical means. Thus, the testing time should not exceed 45 minutes for one session and should be adjusted to the particular child's time capacity.

TESTS USED IN INFANT EVALUATION

Our purpose in this section is not to critique all of the existing evaluation instruments available for use with infants but merely to present a sampling of such instruments.

The Minnesota Preschool Scale

Description

The Minnesota Preschool Scale (MPS) is not designed primarily for use with infants but for the evaluation of children beginning at 18 months of age. It was developed by Florence L. Goodenough, Katherine M. Maurer, and M. J. Van Wagenen at the Institute of Child Welfare, University of Minnesota, in 1938 and revised in 1940. In 1925, the Institute of Child Welfare identified its need for scales to measure the mental abilities of the young child, 6 months to 6 years of age, in order to predict the educational needs of children. The staff of the institute began a study of the experimental use of mental measurements with young children. They felt that the socioeconomic status of the child's family was a strong determining factor in the performance of the child on mental tests. The occupation of the fathers was used to classify children along socioeconomic lines. The institute's staff cautioned, however, that this index was to be used only for the classification of groups and was not to be regarded as a measure for the individual. They used the 1920 census data on the occupations of males in Minneapolis to obtain the groups for standardizing the test.

Technical Information

A total of 900 children, 18 months to 6 years of age, were divided into nine half-year age groups, with 100 in each group. Each group was equally balanced as to sex. There were two forms of the test, A and B, so each group of 100 was further subdivided in order to calculate norms for both forms. The total number of subjects upon which the standardization was based was 1,350.

The 1942 revision of the MPS indicated that the computations for the test's C-scores and IQ scores were based on an erroneous table of standards. Wellman (1949) expressed concern that the maximum IQ on MPS is 152. This was confusing to professionals accustomed to the Binet IQ measurement of 150–200. Furthermore, the small number of items below the age of 3.5 years tended to produce an inflated score for a child below this age. Thus, when a child is retested within 6 months, a decrease in IQ is routinely scored by the very young child.

Olson (1945) questioned the predictive value of the scores from the MPS, due to the differing rate of maturing in girls and boys. Characteristic sex differences emerge at an early age. Therefore, the determination of mental status at an early age and the prediction of mental status at later periods, up to the time of college entrance, is felt to be extremely uncertain with this instrument.

Administration and Scoring

The printed materials for the MPS are organized in a manila portfolio, with abbreviated instructions for each test printed on the series of envelopes that are bound like the pages of a book. In addition to tests on cards in the portfolio, the MPS includes the objects required to complete various tasks. The manual contains detailed instructions for the systemic administration of the test and a great deal of material on "climate-setting" and preferred behaviors on the part of the examiner. Also included are practice items to be used preceding each test. The manual puts great emphasis on the necessity of engaging the child in each task in such a way as to ensure the child's optimal effort toward success.

The MPS is made of 26 separate tests, with scoring instructions printed for each in the manual and on the envelopes in the portfolio containing the test materials. The scores for each test range from 1 to 4 points. The child's chronological age is used to obtain a C-score converted to percentile rank, IQ-verbal, nonverbal, and total scores through manual tables. From a single examination, three scores are obtainable: a verbal score, a nonverbal score, and a combined score. However, it is recommended that only the total or combined score be used for children under 3 years of age.

Summary

Maurer (1946) used an item analysis of the MPS to determine whether items predict ultimate mental ability. She used accumulated data from the Institute of Child Welfare to reexamine at maturity a group of young people originally tested with the MPS at age 6. She retested the members of this group at age 16 or older, using Wells Revision of the Army Alpha Test (based on Binet). Among this group, the results on the comparison of the test scores indicated that nonverbal items were generally predictive, while many verbal items had little or no relation at maturity. Among the items that Maurer found to have high predictive value were imitative drawings, block building, form discrimination, digit span, picture completion, puzzle completion, vocabulary, and understanding of opposites. According to Bayley (1947), the great value of Maurer's research is that it pointed the way to the types of test items that needed to be developed in a preschool test to be able, in fact, to predict mature intelligence at an early age.

The MPS represents an early attempt to evaluate the abilities of the very young child and to predict future performance. At present, however, from the point of view of content, it is out of date, both in the language utilized and in the testing materials included in the kit. In addition, the standardization data are scarce and really cannot be applied to children in an environment nearly 40 years after publication of the test.

Cattell Infant Intelligence Scale

Description

The Cattell Infant Intelligence Scale (Cattell, 1940a) is a downward extension of the Stanford Binet Intelligence Scale (Form L—1937) designed for use with children between the ages of 3 and 36 months. Each age level contains five or more items for assessing the infant's intellectual abilities. Many items are similar to the Gesell tasks and those of the Stanford Binet at the upper age ranges.

Technical Information

Standardization of the scale is based on 1,346 examinations of 274 children between the ages of 3 and 36 months. There is some question as to whether this represents a random sample. Relatively low validity is reported for the ages below 12 months when correlated with performance on the Stanford Binet Form L at 3 years (.10 at 3 months, .34 at 6 months, and .18 at 9 months). Above the age of 12 months, correlations of .56 to .83 are reported. Reliability studies also indicate greater value for ages above 15 months. Although the predictive value of the lower end of the scale is questionable, clinicians at the time the scale was developed considered the test valuable in appraising a child's level of functioning at the time of testing.

Administration and Scoring

The testing time of the scale is approximately 30 to 40 minutes, although there are no specific time limits. All materials used in the evaluation are simple, inexpensive, and designed to appeal to babies and young children. Clear and definite directions for administration are contained in the manual, accompanied by photographs depicting various responses. Test age levels are set at each month for the early ages of 2 to 12 months, increased to 2-month levels for ages 12 to 18 months, and to 3-month levels for ages from 18 to 30 months. Scoring is similar to that for the Stanford Binet (1937). The resulting score is in the form of a mental age that can be converted to an IQ score.

Summary

Following its development, the Infant Intelligence Scale was regarded quite highly as a valuable clinical instrument for evaluating the young child and for use in research. Cattell provided helpful suggestions throughout the manual for evaluating young children. Provisions were made for parental involvement, and there are statements emphasizing the significance and limitations of the test. However, though the test had value at the time of publication, its usefulness now is questionable. Nevertheless, despite technical limitations, the Infant Intelligence Scale represents a good early attempt at infant evaluation.

Gesell Developmental Schedules

Description

The Gesell Developmental Schedules (Gesell & Amatrauda, 1941), published in the format of a book/manual, was developed to measure developmental levels in the four areas of motor skills, adaptive behavior, language ability, and personal/social behavior. Although originally addressed to the medical profession, it has also been widely used in the field of child psychology. Its use is addressed to both normal and "abnormal" infants and young children. The age range considered in evaluation is from 1 to 36 months. The format is relatively uncomplicated, easy to read, and supplemented with many illustrations.

Technical Information

Standardization of the Gesell schedules is lacking; only technical data of the Gesell Institute are available. The technical information is produced by the use of charts depicting the aspects of behavior observed for the key ages of 1, 4, 7, 10, 12, 18, 24, and 36 months. There is little actual information on standardization procedures or statistics involving test use. The original descriptive data are based on white children of the geographical area around the Yale-based Gesell Center.

Administration and Scoring

Administration of the schedules is in the form of observational diagnosis, using as guidelines the behaviors outlined at each age level. The rate of development is summarized by a developmental quotient or D.Q., which represents the proportion of normal development present for a child at a particular age, based on a scale of 100. The D.Q. designates integrated behavior in the four areas evaluated rather than intelligence per se. The D.Q. was claimed to be a constant with predictive value; however, much of the evidence for this claim proved that to be erroneous.

Summary

The Gesell schedules, as well as much of Gesell's other published works, were topics of much controversy, with many legitimate attacks coming from the fields of education and psychology. In some respects, Gesell became as much of a household word as Spock did at a later date. Still, though the influence of Gesell on objective observation is found as the basis of many tests currently available, the Gesell Developmental Schedules suffer from many limitations when viewed as a quantitative assessment instrument.

Griffiths Mental Development Scale for Testing Babies from Birth to Two Years

Description

The Griffiths Mental Development Scale for Testing Babies from Birth to Two Years was originally published in 1951, with a revised edition in 1955. It represents the first infant test standardized on British children. The 260-item test is divided into five subscales—locomotive, personal/social, hearing and speech abilities, eye-hand coordination, and general performance—and a total scale.

Technical Information

The final standardization information for the Griffiths scale is based on a sample of 571 infants from 7 to 70 months of age, selected on the basis of the occupational status of the fathers. The children were divided into age groups so that all age levels evaluated by the test were represented. Between 16 and 31 babies were assigned to age categories by month. Of the original population, 60 infants were reevaluated after 30 weeks. The results of the retesting yielded a correlation of .87 over the time interval.

Administration and Scoring

In the accompanying manual, Griffiths provides detailed directions for the presentation and accurate scoring of the instrument. She also includes helpful recommendations for general testing procedure and a well-explained section on the interpretation of the test results. The individual scores for each of the five categories in the instrument combine to produce a mental age that is computed to a ratio IQ or G.Q., a general intelligence quotient. Neither the administration procedure nor the scoring procedure present undue difficulty.

Summary

The Griffiths scale is considered to be a well-developed test for very young children. However, normative and statistical information for the scale is not extensive. Griffiths herself recommends additional requirements in this regard. It is suggested that the test not be used in countries other than England without alterations, since the language and materials are specifically British in many instances. The instrument has been found to be useful in the evaluation of young babies in England.

Slosson Intelligence Test

Description

The Slosson Intelligence Test (SIT) for Children and Adults (Slosson, 1963) is another test that is not particularly designed for use with infants, but it covers an age range beginning at 2 weeks and ending at age 27 years. It is a short, individual screening device for the purpose of evaluating mental ability. The SIT is fashioned after the Stanford Binet and contains many items from that test.

Technical Information

Standardization data on the SIT are sketchy at best. Given the author's explanation of the normative population, the examiner is left in a quandry as to what population was actually used. There is also a paucity of information from validity studies on the SIT. The SIT reports a high correlation of scores with the Stanford Binet, from .90 to .98. Actually, this is not surprising in view of the fact that the majority of the items on the SIT originated in the Stanford Binet test.

Administration and Scoring

Administration of the SIT is quite easy and takes 15 to 20 minutes. Many items may be credited on parent-report information. The manual provides minimal explanation of behavior characteristics, however. The individual receives credit in the form of a number of months for each correct item. The test is terminated after 10 consecutive failures.

Summary

The SIT is not recommended for use with preschool children. It makes an unusually heavy demand on proficient language abilities. In addition, the test is unsound technically. There is little information regarding the SIT's standardization, reliability, validity, or even rationale.

Denver Developmental Screening Test

Description

The Denver Developmental Screening Test (DDST) (Frankenburg, Dodds, & Fandal, 1969) is a screening device, designed primarily for use in medical centers and hospitals that serve infants and young children. Its purpose is to aid in the early identification of children with developmental difficulties in the areas of language, fine- and gross-motor abilities, and social development. The test's age range is from birth to age 6. Although no elaborate equipment is needed, an accurate understanding of the manual is required. The manual contains precise definitions and descriptions of each behavior evaluated.

Technical Information

The standardization population for the DDST was taken from a cross section of over 1,000 children residing in the Denver, Colorado, area. Whites, blacks, and children of Spanish descent were represented in the population. Family economic status ranged from unskilled labor to the professional fields. Children with diagnosed visual, auditory, neurological, or other impairments were excluded from the population. The distribution of subjects was based on the Denver 1960 census.

Results from using the DDST have been compared with the Stanford Binet and the Mental Scale of Infant Development (1936); available evidence indicates that, compared to the two latter tests, it is not as reliable, valid, sensitive, or selective. Its usefulness with children under 30 months of age is questionable. The most satisfactory results have been shown for children aged 4. The DDST manual contains norms for sex and family occupation groups for each subtest. The test's standardization information is very brief and sketchy.

Administration and Scoring

Administration procedure for the DDST is uncomplicated, and several items may be scored based on parent interview. Items are presented on a score sheet in bars that spread across ages at which a particular behavior is evidenced in child development. Each behavior item is subdivided, indicating percentages of children having achieved or passed an item. The child's age is recorded by a vertical line at the appropriate age level, and items are presented until three errors occur consecutively. Scoring is indicated by pass (P), fail (F), or no familiarity (NO). Items failed above the age line are not considered indicative of delay; items below are tested further.

Summary

Although the DDST appears relatively easy to use, caution should be exercised when crediting items. An examiner using this test should be thoroughly familiar with child development. As the title of the test suggests, it is a screening device and by no means can provide in-depth information concerning the delay that may be suspected.

Ordinal Scales of Psychological Development

Description

The Ordinal Scales of Psychological Development (Uzgaris & Hunt, 1975) provide an evaluation of cognitive function from the Piagetian point of view. Although the test procedure is still in the developmental stages, it may demonstrate new insight into the conceptualization processes of children. The instrument contains seven scales to evaluate vocal and gestural imitation, operational causality, object relations in space, schemes for relating to objects, means for obtaining desired environmental results, and object permanence and prehension.

Technical Information

There is very little technical information available on the ordinal scales.

Administration and Scoring

At this point, the administration and scoring of the ordinal scales are complex and difficult procedures.

Summary

The Ordinal Scales of Psychological Development could prove to be a valuable new approach to preschool and infant assessment.

EVALUATION INSTRUMENTS USED IN THE COMPREHENSIVE SERVICES PROGRAM

Bayley Scales of Infant Development

The Bayley Scales of Infant Development (BSID) (Bayley, 1969) provide the basis of overall evaluation in the psychoeducational component of assessment. The Bayley scales provide a mental measurement index, comprised of cognitive and language-related behaviors; a motor index, made up of fine and large muscle movements and overall body coordination and control; and a behavior analysis scale. The BSID is designed for use with children between 2 and 30 months of age.

Description

The BSID, designed by Bayley and published in 1969, represent the culmination of 40 years of research and clinical practice. The test's mental and motor scales draw heavily on three earlier scales of evaluation that are now out of print: the California First Year Mental Scale (Bayley, 1933), the California Preschool Mental Scale (Jaffa, 1934), and the California Infant Scale of Motor Development (Bayley, 1936). The unpublished 1958 BSID evaluated the first 15 months of life; the 1960 BSID research issue was expanded to include the entire 2nd year to 24 months of age.

The BSID mental scale comprises 163 items that measure cognitive and linguistic abilities. The items examine responses to auditory and visual stimuli, manipulation of objects, social interactive behavior, problem-solving ability, and receptive and expressive language behaviors. Results of the mental scale are expressed as a standard score, the M.D.I. or mental development index.

The motor scale employs 81 items that measure the degree of body control, coordination of large muscles, and fine manipulation skills. Results are expressed as the P.D.I. or psychomotor development index.

The infant behavior record or I.B.R. is in the form of a descriptive rating scale of various social and emotional behaviors displayed by infants. It provides a qualitative measure of the child's social interaction, emotional tone, and general orientation and reaction to the situation of the evaluation session.

Administration Procedure

All materials used in testing with he BSID are provided in the test kit, with the exception of a stopwatch, 8½″ × 11″ paper, facial tissues, stairs, and a walking board. The total average testing time for administration of the mental and motor scales is approximately 45 minutes, rarely exceeding 60 minutes. The order of presentation should be adapted to the responsiveness of the child. The child may be scored for an item demonstrated at any time during the observation period, even though the child failed to demonstrate it satisfactorily when a specific opportunity was available. Any relevant behavior directly observed by the examiner is scorable, even if observed outside the examination room.

In order to administer the BSID adequately, one must be thoroughly familiar with the directions for presenting and scoring items. The mental scale is regularly given before the motor scale because the testing situation changes from sitting to moving about. The BSID testing procedure features age-by-age ordering of the test items; many items are arranged in series in which one basic test procedure or stimulus situation may be scored for several items at different age levels. Items are identified by a situation code. Items in the same situation code group may be observed and scored at one time.

The range of testing is determined by establishing a basal and a ceiling level. The basal level is the item preceding the earliest failure, and the ceiling level is the item representing the most difficult success. The situation codes are useful in the process of seeking a basal level. The manual suggests using a criterion of 10 successive items passed or failed on the mental scale and 6 successive items passed or failed on the motor scale to establish basal or ceiling levels.

Each item is identified in several ways. The item title is descriptive, the item number helps to establish the child's basal level for computing the raw score, the age placement aids in determining where to begin testing, the age range is shown, and the situation codes help to identify related items. Items may be presented by the parent if the examiner feels a behavior can be better elicited in that way.

Scoring

The individual record forms for the mental and motor scales are identified by color—yellow and blue, respectively. Those for the behavior index are white. The BSID use a basal and ceiling item to determine the range of testing. As noted, the basal level is the item preceding the earliest failure, and the ceiling is the item representing the highest level of success. Performance on items is recorded by checking the appropriate column as indicated: pass (P), failure (F), or other (O-omit, R-refused), and RPT (reported by parents). The raw score for each scale is the total number of items passed. Only the items marked P are added into the raw score. Raw scores are converted to the M.D.I. and P.D.I. for the child's appropriate age. Tables are provided in the manual for conversion of raw scores for each of the scales. Each score is an index or normalized standard score. The distribution of raw scores at each age level is converted to a set of normalized standard scores having a mean value of 100 and a standard deviation of 16. For each age group, the lowest standard score generally falls between 55 and 60 points, and the highest score between 140 and 145 points. The resulting M.D.I. and P.D.I. may differ by a few points. However, a difference of 13 points or more may be considered significant. A difference of 20 points or more merits attention. Age equivalents for both scales may be obtained from the norm tables by looking across the rows corresponding to an M.D.I. or P.D.I. of 100 to find the age-group column in which the given raw score is nearest to that obtained by the child. The age given at the head of this column represents the child's age equivalent for the scale.

The manual stresses that an intelligence quotient (IQ) should not be computed based on mental age (MA/CA = IQ). Bayley (1969) sees no evidence to support the interpretation of an IQ score from the BSID.

Further Analysis of Results

An item analysis of the BSID results provides specific information regarding a child's performance. In most cases, a pattern arises that helps to determine areas in which particular emphasis will be necessary in the educational programming. Upon analysis, the infant behavior record lends valuable clues to the infant's temperament, social interactiveness, and the general systems the child applies when faced by various situations. All of this information is necessary to adequately design objectives and a subsequent program that will suit the child's particular strengths, weaknesses, general personality, and life circumstances.

Related Research

The general opinion expressed in the literature is that the Bayley scales fill a long-felt need for a well-standardized and reliable instrument for the assessment of developmental progress in infants. Previous scales based on test items formulated 20 to 40 years ago were standardized on small samples of children from limited geographic and socioeconomic backgrounds. The Bayley scales were standardized according to a stratified sample design that controlled the sex and color within each age group, with further controls related to residence (urban-rural) and education of the head of household.

Although there is general contention that directions in the BSID manual are specific, clear, and logical, it is also agreed that the BSID is difficult to learn how to administer due to the overwhelming amount of information one must keep in mind while giving it. It is assumed that difficulty of administration will decrease with increased practice and familiarity.

Collard (1972) believes that the BSID is a useful tool for the clinician and researcher alike and feels that these scales should prove useful in the recognition and diagnosis of sensory and neurological defects and emotional disturbances and in indicating the possibility of environmental deficits. She states (1972) that "[its] value . . . as a research instrument lies in its careful standardization high reliability, and broad coverage of many aspects of the behavior repertoire of infants, parts of which could be used as subscales in longitudinal studies" (p. 402). Collard (1972) notes that "the test materials are colorful, attractive, durable, washable and have sufficient novelty to be intrinsically interesting to infants and young children and yet are similar to objects with which subjects would be familiar"

(p. 402). However, she criticizes the use of specially constructed stairs and a walking board for testing certain items in the motor scale. She feels that the need for these materials might limit the use of the motor scale because of the difficulty of transporting such items.

Collard (1972) also comments on the chronological order of the BSID items, the use of a situation code, and the use of a color coding in the manual on the test sheets. She feels that all these aspects of the test are helpful. However, she states that it would have been helpful if the age placement of the items had been listed after each item in the situation codes and if these categories were printed on the front and back of a cardboard card that could be consulted by the tester as the test is given.

Collard (1972) concludes:

> The BSID is intermediate between the empirically constructed tests which sample the observed abilities of children in various situations and those tests which may be designed to measure specific mental processes such as memory, object constancy, generalization, learning to solve problems, or learning abstract language concepts. The BSID includes items involving these processes, but does not have sections which measure these processes specifically. (p. 403)

In summary Collard's opinion of the BSID is that, "because of the range of the items, the reliability of the scales, and their careful construction and standardization, the BSID is by far the best measure of infant development available today" (Collard, 1972, p. 403).

Werner and Bayley (1966) reported on a study of 8-month-old infants concerning tester-observer and test-retest reliability of the individual items in the Bayley Revised Scales of Infant Mental and Motor Development. Ninety 8-month-old infants were tested within 1 week of their birthday and observed by a second examiner behind one-way vision screens in the Laboratory of Psychology at the National Institutes of Health (NIH), Bethesda, Maryland, and in six collaborating hospitals. For the purpose of the study, 28 of the 8-month-old infants were tested 1 week later by the same examiners. The results of the study were as follows:

- Test-retest reliabilities were lower than tester-observer reliabilities on the majority of items on both the mental and motor scales.
- Items on the mental scale that had high test-retest reliabilities dealt with object-oriented behavior.
- Items on the mental scale with low test-retest reliabilities were items of a social, interpersonal nature.

- Items on the motor scale that could be observed accurately and were fairly consistent from one testing occasion to another dealt with the independent control of the head, trunk, and lower extremities.
- Items on the motor scale on which infants' performance varied considerably from one week to another were "emerging" items in the area of gross- and fine-motor coordination and items that required assistance by an adult (examiner or parent).

Werner and Bayley (1966) interpreted the results of the mental scale item analysis as indicating that normal infants at 8 months of age are much more variable and more easily inhibited in their social-interpersonal behavior than in their object-oriented behavior. They state that infants who are inhibited by the strangeness of the examiner and situation may be less so a week later, after which the examiner and situation are seen as friendly and familiar. Werner and Bayley (1966) note that, "if for the purpose of screening, we want to single out reliable diagnostic signs on the Mental Scale which reflect a suitable level of maturation, we might put more confidence in the constancy of object-oriented behavior" (p. 47). In examining the results of the motor scale item analysis, they comment that, while the infant, once matured to a certain level, cannot help but keep the head balanced, sit, stand up, or walk alone, the child can resist cooperation on items requiring interaction with an adult. In addition, they note that fine motor coordination items that show low test-retest agreement, such as "partial finger prehension" and "neat pincer," are likely at this stage to mature very quickly within 1 week, the time between test and retest.

Willerman, Broman, and Fiedler (1970) reported on a study that explored the relation of the research form of the Bayley Scales of Mental and Motor Development to 4-year Binet IQ as a function of social class. The subjects for the study were 3,037 white children born at Boston Lying-in Hospital (BLH). At 8 months of age, the infants were routinely brought to BLH or Children's Hospital Medical Center (CHMC) and administered the collaborative research form of the Bayley Scales of Mental and Motor Development. At four years of age, the children returned to CHCM and were given the abbreviated version of the Stanford Binet Intelligence Scale, Form L–M.

The major finding of the study was that infant developmental status interacts with socioeconomic status (SES) in the incidence of low 4-year IQ. The results indicated that retarded infant development is associated with disproportionally poorer intellectual performance in the context of higher SES and that retarded low-SES infants are more vulnerable to the adverse effects of their environment. Conversely, the results indicate that advanced infant development can minimize the occurrence of low IQ among low-SES individuals.

The results failed to indicate what influences accelerated infant development. Willerman et al. (1970) state that their data indicated a very poor relationship between social class and test performance in infancy. "The genetic or environmental influences which lend to accelerated infant maturational status remain a mystery" (p. 75). The authors further note that, among high-SES groups, the study results suggest that the infant test is a poor predictor of later intellectual status, since infant developmental status bore little relation to 4-year IQ. "The process by which poorly developed infants from high SES environments overcome their deficits is unclear" (p. 75). They conclude that the fact that high SES can mask deficits points to the need for taking SES into account in grouping the effects of infant experience, such as perinatal stress. They further conclude that poverty, which produces a higher incidence of perinatal morbidity as well as mortality, will amplify the IQ deficit in poorly developed infants.

Gannon (1968) reported a study that correlated six measures of performance on the Bayley Scales of Mental and Motor Development at 8 months with 48-month Stanford Binet IQs and the Graham-Ernhart Block Sort Test (G-E BST), a concept-formation test. The study was based on data from the Charity Hospital (New Orleans) Child Development Study population. A total of 384 children who had been tested at both 8 months and 48 months were included in the study.

The results indicated that all but one of the six measures correlated significantly with IQ, while three were predictive of block sort scores. Scores derived from item analyses of the Bayley scales and the 48-month tests also yielded significant correlations with later performances. Weighing items did not substantially increase relationships. Gannon (1968) stated that "these results are similar to previous data: there are statistically, but not practically, significant correlations between infant and preschool test performances" (p. 1199). He concluded that extreme caution should be taken in interpreting infant-scale performance except for the purpose of providing tentative evidence of contemporary developmental progress. He does not advocate the use of the test to predict IQ at a later age.

Kohen-Raz (1976) reported on a scalogram study based on empirical data as collected through routine administration of the Bayley Infant Scales of Mental Development. The purpose of the study was to break the mental scale down into subscales or scalable sequences. Five scales emerged, designated according to the prominent type of infant behavior measured by them: eye-hand, manipulation, object-relation, imitation-comprehension, vocalization-social contact-active vocabulary. Kohen-Raz concluded that scalable sequences of infant behavior, as measured by items of the Bayley mental scale, are well demonstrated.

Summary

For the purpose of evaluating the overall development of infants, the most appropriate instrument at this time appears to be the Bayley Scales of Infant Development. The BSID represent a well-designed progression of developmental behaviors that can indicate a general mental and general motor level of functioning. Item analysis can determine specific areas of delay within the two general scales. The social behavior summary presents valuable examples of the child's interactive behavior, with the examiner, the attending parent, and objects in the environment. Statistical information on the BSID is quite extensive, and the Bayley scales are still being used in various research studies to determine further uses and the usefulness of the instruments. Used with caution and supplemented by observation and informal evaluation, the Bayley scales are exceedingly valuable to the infant interventionist.

Developmental Programming for Infants and Young Children

Developmental Programming for Infants and Young Children: Assessment and Application, Volume 1 (Rogers & D'Eugenio, 1977), provides a supplement to the BSID. Since many of the items contained therein are similar to those in the BSID, scoring can be done simultaneously. The rationale for using this additional instrument is that the developmental program assessment volume categorizes behaviors more precisely than the BSID. There are six subscales in the instrument. Although the Bayley scales serve as the standardized evaluation measure, they yield two scores that represent a summation of behaviors. Since information gained from the assessment is to be used in the implementation of an intervention program for parents and child, a clear and precise breakdown of behaviors for the development of consequent objectives is deemed necessary. The cumulative score produced by the BSID does not provide specificity of information for this purpose.

Description

The Developmental Programming for Infants and Young Children, the overall program edited by D. Sue Schafer and Martha S. Moersch (1977), is comprised of three components or "volumes." Volume 1, with which we are concerned, is titled Assessment and Application. This is the evaluation component of the program used in conjunction with Volume 2 titled The Early Intervention Developmental Profile (EIDP). There are 274 items representing six developmental areas.

1. perceptual/fine motor
2. cognition
3. language
4. social/emotional
5. self-care
6. gross motor

These items, arranged in developmental sequence, parallel the basic areas of concentration in the Comprehensive Services Program (in the EIDP, audition is not considered separate from other areas). The profile is of great assistance in presenting information concerning functioning levels for the child under age 36 months of age. The authors indicate that the purpose of the profile is not to diagnose disabilities or to predict performance but to describe strengths and weaknesses in current functioning.

Administration Procedures

Since this is not a test kit, no materials are provided. A list of items is included in the manual, all of which are contained in the BSID kit. Suggestions in the manual are made for the sequence of observing behaviors, however variations are permissible. Therefore, joint use with the BSID works very well.

Scoring Procedures

Scoring techniques are provided for each profile item. A score of pass (P), fail (F), emerging skill (ES), or omitted item (O) is possible. Scores are recorded on a profile graph. The resulting developmental level does not indicate mental age but provides a graphic illustration of the child's performance in the various areas examined. Details for scoring and plotting information on the profile graph are contained in the manual section.

Reliability and Validity Information

The EIDP has not been standardized. Therefore, the items selected and assigned to specific age ranges were based on standardization and research of other instruments. For original items, mostly projection-based, age norms were based on Piaget's (1954) original suggestions. Nonstandardization is rationalized by emphasizing that the purpose of the profile is to supplement standardized instruments when diagnosis is required. The profile offers only a "general estimate."

Correlation coefficients are generally high with evaluation instruments currently in use. The highest was .96 for the BSID mental index and the

EIDP social and cognitive profiles. The EIDP perceptual/fine-motor profile and gross-motor profile also showed high correlations when compared with the BSID motor index (.84 and .95, respectively); this involved scores for 14 children.

A tester-observer paradigm was used to examine inter-rater reliability. The range of agreement between tester-observer was from 80 to 97 percent, with a mean of 89 percent agreement overall. Children's scores on the profile were also examined over time at 3- and 6-month intervals following initial evaluation. Correlations between the first testing and subsequent sessions were found to be uniformly high.

Summary

Developmental Programming for Infants and Young Children can serve as a helpful, informal evaluation instrument in support of the Bayley scales as well as a valuable record-keeping device for charting progress of the young child in an intervention program. Items may be integrated into specific objectives for children. Coordinating activities offered in the program provide excellent basic suggestions for activities to demonstrate to parents or to require parents to carry out within the home program. In addition, the program's evaluation and follow-up suggestions are felt to be open and flexible enough to be used in a variety of settings.

EVALUATING THE CHILD OVER 2½ YEARS OF AGE

The preschool child over 30 months of age requires a somewhat different approach in the assessment domain. By this age, the child has established some basic foundations of growth and is in the process of perfecting early skills in the various developmental areas. In many ways, this age group is much easier to evaluate, in other ways it is not.

The baby, subject to basic limitations in movement and expression, progresses rapidly to independence as the infant gains increased self-control and consequently control over the environment. The difference between the 3-year-old and the 3-month-old is phenomenal. By 30 months, the average child has increased four times in birth weight and nearly doubled in height. The child is moving from "activity-oriented intelligence" to more symbolic thought processes (Lefrancois, 1973). The normally developing child can comprehend spoken language quite well and is able to express feelings and desires.

The preschool child is also somewhat more flexible in regard to environmental surroundings. We find, for example, that once a child has a chance to inspect and feels assured with a new room setting, he can be evaluated in a rather wide variety of settings, provided blatant distractions are not present. Often the presence of a friendly stuffed animal can also help during testing. It is important for the examiner to recognize and capitalize on these factors. They can definitely serve as either distinct advantages or hindrances in evaluating infants and preschool children.

The concerns expressed in relation to evaluating the infant hold true also for the older preschool child. To recapitulate, they may be summarized as follows:

- Performance on various evaluation instruments represents the child's present functioning level and should not be used as a predictor of future performance.
- Test selection must be based on a thorough understanding of the test purpose, content, reliability, validity, and appropriateness.
- The examiner administering the test should be able to demonstrate proficiency in testing, both from a personal and a technical frame of reference.
- The individual child remains the paramount issue during evaluation. Accommodations to allow the child's realistic performance should be ensured.
- The testing environment should be made conducive to security and success for the child.

In addition, the examiner must bear in mind that the individuality of experience of the older preschool child may be much greater than that of the infant (Safford, 1978). The child at age 3 has a repertoire covering a wide variety of experiences and interactions in the child's past and present environment.

Another issue relates to children who exhibit various delays. A delay of 2 months at infancy could mean a delay of a full year by age 3. The gap in developmental retardation can often widen with increased age. The examiner may have a normal-sized three-year-old with abilities and interests of a much younger child; this situation will affect the entire assessment process.

The importance of play is pertinent to the preschooler. Play is the universal activity of the young child (and will be discussed in detail in the intervention section of this book). Indeed, it provides the best means to develop rapport and observe child behavior in a relaxed and pleasurable setting.

TESTS USED IN EVALUATING PRESCHOOL CHILDREN

A large number of evaluation instruments are designed to test one or several developmental areas in the preschool years between the ages of

2½ and 6 years. Since our purpose in this chapter is to examine the overall or psychoeducational evaluation of preschool children, however, only tests that involve a multiskill examination or tests of intelligence will be presented here. Language evaluation instruments will be examined in the following chapter. The Slosson Intelligence Test (SIT) and the Minnesota Preschool Scale (MPS) have already been discussed and will be omitted here, although they are designed to evaluate abilities within the age range of 2½ to 6 years.

Wechsler Preschool and Primary Scales

Description

The Wechsler Preschool and Primary Scale of Intelligence (WPPSI), developed by David Wechsler (1967), is designed to measure the youngest population assessed by the three Wechsler scales. The Wechsler-Bellevue Intelligence Scale (1939), the original test, was designed for use with adults. In 1949, the Wechsler Intelligence Scale for Children (WISC) was published, based on the format and content of the original adult measure. Wechsler revised his adult scale in 1955; this became the Wechsler Adult Intelligence Scale (WAIS), which still exists in that form. In 1967, the WPPSI was introduced to provide a measure for the preschool child between the ages of 4 and 6½ years. The most recently updated member of the Wechsler family is the Wechsler Intelligence Scale for Children, Revised (WISC-R), the original WISC revised and restandardized in 1974.

The WPPSI has two scales, as do the other Wechsler scales: a verbal scale and a performance scale. These combined scales result in a full scale whose results are interpreted as an overall IQ score.

The verbal scale is made up of five main subtests and one supplementary test that is not used in establishing IQ tables. Generally, the verbal-scale subtest requires responses in the form of oral communication to a specific question or statement of a problem.

The first verbal subtest is on *information*. It examines the child's ability to answer factual questions that relate to experiences common to young children. The *vocabulary* subtest evaluates the child's ability to define words. The subtest on arithmetic is concerned with the ability to solve simple mathematical problems. It contains counting items and arithmetic operations. The subtest on *similarities* requires the child to determine relationships between words via analogies. The subtest on *comprehension* evaluates "social cognition" or the reasons why particular things are done. This subtest is connotative in nature. Finally, the supplementary subtest on the verbal scale is *sentences*; it requires the child to repeat verbatim sentences read by the examiner.

There are also five performance subtests with a supplementary category. Generally, these require some type of manipulation or problem-solving activity. Although no verbal responses are required, comprehension of directions is necessary.

The *animal house* subtest requires the child to associate four pictured animals with four different colored pegs and to match them within a designated time limit. The administration of this subtest a second time constitutes the supplementary subtest on the performance scale. The *picture-completion* subtest involves identification of a missing part of a pictured object. The *mazes* subtest requires the child to trace a path through increasingly difficult maze puzzles. The subtest on *geometric designs* assesses the child's ability to copy geometric designs. The final performance subtest is on *block design*. A stimulus design is presented, and the child's task is to reconstruct the design with manipulative blocks.

Technical Information

The WPPSI was standardized on a population of 1,200 children considered to be representative of the 1960 census, based on age, sex, geographic region, rural-urban residency, race/color, and occupation of the father. Reliability evidence is good and is explained in detail in the manual.

Several validity studies have been conducted with the WPPSI. The correlation between performance on the WISC-R and the WPPSI full scale score for 6-year-olds was .82. Among the individual subtests, the WPPSI verbal and performance categories correlated highly with parallel subtests on the WISC-R. However, validity studies with other instruments—the McCarthy Scales of Children's Abilities (MSCA) and the Stanford Binet (Form L–M)—were somewhat lower. For subjects aged 6 to 6½, the coefficients of correlation were .71 for the general cognitive index of the MSCA and .73 for the Stanford Binet.

Administration and Scoring

Complete administrative directions are presented in the WPPSI manual, and the score sheet contains various clues pertaining to each item. The test is lengthy and requires some study of testing procedure to allow for a smooth administration. Subtests are presented in an order that intermingles verbal and manipulation subtests.

Scoring on the WPPSI is done by assigning a number score to each item as directed by the manual. Scores for each subtest are added into a total raw score for that subtest. Raw scores are converted to scale scores, which in summation yield the verbal, performance, and full scale IQ scores. The scoring is an involved process and should be carefully computed.

Summary

The WPPSI is still widely used by psychologists in evaluating preschool children. The test is limited in that the lower range is at age 4 while much current emphasis is on evaluation of the much younger child. There is also some question as to the actual value of a global IQ score. Additional information can be gained through use of item analysis on individual subtests.

Stanford Binet Intelligence Scale

Description

The oldest and best known test of intelligence is the Stanford Binet. Its story begins in 1905, when the test's first edition was developed by Alfred Binet in France. Since that time the test has undergone a series of revisions—in 1908 (renamed the Binet Simon Scale), 1911, 1916 (revised by Louis Terman for use in the United States; the Stanford revision and extension of the Binet-Simon Scale), 1937, 1960, and 1972 (normative edition by Terman and Merrill). Each of these editions, including the latest, have been the topic of much discussion.

The Stanford Binet is comprised of items that increase in difficulty from the 2-year level to the adult superior level. The items represent a wide range of behaviors. Originally the test was on an age-scale; this was dropped in the 1972 revision.

Technical Information

The Stanford Binet, normative edition (Terman and Merrill, 1973), was standardized on a sample of 2,100 subjects from seven community settings with approximately 100 representatives for each age level. The defining characteristics of the population, however, are not contained in the manual. The reliability of the 1972 edition is based on the reliability of the earlier test versions, actually as updated in the 1937 edition. The same is true regarding validity.

Administration and Scoring

The Stanford Binet items are administered in order, once basal level is established according to instructions supplied in the manual. The ceiling on the test is the lowest age level at which all items are failed. Credit in terms of months is given and summed to equal a mental age, which is converted to an IQ score.

Summary

Throughout its history, the Stanford Binet has been the subject of much discussion. The newest edition may be somewhat more questionable than earlier revisions, due to the lack of necessary data regarding the normative sample, reliability, and validity. In its use with preschool children, it is questionable whether a global IQ score (as with the WPPSI as well) is really of much assistance when the purpose of evaluation is to gain information to promote appropriate intervention. An item analysis, categorizing items into particular areas of development, would present some of this information. However, this could be quite time consuming and there would be much overlap.

Columbia Mental Maturity Scale

Description

The Columbia Mental Maturity Scale (CMMS) (Burgemeister, Blum, & Lorge, 1972) was developed as an individualized testing instrument involving a minimum of required verbal responses. It was originally published in 1954, with revisions in 1959 and 1972. The 92-item test has an age range from 3 years, 6 months to 9 years, 11 months. Its purpose is to evaluate reasoning ability. The items are presented on cards with three to five illustrated drawings. The child is required to classify and relate the drawings by indicating through pointing which of the choices is unrelated or different.

Technical Information

Standardization data for the 1972 revision of the CMMS are based on a population of 2,600 children, proportionately represented based on the 1960 U.S. Census. However, in the normative sample, there were actually more children from large cities than was representative of the general population. The population was stratified, based on age, sex, race, geographic area, and occupation of father.

The CMMS's reliability information in the manual indicates internal consistency coefficients from .85 to .91. Three different age groups were involved in another study of the test's test-retest reliability. The children in the groups showed an average gain of 4.6 age-deviation score points between testing sessions. The reliability scores were from .84 to .86.

The early versions of the CMMS were not considered highly valid measures (Estes, Kodman, & Akel, 1959). The 1972 edition seems to have improved the test somewhat. Correlations with the Stanford Achievement Test (1964) are reported to range from .31 to .61 and with the Elementary I level of the Otis Lennon Mental Ability Test from .62 to .69. A correlation of .67 is indicated with the Stanford Binet Intelligence Scale—Form L–M.

Administration and Scoring

Administration of the CMMS is quick and easy. Children are provided with three example items before actual scoring begins. The total number of correct items equals the raw score, which may be converted, by tables contained in the manual, to age-deviation scores (standard scores), stanines, percentile ranks, and a maturity index (similar to a mental age). The symbols U and L are used to indicate upper and lower ranges of a particular age level.

Summary

The CMMS appears to be sound in regard to standardization and technical issues. However, caution should be exercised in generalizing from the test's results, since there is not a complete representation of developmental areas or intellectual ability in the test. The authors emphasize that the CMMS provides an estimate of reasoning ability and is not an absolute measure of intelligence. Item analysis is helpful in determining particular classification or discrimination strategies a child might use.

Peabody Picture Vocabulary Test

Description

A widely used test in the measurement of children's intellectual ability is the Peabody Picture Vocabulary Test (PPVT) (Dunn, 1965). The test's age range is from 2 years, 6 months to 18 years. The PPVT is comprised of plates illustrated with four drawings. There are two forms of the test that vary in the stimulus word for each item.

Technical Information

The PPVT was standardized on the white population residing in the geographic area of Nashville, Tennessee, which limits generalization somewhat. The normative sample was made up of 4,012 individuals representing the age ranges from 2½ to 18 years. The PPVT manual contains a large report on reliability studies as well as reports computed for the standardization sample. All are comparable, ranging from .67 to .84. There are also many validity reports with various correlations reported for different populations. Correlations of the PPVT with the WISC total-scale IQ range from .43 to .92. None are reported for PPVT with the WPPSI.

Administration and Scoring

The PPVT test procedure is untimed but can be completed in about 15 minutes. The examiner says the stimulus word for each item, and the child indicates the correct choice by pointing to the appropriate picture. Testing continues until six consecutive errors are made. The raw score is the total number of correct items, which is converted to mental age and deviation IQ with a mean of 100 and a standard deviation of 15.

Summary

Much caution should be exercised in the use of the PPVT as an intelligence test, since it measures only the child's receptive language, and a small proportion of it at that. Although technically it appears to outdo other picture vocabulary tests, it is not generalizable due to the normative sample limitations. Its value, often overrated, is in its use as a screening device.

Nebraska Test of Learning Aptitude

Description

Since our focus population is made up of children with hearing and/or language deficits, we will examine two testing instruments designed for use with the hearing-impaired individual. The first is the Nebraska Test of Learning Aptitude (NTLA) (Hiskey, 1966). Originally developed in 1941, with revisions in 1957 and 1966, the NTLA is an individually administered instrument, designed to evaluate the learning aptitude of individuals within the age range of 3 to 16 years. The NTLA manual contains two sets of administrative directions for twelve subtests; one contains verbal directions, and the other employs pantomime and gesture. Test items progress in difficulty for each subtest. Not all of the subtests are administered to any one individual. Figure 4–1 illustrates the subtests included in the test and the age range to which they are given. The NTLA is a performance test and there are no verbal responses required. The child is requested to point to the correct answer or manipulate various materials according to examiner instruction.

Figure 4–1 Subtests of the Nebraska Test of Learning Aptitude

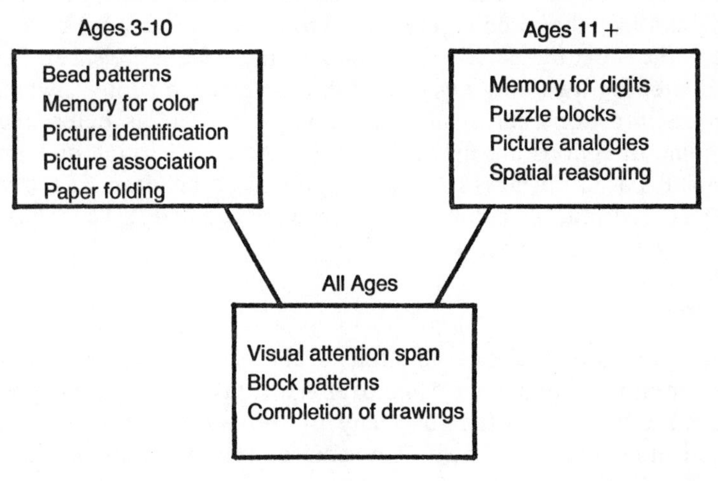

Technical Information

The original NTLA form was normed on hearing-impaired students enrolled in a midwest state residential school for the hearing-impaired and a one-day program in Lincoln, Nebraska. Norms for the hearing population were added in the 1957 revision. Hiskey also added additional items and a spatial relations subtest to his earlier version. The revised test was administered to both hearing and hearing-impaired children aged 2½ to 17½ years who were selected on the basis of parent occupational level in relation to 1960 U.S. Census data.

Information about the nature of NTLA's normative samples is sparse, as is information on the reliability and validity of the test. There are no subtest reliabilities but there are reported split-half reliabilities of .95 (hearing impaired, ages 3–10), .92 (hearing-impaired, ages 11–17), .93 (hearing, ages 3–10), and .90 (hearing, ages 11–17). Concurrent validity data and correlations of learning ages of the subtests with the total test median learning ages are also available. Hiskey's 1966 revision of the test reports concurrent validity coefficients of .82 between the NTLA and WISC IQs for 52 hearing children aged between 5 and 11 years. Hiskey also reports correlations between NTLA and Stanford Binet IQs of .86 for 99 hearing children aged 3 to 10 and .78 for 50 hearing students aged 11 to 17. Technical data on the NTLA are clearly limited.

Administration and Scoring

Administration of the NTLA requires a good understanding by the examiner of the directions, materials, score sheet, and basic test format. Testing can usually be completed in 30 to 45 minutes. Subtests are presented in the order indicated in the manual and on the score sheet. Scoring is conducted by awarding designated points for each subtest, which are converted into age equivalents, and a median score is determined. If pantomime directions are used, a learning age and learning quotient are developed, based on norms for hearing-impaired children. If the verbal directions are used, the child receives a mental age and IQ score based on the hearing sample norms.

Summary

In addition to its technical limitations, the NTLA presents unrealistic results for children under age 5 and over age 12; the scores are depressed. The picture materials used for many of the subtests are very poorly designed and unexciting. The NTLA requires extreme caution in interpretation. We do not recommend its use with preschool children.

Leiter International Performance Scale

Description

Originally published in 1929 by Pursel Leiter for the purpose of assessing the intelligence of children with limited verbal abilities, the Leiter International Performance Scale (LIPS) has undergone six revisions (1934, 1936, 1938, 1940, and 1948). In 1950, Grace Arthur published an adaption of the test, the Arthur Adaptation of the Leiter International Performance Scale (AALIPS). The 1948 revision and the AALIPS are both individually administered tests; the materials for both are the same. The AALIPS evaluates an age range from 2 to 12 years; the 1948 LIPS, containing additional items, extends the range to age 18. Generally, the test's items require perceptual organization and discrimination.

Technical Information

Normative data as described in the manual are inadequate for both scales. The information indicates the sample is from a middle-class, midwestern, metropolitan background with few representatives from either end of the socioeconomic continuum. There is no information concerning the norming of children for whom the test was originally designed. Correlations between the AALIPS and the Stanford Binet for children ages 4 through 8 range from .69 to .93. Correlations with the WISC performance scale range from .79 to .80.

Administration and Scoring

Administration of the Leiter scale involves some practice. Confusing and poorly illustrated manual directions make interpretation of administrative procedure difficult. The procedure involves the use of a response frame and two trays of response blocks and corresponding stimulus cards. The examiner places a stimulus card in the frame and pantomimes instructions. The child then places appropriate blocks in the frame. Scoring presents a problem because correct answers are not provided; therefore, the examiner must make a subjective opinion regarding correctness. Credit received for items passed in subtests is in the form of months, which, when summed, equals a mental age, which can be converted to an IQ score.

Summary

The Leiter scale presents several problems, both technically and managerially. In addition, scores for children under age 6 tend to be depressed. Much caution should be exercised in the use of this test.

THE EVALUATION INSTRUMENT USED IN THE COMPREHENSIVE SERVICES PROGRAM

McCarthy Scales of Children's Abilities

In the Comprehensive Services Program, the McCarthy Scales of Childen's Abilities (MSCA) (McCarthy, 1972), serve as the basic evaluation instrument for use with children over 30 months of age. The MSCA, developed by Dorothea McCarthy and published in its present form in 1972, represents an attempt to fill the clinical-diagnostic gap. It assesses children at a younger age than the WPPSI, beginning at age 2½, where the Bayley scales terminate. The McCarthy scales were designed to assess what the author felt were important areas in the development of preschool children.

Description

The MSCA were designed as an evaluation instrument for use with children within the age range of 2½ to 8½ years. It is divided into 6 component scales, which are comprised of 18 individual subtests that explore a large range of child behavior. Each scale provides a raw score conversion to a scaled score or index, based on the child's chronological age.

The MSCA *verbal scale* is made up of six subtests designed to indicate the child's facility with language, both comprehension and production. The subtests involve such tasks as memory for pictures, comprehension and definition of vocabulary, and concept awareness. The various subtests provide an indication of a child's general, overall language-functioning abilities. The other five scales are also based to various degrees in a language context. In other words, some facility in communication and language awareness is also necessary to complete the various tasks in other scales' subtests.

The *perceptual performance scale* requires no verbal expression by the child. However, the child must exercise receptive ability in understanding the spoken directions of the examiner. The subtests contained in this scale are puzzle formations; imitative block building; imitative tapping sequence; orientation to left and right; design imitation; creative drawing of a person; and conceptual grouping of items based on variables of shape, size, and color. This scale has seven subtests.

The *quantitative scale* examines the child's awareness of numbers and comprehension of quantitative language through four subtests, which, as noted, are dependent on a certain facility in language.

The *general cognitive scale*, unlike the other scales, is actually a composite score representing all of the subtests in the verbal, perceptual, and quantitative scales. Its task is to measure general cognitive abilities of the child, producing a general cognitive index (GCI) comparable to, but not actually, an IQ score.

The *memory scale* is somewhat similar in format to the general cognitive index in that it is represented by subtests from other scales. However, the general cognitive index considers all of the represented subtests, while the memory scale is concerned only with those subtests, six altogether, that entail a memory component. These subtests include the memory-for-pictures task, the imitative tapping sequences, and the subtest on memory for numbers in sequence.

Finally, the *motor scale* evaluates in five subtests the child's ability to perform various large- and small-muscle activities. Actually, all of the subtests contained in the perceptual performance scale involve the ability to manipulate or control movement in some way; however, only two of those subtests are regarded as overlapping in scoring. The interrelationship of the various scales is illustrated in Figure 4–2.

Administration and Scoring

All of the necessary materials for test administration, except a stop watch, are contained in the MSCA testing kit. All of these materials are

Figure 4–2 Subtests of the McCarthy Scales of Children's Abilities

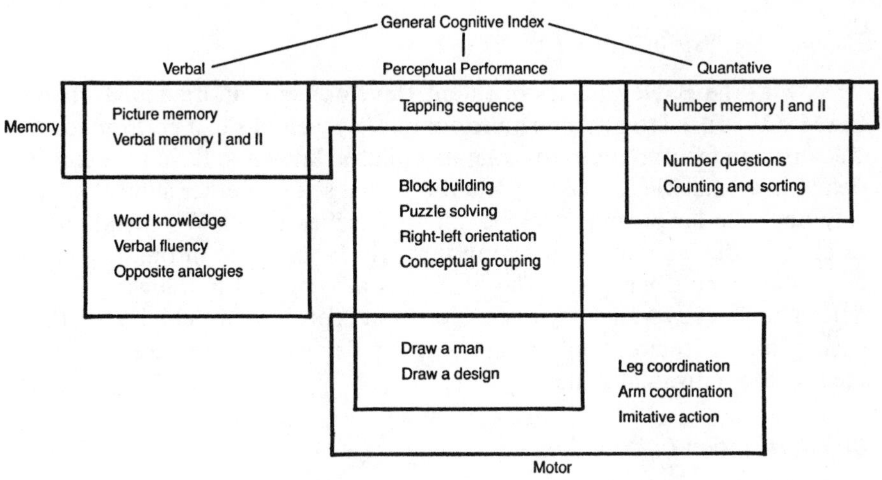

generally interesting to young children. Testing time is approximately 45 minutes. The order of presentation varies with the scales involved and provides a good balance of tasks requiring manipulative and verbal activities as well as variation in difficulty.

The MSCA is relatively easy to administer, with clear and explicit directions provided in the manual and a well-designed scoring form that provides brief directions. Test items within each subtest are arranged in order of increasing difficulty. The score sheet and manual indicate suggested ages to begin testing for each subtest as well as the number of errors that constitute termination of the administration. Although it is suggested that the subtests be administered in the order indicated on the score sheet, subtests can be reordered when deemed necessary without affecting the overall test performance of the child.

The scoring, though technically complicated with various weighted scores, is not difficult in practice because of the step-by-step recording procedure illustrated on the scoring sheet and the clear manual directions. Simply stated, raw scores for items are totaled and then weighted, based upon their importance. The weighted raw scores are distributed among the various scales as directed in the manual and scoring sheet, where they are then summed to yield composite raw scores. These composite scores are then transformed into normalized standard scores from a table arranged according to age of subject. These scores or indexes permit direct comparison across the five scales. The general cognitive index is a special composite of three scales with a normalized standard score conversion of its own.

Further Analysis of Results

As with the Bayley Scales of Infant Development, an item analysis of the MSCA is used to evaluate more completely a child's test performance. Because the tests are used to examine children known to have a language delay, it is valuable to look beyond the verbal scale to other subtests that rely on some language proficiency. This clarifies the child's results and often provides us with information that will be of value in the language evaluation (see Chapter 5). The MSCA is also helpful in allowing us to determine if an overall delay of development is present in a child, as in the case of mental retardation, and in targeting delay in specific areas examined by the individual scales.

Standardization Information

The MSCA was normed on a population of 1,032 children, about evenly divided between girls and boys and representative of the major demographic characteristics of the national population as recorded in the 1970 census. At least 100 children at each age level from 2½ to 8½ years of age were tested, with only severely handicapped individuals excluded. The standardization sample thus was intended to reflect a normal population in the given age range. It is presumed to be free of discriminatory factors relating to race, sex, or socioeconomic status.

The average reliability coefficient for the general cognitive index is .93, based on split-half test comparisons. For the other scales, reliability ranges from .79 to .88, with the motor scale being least reliable at the upper age levels. The standard error of measurement for all scales across the ten age groups was approximately 4 to 5 points. For convenience, the scales are arranged so that the general cognitive index has a mean of 100 and a standard deviation of 16, while the five other scales have a mean of 50 and a standard deviation of 10.

The validity of the MSCA items, subtests, and scales is still being researched. In the original standardization, McCarthy reports a comparison of MSCA scores with WPPSI and Stanford Binet scores for 36 children with a mean age of about 6 years old. The correlation of MSCA scale scores with the WPPSI verbal, performance, and full scale IQ and the Stanford Binet IQ was not strong. However, the general composite index correlated with the WPPSI full scale at .71 and with the Stanford Binet at .81. Subsequently, Gerken (1978) compared preschool MSCA GCI scores with Stanford Binet IQ and found that, though the scores correlated significantly, 40 of the 44 subjects scored absolutely higher on the Stanford-Binet. Finally, significant positive correlations have been reported between the MSCA and the WISC-R by Davis and Slettedahl (1976) and Goh and Youngquist (1979).

Most of the continuing validation and interpretation of MSCA scores has been due to the work of Alan S. Kaufman, who assisted McCarthy with much of the technical development of the test (Kaufman, 1976; Kaufman & Dicuio, 1975; Kaufman & Kaufman, 1973; Kaufman & Kaufman, 1977a; Kaufman & Kaufman, 1977b). Of the several technical questions that remain unanswered concerning the use and interpretation of the MSCA, two questions in particular have received much attention. The first concerns the use of the MSCA with black children in the face of an acrimonious testing controversy leading to ongoing litigation. The second question arises out of the suggestion made by McCarthy and others (e.g., Kaufman) that the MSCA is capable of more sensitive detection of learning disabilities.

Related Research

A matter of much contemporary concern and stirring debate regarding standardized test instruments is the development of nondiscriminatory factors regarding sex, race, region, and socioeconomy. Two analyses done on black-white differences on the MSCA (Kaufman & Dicuio, 1975; Kaufman & Kaufman, 1973) show no evidence of unfairness to black children. In the study by Kaufman and Dicuio, a separate factor analysis of the MSCA for blacks and whites was conducted to assess construct validity for each race and to assess the degree of congruency of factors between blacks and whites. Both blacks and whites responded well to the scale structure of the MSCA, and construct validity was determined for different age groups for both blacks and whites. The overall conclusion was that the test measured abilities independent of race.

In the study by Kaufman and Kaufman (1973), there was a discrepancy between the oldest group of blacks and whites on the general cognitive index, with whites scoring about a .5 standard deviation better, but no significant differences were indicated between the youngest and middle age groups. Also, the results showed better black coordination on the motor scales for the middle age group but nothing significant for the youngest and oldest children. Overall, it can be concluded that there is no race discrimination in favor of white children in performance on the MSCA cognitive scales (Kaufman & Kaufman, 1973).

Additional studies investigating the possibility of sex discrimination factors on the MSCA have been conducted. Kaufman and Kaufman

(1977a) compared boys' and girls' scores on the MSCA. Although there were slight differences in scores favoring the girls on all scales, they were considered insignificant. They concluded that there is "no obvious bias in favor of either sex" (p. 362) and that "the McCarthy scales provide fair measurement of both sexes" (p. 365).

The Kaufman data also have provided added and needed support for the independence of the factors suggested by the different subtest scales. Since the MSCA was intended to be a diagnostic instrument in which pattern of performance on the various scales was to have programming as well as heuristic value, it has been important to discover what kinds of patterns and discrepancies are significant. However, any analysis of discrepancy would be useless if there could be no confidence that the factor structure of the scales supported the theoretical model. Kaufman (1976) completed his analysis of the factor structure of the MSCA, using the standardization population, and concluded that the same factors appeared at each age level.

On the question of profiles, Kaufman (1976) analyzed the scatter of the normal scores from the standardization population. He found that a mean of 14.4 (i.e., 1.5 S.D.) points difference existed between the highest and lowest scale score. If the motor scale was removed, the discrepancy or scatter difference was still 11.9 points on the average. Of the sample, 30 percent had at least one scale score deviating significantly, and 9 percent had three or more scores deviating significantly from the child's own mean score. Motor ability was most frequently different from the child's mean, and memory was least likely to deviate. Ysseldyke and Samuels (1973) computed a table of statistically significant scale-index differences for the 5 and 1 percent levels of confidence. This table permits much more confident analysis of score scatter than the table of mean significant differences supplied by McCarthy in the manual.

On the question of the MSCA's ability to detect learning disabilities, Kaufman and Kaufman (1977b) have suggested while learning-disabled children by definition score at or near the mean on IQ measures, they score 15 or more points below the mean on the general composite index. If this suggestion is correct and corroborated by empirical evidence, the MSCA will emerge in a new and powerful light. Goh and Youngquist (1979) have recently reported that learning-disabled students who score at or near the mean on the WISC-R do score significantly lower on the general composite index. However, it is not yet clear how much of this discrepancy is due to simple low achievement by learning-disabled students and how much is based on some greater sensitivity of the MSCA to deficiencies inherent in learning-disabled children.

Summary

Reviews of the MSCA reflect, for the most part, commendations, praise, and pledges of support for the scales. However one of the most common complaints is about the amount of time involved in the scoring, which is relatively complex (Davis, 1974). Still, Davis comments that the McCarthy scales are probably the best test available to date for assessing young children's mental abilities. The McCarthy scales are being used increasingly in school systems because the test is an eclectic instrument that covers more information than the Stanford Binet and is more appealing to children than the Wechsler scales. In addition, technically, there is no fault in the MSCA.

The MSCA may, therefore, prove to be a powerful tool in the diagnostic regimen. It has accounted for itself well so far in the increasing number of empirical studies undertaken to examine its structure, theoretical foundations, and interpretive claims. Its administrative simplicity and attractiveness to children are additional strong arguments for its continued, though naturally, cautious use.

GENERAL PROCEDURES IN PSYCHOEDUCATIONAL EVALUATION

Preliminaries

During the audiological evaluation, a member of the educational staff is present to observe the child during the actual testing session and to participate in the conference immediately following. Information is gathered regarding the child's behaviors in the test situation, toward the audiologist, and toward the attending parent. A joint conference allows the sharing of information from the audiologist and interventionist with the family and eliminates endless repetition of questioning by professionals. Pertinent background knowledge can be obtained by all participants at one time, and the staff can present a consistent and unified set of information.

During the conference, an appointment is set for the psychoeducation and language-evaluation components. It is preferable to schedule the child again within the next week, unless there is need for intermediary medical attention that might affect the child's performance in further evaluation. An appropriate time and test setting are discussed thoroughly with the parents, and decisions are based on what is determined to be most conducive to the child's comfort and well-being. Also, the general purpose and procedure of the forthcoming evaluation are explained.

The Testing Session

Since the time and place of evaluation has been carefully set, the promptness of the examiner's appearance is absolutely necessary. All arrangements of testing equipment and materials are completed before the scheduled time. The evaluation is completed by a two-member team. This has at least two important advantages. First, one team member can score and cue the other as to item sequence. The "free" member is able to interact totally with the infant or child without having to contend with score sheets, and so forth. The second advantage is that two people tend to ensure greater objectivity in scoring such areas as the behavior index on the BSID and in summarizing observations during the evaluation session.

Of course, the testing environment is determined by each individual child based on the concerns discussed earlier in this chapter. If the evaluation is done outside the home, the child is allowed a few minutes to survey the testing room. "Friends," such as stuffed animals, are permitted as long as no distraction is evidenced. Often the presence of some favorite toy is actually an aid to the examiner in urging a child's participation in the tasks.

Parent Involvement

Parent participation is an individual matter. The parents are encouraged to observe and to actually be with the child during the testing. They can serve as a valuable aid in encouraging participation and in providing information during the session. Some parents, however, prefer not to observe or participate, and that choice should be respected.

Follow-up Conference

After the testing session is completed, an informal conference is held with the parents to discuss in general the overall situation. This is helpful for both examiner and parents in understanding what occurred and in answering questions regarding the tests and the child.

Reporting

Reports are prepared in written form on the same day as the evaluation as a joint effort by the scorer and examiner. If the testing is completed at the center, the audiologist is present as an observer (from an observation booth), and this professional's input is also considered. Reports of the total assessment are presented to parents and thoroughly discussed within one week of assessment completion.

ONGOING ASSESSMENT

As an integral aspect of the educational process, assessment, including psychoeducational evaluation, must be ongoing in order to gather continually new and vital information regarding the child's progress. Initial assessment provides a foundation of information to begin educational or interventional programming, but actual growth can be determined only through a program of continued monitoring. Indeed, Meyen (1972) suggests that the initial assessment should be viewed as a beginning step in a continuous assessment program. Continuing evaluation via both formal and informal approaches, coupled with frequent audiological and language monitoring, will provide staff and parents with evidence of progress and of deficient areas in the child's program. Initial recommendations can be modified as evidence of the child's needs and accomplishments is revealed. Wallace and Larsen (1978) state that assessment becomes "subsumed" in the educational process and is inseparable from other instructional procedure. Assessment when viewed as an ongoing component in the educational process becomes a system of assessment. Haring, Hayden, and Beck (1976) have outlined five aspects denoting a positive assessment system:

1. administration by a qualified examiner
2. quantified scoring and high inter-rater reliability
3. developmental progress as the basis
4. presentation of evolving growth
5. promotion of intervention efforts

These five aspects define the basic framework that should underlie an evaluation process. Each component is important in its own right, but also serves to interact with, and to strengthen or weaken the value of, the others.

PROGRAM EVALUATION

Program evaluation is implicit in the evaluation of the child. In fact, if assessment is viewed as a continuous process, program evaluation becomes an inseparable part of that process. Over time, children will display changes that are due partly to maturational progress and, hopefully, partly to the intervention program.

Safford (1978) presents two essential reasons for relating child progress to program impact. First, programs require an investment of time, energy, and money, by both parents and professionals. Therefore, accountability for such expenditure is demanded on at least a moral level. The program must be deemed to be justified. Second, evaluation can aid in indicating the benefits in program components as well as in ferreting out aspects that may be ineffectual. The program can then be modified to benefit the needs of the child.

The purpose of assessment in the accurate and objective determination of a child's characteristics cannot be viewed as separate from the design and implementation of a program of instruction based on objectives derived from that assessment (Blanco, 1972). Constant reevaluation of the child results in reevaluation of objectives, techniques, and strategies employed to implement the objectives of the program. The fact is that the true evaluation of a program occurs when the child performs certain goal behaviors not only in the structured circumstance of formal testing but in the day-to-day normal environment of the program setting (Kamii, 1973).

SUMMARY

Psychoeducational or developmental evaluation is an important consideration in overall assessment. It can provide the interventionist with pertinent knowledge regarding the child's general abilities as well as performance in specific areas of growth. However, great care must be taken to ensure that the testing instrument is appropriate for the child, that the examiner is keenly aware of both the client and the instrument, and that the information derived from the evaluation can supply relevant information for the programming of the child.

REFERENCES

Arthur, G. *Arthur adaptation of the Leiter International Performance Scale*. Chicago: C. H. Stoelting, 1950.

Bayley, N. *California First Year Mental Scale*. Chicago: C. H. Stoelting, 1933.

Bayley, N. *California Infant Scale of Motor Development*. Chicago: C. H. Stoelting, 1936.

Bayley, N. Review of *Intellectual status at maturity as a criterion for selecting items in preschool tests* by K. M. Maurer, 1946. *Journal of Educational Psychology*, 1947, *47*, 314–315.

Bayley, N. *Bayley Scales of Infant Development*. New York: Psychological Corporation, 1969.

Blanco, R. *Prescription for children with learning and adjustment problems*. Springfield, Ill.: Charles C Thomas, 1972.

Burgemeister, B., Blum, L. H., & Lorge, I. *Columbia Mental Maturity Scale*. New York: World Books, 1972.

Cattell, P., *Cattell Infant Intelligence Scale*. New York: Psychological Corporation, 1940. (a)

Cattell, P. *The measurement of intelligence in infants.* New York: Psychological Corporation, 1940. (b)

Cazden, C. The situation: A neglected source of social class differences in language use. *Journal of Social Issues,* 1970, *26,* 35–60.

Collard, R. R. Review of the *Bayley Scales of Infant Development.* In O. K. Buros (Ed.), *Seventh mental measurement yearbook* (Vol. 1). Highland Park, N.J.: Gryphon Press, 1972.

Davis, E. E. Review of MSCA. *Measurement and Evaluation in Guidance,* 1974, *6,* 251–254.

Davis, E. E. Concurrent validity of the McCarthy Scales of Children's Abilities. *Measurement and Evaluation in Guidance,* 1975, *8,* 101–104.

Davis, E. E., & Slettedahl, R. W. Stability of the McCarthy scales over a one year period. *Journal of Clinical Psychology,* 1976, *32,* 798–800.

Doll, E. A. *Preschool attainment record.* Minneapolis, Minn.: American Guidance Service, 1966.

Dunn, L. M. *Peabody Picture Vocabulary Test.* Circle Pines, Minn.: American Guidance Service, 1965.

Estes, B. W., Kodman, F., & Akel, M. The validity of the Columbia Mental Maturity Scale. *Journal of Consulting Psychology,* 1959, *23,* 561–563.

Fallen, N. *Young children with special needs.* Columbus, Ohio: Charles E. Merrill, 1978.

Frankenburg, W. K., Dodds, J. B., & Fandal, A. W. *Denver Developmental Screening Test (DDST).* Denver, Colo.: Ladoca Project and Publishing Foundation, 1969.

Gannon, D. J. Relationship between eight month old performance on the Bayley Scales of Infant Development and forty-eight month intelligence and concept formation scores. *Psychological Reports,* 1968, *23,* 1199–1205.

Gerken, K. C. A comparison of the Stanford Binet Intelligence Scale and the McCarthy Scales of Children's Abilities with preschool children. *Psychology in the Schools,* 1978, *15,* 468–472.

Gesell, A. *The first five years of life.* New York: Harper and Row, 1940.

Gesell, A., & Amatrauda, C. S. *Developmental diagnosis: Normal and abnormal child development: Clinical methods and practical applications.* New York: Paul Hoeber, 1941.

Goh, D. S., & Youngquist, J. A comparison of the McCarthy Scales of Children's Abilities and the WISC-R. *Journal of Learning Disabilities,* 1979, *12,* 344–348.

Goodenough, F. L., Maurer, K. M., & Van Wagenen, M. J. *Minnesota Preschool Scale.* Circle Pines, Minn.: American Guidance Service, 1940.

Griffiths, R. *Mental Development Scale for Testing Babies from Birth to Two Years.* London: Child Development Research Center, 1955.

Haring, N. G., Hayden, A. A., & Beck, G. R. General principles and guidelines in programming for severely handicapped young children and adults. *Focus on Exceptional Children,* 1976, *8,* 1–14.

Hiskey, M. *The Nebraska Test of Learning Aptitude.* Lincoln, Nebr.: Union College Press, 1966.

Jaffa, A. S. *California Preschool Mental Scale.* Berkeley, Calif.: University of California Press, 1934.

Kamii, C. An application of Piaget's theory to the conceptualization of a preschool curriculum. In R. K. Parker (Ed.), *The preschool in action.* Boston: Allyn & Bacon, 1973.

Kaufman, A. S. Are the profiles of normal children flat? *Psychology in the Schools*, 1976, *13*, 284–285.

Kaufman, A. S., & Dicuio, R. F. Separate factor analyses of the McCarthy scales for groups of black and white children. *Journal of School Psychology*, 1975, *13*, 10–17.

Kaufman, A. S., & Kaufman, N. L. Black-white differences at ages 2½–8½ on the McCarthy Scales of Children's Abilities. *Journal of School Psychology*, 1973, *11*, 196–206.

Kaufman, A. S., & Kaufman, N. L. *Clinical evaluation of young children with the McCarthy scales*. New York: Grune & Stratton, 1977. (a)

Kaufman, A. S., & Kaufman, N. L. Research on the McCarthy scales and its implications for assessment. *Journal of Learning Disabilities*, 1977, *10*, 284–291. (b)

Kerlinger, F. N. *Foundations of behavioral research*. New York: Holt, Rinehart, and Winston, 1973.

Kohen-Raz, R. Scalogram analysis of some developmental sequences in infant behavior as measured by the Bayley Scales of Infant Development. *Genetic Psychological Monographs*, 1976, *76*, 3–21.

Lefrancois, G. R. *Of children: An introduction to child development*. Belmont, Calif.: Wadsworth Publishing Co., 1973.

Leiter, P. *The Leiter International Performance Scale*. Chicago: C. H. Stoelting, 1929.

Maurer, K. M. *Intellectual status at maturity as a criterion for selecting items in preschool tests*. Minneapolis: University of Minnesota, 1946.

McCarthy, D. *McCarthy Scales of Children's Abilities*. New York: Psychological Corporation, 1972.

Meyen, E. L. *Developing units of instruction: For the mentally retarded and other children with learning problems*. Dubuque, Iowa: William C. Brown, 1972.

Nunnally, J. *Psychometric theory*. New York: McGraw Hill, 1967.

Olson, W. C. Review of *The mental growth of children from two to fourteen years* by F. L. Goodenough and K. M. Maurer. *American Journal of Psychology*, 1945, *58*, 151–152.

Piaget, J. *The construction of reality in the child*. New York: Basic Books, 1954.

Rogers, S. J., & D'Eugenio, D. B. *Developmental Programming for Infants and Young Children: Assessment and Application*. In D. S. Schafer and M. S. Moersch (Eds.), *Developmental programming for infants and young children. Vol. 1*. Ann Arbor, Mich.: University of Michigan Press, 1977.

Safford, P. L. *Teaching young children with special needs*. St. Louis, Mo.: C. V. Mosby, 1978.

Salvia, J., Ysseldyke, J. E. *Assessment in special and remedial education* (2nd ed.). Boston: Houghton Mifflin, 1981.

Salvia, J., Ysseldyke, J. E., & Lee, M. 1922 revision of the Stanford Binet: A farewell to the mental age. *Psychology with Schools*, 1975, *12*, 421–422.

Schafer, D. S., & Moersch, M. S. (Eds.). *Developmental programming for infants and young children* (3 vols.) Ann Arbor: University of Michigan Press, 1977.

Slosson, R. L. *Slosson Intelligence Test for Children and Adults (SIT)*. East Aurora, N.Y.: Slosson Educational Publications, 1963.

Terman, L., & Merrill, M. *Stanford Binet Intelligence Scale* (1972 norms ed.). Boston: Houghton Mifflin, 1973.

Uzgaris, I., & Hunt, J. McV. *Assessment in infancy: Ordinal Scales of Psychological Assessment*. Urbana: University of Illinois, 1975.

Wallace, G., & Larsen, S. C. *Educational assessment of learning problems: Testing for teaching.* Boston: Allyn & Bacon, 1978.

Wechsler, D. *The Wechsler Adult Intelligence Scale (WAIS).* New York: Psychological Corporation, 1955.

Wechsler, D. *The Wechsler Preschool and Primary Scale of Intelligence (WPPSI).* New York: Psychological Corporation, 1974.

Wechsler, D. *The Wechsler Intelligence Scale for Children, Revised (WISC–R).* New York: Psychological Corporation, 1974.

Wellman, B. L. A critique of the Minnesota Preschool Scale. In O. K. Buros (Ed.), *The third mental measurements yearbook.* Highland Park, N.J.: Gryphon Press, 1949.

Werner, E. E., & Bayley, N. The reliability of Bayley's Revised Scale of Mental and Motor Development during the first year of life. *Child Development,* 1966, *37,* 39–59.

Willerman, L., Broman, S. H., & Fiedler, M. Infant development, preschool I.Q., and social class. *Child Development,* 1970, *41*(1), 69–77.

Ysseldyke, J., & Samuels, S. Identification of strengths and weaknesses on the McCarthy Scales of Children's Abilities. *Psychology in the Schools,* 1973, *10,* 304–307.

SUGGESTED READINGS

Anastasi, A. *Psychological testing.* New York: Macmillan, 1976.

Buros, O. K. (Ed.). *Mental measurement yearbooks* (Vols. 1–7). Highland Park, N.J.: Gryphon Press 1938–1972.

Cronback, L. J. *Essentials of psychological testing.* Englewood Cliffs, N.J.: Prentice Hall, 1970.

Gronlund, N. E. *Measurement and evaluation in teaching.* New York: Macmillan, 1976.

Kerlinger, F. N. *Foundations of behavioral research.* New York: Holt, Rinehart, and Winston, 1973.

Chapter 5

Language Evaluation

M. Suzanne Hasenstab

The ability to communicate, verbal competence, and speaking proficiency have been the badge of education, intelligence, and social acceptance for centuries. Social class has clearly been based on how one speaks. Historically, those who are unable to communicate via acceptable standards of verbal expression have been considered socially inferior, mentally deficient, or even insane. They have been institutionalized, reduced to begging, or even put to death.

The evidence of communication problems in the form of language delay is observable at an early age, in fact, within the first year of life. Early researchers concerned with child development (Doll, 1966; Gesell, 1940, 1956) began to note milestones in various areas of child growth. One of these areas was language and speech development. Cognitivist theory (Piaget, 1926, 1952; Vygotsky, 1962) pointed out the relationship between language and the child's developing understanding of the world. Finally, linguists began to decipher the components of language and their governing rules (Berko, 1958; Chomsky, 1957, 1965; Chomsky & Halle, 1968; McNeill, 1970).

In the 1960s and 1970s, educators and psychologists began to examine child language as more than a series of milestones that a child passes through at various ages. They discovered that children acquire rules for the generation of words, phrases, and sentences in a predictable order (Bloom, 1970; Brown, 1973; Brown & Bellugi, 1964; Menyuk, 1969). It is now possible to determine not only if a child demonstrates a language delay, regardless of cause, but to ascertain the extent and areas of language development that are involved.

CONCERNS AND CONSIDERATIONS IN LANGUAGE EVALUATION

The third component of assessment in the Comprehensive Services Program is language evaluation. In language evaluation we are concerned

1 as a language user within the communication world. This leserves an in-depth examination apart from, and in addition to, the psychoeducational evaluation. In language evaluation, we are already aware that the child exhibits some type of language problem (that is usually why the child has been referred in the first place). This fact has been borne out in performances on the Bayley Scales of Infant Development (Bayley, 1969) and the McCarthy Scales of Children's Abilities (McCarthy, 1972). In other words, the item analysis on the Bayley scales indicates that linguistic tasks are deficient, or the verbal scale on the McCarthy test is depressed for the child's age or in relation to other developmental areas.

Definition of Language

Language, for our purposes, is centered in a model of communication. It is through communication, or human interchange, both verbal and written, that the child will learn the bulk of information afforded by the environment during a lifetime. Language is made up of interrelated components that develop in conjunction and in support of one another. One component that has received much attention in the past is *phonology*, or the representation of meaning, through the articulation and production of segmental and suprasegmental phonemes. Phonology is demonstrated in spoken language. A second component is *syntax*, which has received much attention from professionals studying language since Chomsky's early work in the late 1950s. Syntax is the order or patterning of language as represented in spoken or written language. Closely associated with syntax is *morphology*, which deals with the inflection of language. *Semantics*, or meaning in language, is associated with the concepts and ideas formulated and understood by the language user. Semantics is carried via phonology, syntax, and morphology in both verbal and written language.

A final component is *pragmatics*, or the function of language, which is the orchestration of all the component parts in actual language use. As Muma (1978) has so aptly stated, pragmatics is comprised of the rules we each know and use to determine "*who* says *what* to *whom, how, why, when*, and *in what situations*" (p. 137). We are currently in a period of intense interest in the pragmatic component of language. Syntax, phonology, and semantics have all previously been spotlighted by researchers and practitioners. Now we have reached the "age of pragmatics." The involvement is an exciting one because it requires a high level of operation or synthesis of the component parts (syntax, phonology, lexicon) into meaning and context.

It is not the purpose of this chapter to delve into theory and elaborate discussion of the language components, but a firm understanding of these components is essential for the reader to grasp completely the evaluation process. Suggested readings at the end of the chapter will add further clarity.

Purpose of Language Evaluation

Based on the foregoing definition of language and its components, the purpose of language evaluation is to determine the extent of an individual child's language delay and in what particular area the problem occurs (there could, of course, be problems in all components). An accurate picture of the child's language abilities and deficits will provide the basis of an individual language development program in the child's educational setting.

A major objective in language assessment is to indicate as specifically as possible the level of the language acquisition process at which the child is presently functioning in order to facilitate appropriate language instruction. Nebulous assessment information is of little or no value in determining the educational needs of a child. In assessment procedure, the results must indicate the particular areas of the child's language development stage which are delayed. These areas must be indicated in such a way that the teacher/clinician can target specific and appropriate objectives, materials, and activities to benefit the child. In the assessment and evaluation of language, the examiner must investigate the regularities in the linguistic system that will provide information regarding hypotheses and rules employed by the child in the generation of language. All measures of language have as their goal the evaluation of language performance. They all make certain assumptions regarding a child's linguistic competence or knowledge of the language system. In this context, it is assumed that a relatively accurate representation of language knowledge and use can be inferred.

Another objective in language assessment and evaluation is related to the fact that language is a process and is therefore ongoing. Thus, language measures should be able to provide information indicating progress, rate of acquisition, and completeness over time. Because language is profoundly complex, language evaluation must also be complex if it is to provide a total description of the child's facility with the process.

Assumptions for Language Evaluation

The strategies of language analysis are based on several assumptions that together comprise a model of language acquisition:

- Language acquisition is developmental.
- Hearing-impaired children and most language-delayed children are more similar to than they are different from normal in the acquisition process.
- Hearing-impaired children and most language-delayed children have the potential for acquiring language and its various communicative functions in speaking/signing, reading, writing, and thinking.
- Language systems are rule-governed and observations of instances of these rules can assist the diagnostician in formulating a hypothesis regarding a child's language system.
- Language acquisition is a hypothesis testing process.
- The sequence of language acquisition is fairly stable while the rate is variable.
- Pragmatic, semantic, syntactic, and phonologic components are interactive in language/communication acquisition.

The current effort is to determine the pragmatic aspects of language or the role of context in language acquisition in order to synthesize it with phonologic, syntactic/morphologic, and semantic information. During the first years of life, the young child acquires considerable knowledge of the pragmatic and semantic functions of language. The child expresses this knowledge nonverbally or couples it with situational cues before using grammatical relations (Bates, 1976; Bruner, 1975; Dore, 1974; Greenfield & Smith, 1976; Halliday, 1977). Early communicative intents are expressed first through gesture, then there is a movement toward "language proper," or a much more representational or symbolic use of language.

Need for Language Evaluation

In one form or another, language, through communication and reading, forms the foundation of the educational career for all students. Unless language is developed and utilized, both receptively and expressively, the child will be unable to meet successfully the educational challenges of our schools. Bangs (1968) points out that children often suffer devastating consequences of school failure because language difficulties were not detected and appropriate intervention was not employed at the preschool age. A student must be able to comprehend and use visual and auditory linguistic information.

Issues in Language Evaluation

As in psychoeducational evaluation, the evaluation of a child's linguistic ability presents some pertinent concerns. Some of these concerns are shared with other areas. The consideration of test selection and examiner qualification apply to language analysis as well as to psychoeducational testing. Furthermore, the test setting, which may be vital to securing optimal results, must not be neglected. The child, equipped with a particular experiential background, current environment, and individual abilities, is still the focal point. Finally, there is the concern regarding the philosophy of what language evaluation actually is and what is to be assessed.

Characteristics Common to Children with Language Delay

The following characteristics are found in both hearing and hearing-impaired children who exhibit language delay:

- exclusive use of nouns and nonuse of other functional language aspects
- restricted system in syntax to base level sentences, little or no use of transformations
- limited vocabulary and meaning and comprehension due to representational problems in semantics
- time delays in the processing of auditory or visual information
- difficulties in focusing on language due to environmental distractibility
- large comprehension-production gap
- difficulty in modification of language across persons or situations
- inflexibility in use of patterns and structures of language
- failure to move from lower levels of language acquisition

The use of language by hearing-impaired and language-delayed children has been examined in considerable detail. Specific areas covered include syntax (Russell, Quigley, & Power, 1976), semantics (Scroggs, 1977; Skarakis & Prutting, 1977), pragmatics (Kretschmer & Kretschmer, 1978), and phonology (Ling, 1976).

REVIEW OF LANGUAGE EVALUATION INSTRUMENTS

Checklists

There are various approaches to the evaluation of language. The checklist method, employed in such tests as the Scales of Early Communication Skills for Hearing Impaired Children (Moog & Geers, 1975), the Communication Evaluation Chart (Anderson, Miles, & Matheny, 1963), and the Verbal Language Development Scale (Mecham, 1958, 1971), lists items relating to language behaviors in a developmental order with several examples offered for each level. The problem with the existing checklists is that the behaviors are general and language components are not differentiated. Also several of these tests, such as the Verbal Language Development Scale (Mecham, 1958, 1971) and the Receptive Expressive Emergent Language Scale (Bzoch & League, 1971), are conducted via an interview technique. Although parent or other informant comments and information are helpful in gaining a complete picture of a child's functioning or background, the examiner must be wary of biased commentary.

Intelligence Tests

Another approach in language evaluation is through standardized intellectual and developmental evaluation. Tests using this approach include language-related items, for example, the McCarthy Scales of Children's Abilities (McCarthy, 1972), the Wechsler Preschool and Primary Scale of Intelligence (Wechsler, 1967), the Bayley Scales of Infant Development (Bayley, 1969), and the Stanford Binet (Terman & Merrill, 1973). The items, however, reflect a part of the child's overall intellectual or developmental level, not specifics regarding language abilities or deficits. As pointed out in the preceding chapter, the central goal of evaluation in that general realm is overall or developmentally related. Therefore, the above tests may indicate difficulty in the area of language either in a subscale score or index or through an item analysis, but they do not specifically describe the depth and involvement of the deficiency.

Screening Tests

Some tests are designed specifically as screening tests, for example, the Bankson Language Screening Test (Bankson, 1977), the Stycar Language Test (Sheridan, 1976), the Vane Evaluation of Language Scale (Vane,

1975), and the Preschool Language Screening Test (Hannah & Gardner, 1974). These tests may be effective in varying degrees in locating children with language delay. Most of them, however, are for children above age 2. Furthermore, their purpose remains that of a screening device, not one of in-depth evaluation of a language problem, its extent, and the areas affected. Low scores obtained on screening tests indicate a need for further in-depth and comprehensive evaluation.

Tests of Language Development

Several tests have been proposed to assess early language in depth, for example, the Reynell Developmental Language Scales (Reynell & Huntley, 1979), the Utah Test of Language Development (Mecham, Jex, & Jones, 1967), the Preschool Language Scale (Zimmerman, Steiner, & Evatt, 1969), the Illinois Children's Language Assessment Test (Arlt, 1977), the Houston Test for Language Development, Parts I and II (Crabtree, 1958, 1963), and the Test of Language Development (Newcomer & Hammill, 1977). Whether they meet this goal or not is debatable. The Reynell Developmental Language Scales, which may well prove to be a reliable and valid measure, are designed for specific use with British children. The other tests, whatever their ostensible purpose, sample only general language behaviors at various age levels. They do not provide an extensive in-depth analysis of language specific to the component parts, especially within a natural setting.

One test that deserves special mention is the Sequenced Inventory of Communication Development (Hedrick, Prather, & Tobin, 1975). This is a well-designed test that is highly pragmatic in its view of language. It has, in fact, proved to be a valuable measure of the general development of communication. However, it is not specific enough to indicate precisely what a particular child's language performance is in regard to the various language components.

Two other tests that are somewhat unique in their approach are the Environmental Language Inventory (ELI) (MacDonald & Blott, 1978) and the Environmental Pre-Language Battery (EPB) (Horstmeier & MacDonald, 1978). The ELI analyzes the semantic/grammatical production rules of early utterances through imitation, conversation, and a free play setting. The EPB is designed to assess preliminary language skills of children (or adults) functioning at one-word utterances or below. Both the ELI and EPB require adequate knowledge of the testing procedure. An advantage in their use is that they are the basis for a therapy model. The results determine training objectives; therefore assessment is followed by programming. They also make available a parent program.

Evaluation of Performance in Specific Language Areas

Other testing instruments that purport to assess language development include measurements of aspects of syntax, such as the Northwestern Syntax Screening Test (NSST) (Lee, 1971) and the Carrow Elicited Language Inventory (CELI) (Carrow, 1974). The NSST tends to penalize the child as a language generator and, as such, does not provide the opportunity for the child to generate syntax within a semantic context. Similarly, the CELI prohibits observation of the child's spontaneous use of syntactic structures, in that it relies on imitative responses from the child. Both of these instruments measure only specific, and rather isolated, aspects of sentence patterning, thus giving a fragmented view of the syntactic structures within the child's linguistic repertoire. Other tests involving sentence repetition tasks have this same difficulty.

Sentence Repetition Tests

Generally, sentence repetition tests involve an elicited imitation of sentences arranged in increasing difficulty and complexity as a form of expressive and receptive language evaluation. This format has been used by several professionals in the study of child language (Carrow, 1974; Fraser, Bellugi, & Brown, 1963; Menyuk, 1964; Zachman, Huisingh, Jorgensen, & Barrett, 1976, 1977). A sentence repetition test is centered on the examination of linguistic structures that are used infrequently in a child's repertoire. The general procedure with sentence repetition is to present a sentence to a child and request that it be repeated immediately. The assumption underlying this approach is that the child will imitate only those structures that are comprehensible and that can be produced spontaneously. The child will "filter" incoming messages through the available language-processing strategies and will imitate or repeat the stimulus sentence at the level of linguistic functioning current to the child. It is assumed that, if the child produces an utterance, it is comprehended.

There is disagreement regarding the value of sentence repetition tests. The fact is that, in an elicited imitation-performance setting, memory skills are involved, as well as variability among children's behavior. Another concern arises in the interpretation of utterances as they would appear in discourse. For example, a child may answer a question presented in a sentence repetition test rather than repeat it, as is required by test procedure. Perhaps the best use of sentence repetition tests is in supplemental language evaluation to augment information already secured.

Tests of Auditory Comprehension

Auditory comprehension tests as measures of language reception have been used in such instruments as the Assessment of Children's Language Comprehension (ACLC) (Foster, Gidden, & Stark, 1973), the Test for Auditory Comprehension of Language (TACL), (Carrow, 1973b), and the Screening Test for Auditory Comprehension of Language (STACL) (Carrow, 1973a). The ACLC is in reality a test of auditory retention, while the TACL and STACL rely on the auditory comprehension of specific syntactic and morphological components of language devoid of situational contexts. Although the Illinois Test of Psycholinguistic Abilities (Kirk, McCarthy, & Kirk, 1968) refers to psycholinguistics in its title, it in fact measures auditory and visual skills relating to perception, memory, and discrimination. Although these skills are associated with language in a general way, they are more in the domain of cognitive functioning.

Several picture vocabulary tests discussed in the preceding chapter will not be reexamined in this section, except to say that these tests are a measure of a child's understanding of vocabulary out of context and fail to take into account recent advances in knowledge concerning language development and assessment. Examples of picture vocabulary tests, in addition to those mentioned earlier, are the Language Facility Test (Darley, 1977) and the Michigan Picture Language Inventory (Wolski & Lerea, 1962)

Language Samples and Analyses

One approach to the evaluation of language that is receiving increasing attention and use is based on the securing of a sample of utterances produced by a child and the consequent analysis of those utterances. Use of a language-sample analysis procedure permits the examiner to observe and record aspects of a child's communication abilities, including characteristics of communication interaction and the specific aspects of language expression (phonology, syntax, semantics, morphology). Bloom and Lahey (1978) emphasize that, in order to determine what behaviors are part of a child's language repertoire, it is necessary to observe the child's language according to content, form, and use. The more varied the context in which a child is observed, the better the chance of obtaining information that is representative of the child's knowledge of language. With a language-sample approach, a child may be observed in several different situations and settings. A sample can be recorded through direct interaction between the child and the examiner or through monitoring the child in conversation with another person. The overall goal is to discover the child's use of language in day-to-day living, and the setting should reflect this aspect.

There is a variety of opinion regarding the gathering of a language sample. Although there is agreement that the sample should represent the child's linguistic ability realistically, there are differences of opinion as to whether samples should be derived from predetermined stimuli, such as pictures, or through the child's spontaneous interactions. Generally, the less structured and less adult-oriented the setting, the more observable becomes the language, particularly natural language. Pictures have been shown to be the least effective way to elicit a natural sample of language usage.

Another issue surrounding the use of language samples concerns the number of utterances necessary to give adequate representation to a child's use of language. The number of such utterances that have been suggested range from 10 to 150. The issue has clearly not been resolved. It would seem logical however, that the number should depend on the time available and the age of the child.

Language sampling is effective as an ongoing process of language evaluation. Therefore, examples of language behaviors can be observed in a variety of contexts and the utterances accumulated over a short time period. Ten utterances by a 3-year-old collected in four or five settings over a period of 1 day would probably produce more valuable information than 50 utterances obtained through an examiner-child interaction in which the adult places constraints on the freedom of the child's expression simply by the formality of the situation.

Developmental Sentence Analysis

Various forms of language-sample analyses have been developed. The system known as Developmental Sentence Analysis (DSA), designed by Laura Lee (1974), is comprised of two separate procedures: developmental sentence types (DST) and developmental sentence scoring (DSS). The purpose of DST is to account for sentences occurring in the earlier stages of language development. The procedure is used if more than 50 percent of the sample produces utterances that are presentences, that is, productions by the child that do not contain a noun and verb in a subject-predicate relationship. DST requires a sample of no less than 100 utterances, which are classified into three categories of single words, two-word combinations, and nonsentence constructions of more than two words. The utterances are then described in one of five ways:

1. noun-phrase elaborations
2. designative utterances

3. descriptive statements
4. verb elaborations
5. fragments

The central purpose of DST is to provide the examiner with information on the particular structures that a child employs, thus determining a starting point for intervention through a language program.

In DSS, the second DSA procedure, a minimum of 100 utterances is also required, of which at least 50 percent must be true sentences with subjects and predicates. The sentences are analyzed according to eight syntactic/morphological features.

1. indefinite pronouns and noun modifiers
2. personal pronouns
3. main verbs
4. secondary verbs
5. negatives
6. conjunctions
7. interrogative reversals
8. wh-questions

Scoring credit is awarded for correct and attempted productions of a particular form. For example, an attempt mark would be noted if a child uttered, "Her wants it," rather than, "She wants it."

Though a relatively simple procedure, DSS has been criticized on several points. One criticism concerns the fact that DSS does not account for utterances that express syntactic understanding, nor does it allow for the fine-feature discrimination necessary to detect subtle differences in child language knowledge. Kretschmer and Kretschmer (1978) indicate that there is no provision with DSS for the specification of deviations from normal linguistic use. Moreover, both DSS and DST are concerned only with the syntactic or morphological aspects of the child's language.

Language Sampling Analysis

In 1974, Tyack and Gottsleben developed a system of Language-Sampling Analysis (LSA) in which the obtained utterances are assigned to one of five linguistic levels based on a word-to-morpheme index. Subsequently, the child's productions are assigned to categories to determine if the child is using expected structures at the child's word-morpheme level. The procedure can be summarized in five basic steps:

1. Words and morphemes are counted in each sentence.
2. The word-morpheme index is computed by determining the mean number of words per sentence and the mean number of morphemes.

3. The sample is then assigned to a language level.
4. Forms and constructions are sorted into classifications.
5. Baseline and goal analysis is completed for the LSA results.

After the analysis is completed, the data are summarized on a form provided by the authors of the system. This information is then used to devise individual lanaguage programming for the child evaluated.

As with the DSA approach, the LSA procedure is well-explained and relatively easy to master after several attempts. However, LSA, like DSA, also makes little provision for describing semantic or pragmatic difficulties in language.

Applied Linguistic Analysis

The procedure of Applied Linguistic Analysis, designed by Hannah (1979) for analyzing language samples, also stresses the syntactic aspects of language. It involves the recording and transcribing of utterances and then the categorization of the utterances into seven different classifications.

1. embedding
2. conjoining
3. simple transform
4. simple sentence/linear expansions
5. basal sentence
6. minor sentence unit (such as an answer to a question)
7. restricted forms (including fragments and incomplete units)

Hannah's procedure can be applied to children who are of preschool age or who are unable to produce the required 50 utterances needed for the more complex categories. The procedure in such a case involves only four classes:

1. single words or morpheme relations
2. holophrastic productions
3. two- and three-word combinations (N + V, N + V + N, etc.)
4. basal sentences

After the classification of the utterances, as appropriate, the examiner selects rules that correspond to each utterance. Tables are provided for this purpose. A certain number of points are awarded for each item in each classification. The total number of points may then be compared to norms provided by Hannah. Percentages are established to determine which categorical areas should be targeted for language training.

Hannah's system is perhaps the most inclusive of the procedures we have described. It capitalizes most effectively on the information that has been produced as related to transformational grammar and the development of syntax. But the fact that it does not address semantics and pragmatics limits its use with hearing-impaired children or those with language delay evident in these components.

Observing Semantics Through Language-Sample Analysis

We have indicated that one of the difficulties with the three systems we have described is that they are not concerned with the semantic component of language. However, there are two procedures, now in popular use with the evaluation of language, that do extend to the semantic component. The first, Language Sample Analysis by Bloom and Lahey (1978), illustrated stages of language development based on semantic/syntactic relationships. It progresses from single-word use through two- and three-word utterances, embedded relations, grammatical morphemes, successive utterances, syntactic connectives and modals, to relative sentences. Obviously more complex than a simple syntactic analysis, Bloom and Lahey's system has been quite effective in describing child language ability according to the aspects of syntax and semantics as they relate to the child's use of language.

The second procedure, developed by Kretschmer and Kretschmer (1978), is a system for analyzing language samples that provides perhaps the most in-depth and complete coordination to date of known information regarding language. This procedure involves an extremely sophisticated explanation of how an individual uses language syntactically and semantically within a context of discourse. It is quite appropriate for the evaluation of language of most hearing-impaired individuals of school age or older.

Summary

Language samples and language-sample analysis appear to provide the most realistic way in which to evaluate the language of young children. By observing the child as a language user, valuable information can be ascertained for the purpose of forming an appropriate language program that capitalizes on the linguistic function that the child already portrays and indicates those areas in which intervention should be applied.

LANGUAGE EVALUATION INSTRUMENTS

In the remainder of this chapter, we present various language evaluation instruments, some of which have been mentioned earlier. A short description of each test is provided, together with test and normative and scoring information and a brief summary on the effective use of the test with preschool children, especially those with hearing or language difficulty.

Arizona Articulation Proficiency Scale

Description

The Arizona Articulation Proficiency Scale (AAPS) (Janet Barker Fudala, Western Psychological Services, 1974) attaches a numerical value to misarticulated phonemes, according to the sounds' frequency of occurrence in American English. The frequency value was determined by the number of times a sound would most likely occur in 100 speech sounds, based on studies done at Bell Laboratories. The test also provides an age level for the mastery of each sound.

Technical Information

Age norms were derived from 702 "average" children in the Seattle, Washington, public schools from age 3 years to 11 years, 11 months, excluding those with substantial deprivations in hearing, mental ability, neurological functioning, or emotional stability. No information regarding ethnic or racial distribution was reported. A reliability coefficient of .96 was obtained by 19 public school clinicians testing 105 children. The test-retest interval was 1 week. Support for test validity is shown by the correlation of .92 between AAPS scores and a subjective judgment of defective articulation made by 10 speech clinicians in recorded conversational samples of 45 children.

Administration and Scoring

The AAPS consists of 48 standard picture cards to be named by the child. The examiner may present a clue or may model the item if it is not immediately identified. Two additional stimulus pictures may be used to elicit spontaneous speech for comparison. Vowel, as well as consonant production, can be evaluated with the test.

In scoring the AAPS, only errors are recorded. Each error has a numerical value and a referential age level at which 90 percent of the normative sample mastered the sound. The derived total score is interpreted according to a continuum of intelligibility. The test includes a formula for computing the degree of speech improvement between test and retest performance.

Summary

The AAPS generally takes somewhat longer than other tests to administer and score, but it is felt to provide valuable information as a basis for long-term therapy planning and accountability in reporting progress. Further standardization measures and refinement of the weighing of intelligibility values are needed. As with other standardized articulation tests, it may prove of more value with older clients than with very young hearing-impaired or language-delayed children, for whom language is of prime importance rather than articulation per se.

Assessment of Children's Language Comprehension

Description

The Assessment of Children's Language Comprehension (ACLC) (Rochana Foster, Jane J. Gidden, & Joel Stark; Consulting Psychologists Press, 1969, 1973) attempts to pinpoint the grammatical level at which the child fails to encode and retain words. It can also aid in the identification of the types of items that are difficult for the child to comprehend. Words in test items, or "critical elements," are taken from the semantic classes of agent, action, object, attribute, and relations. Test items consist of combinations of one to four of these critical elements. The ACLC is primarily an individual test, but a group screening form is also available.

Technical Information

Normative data for the individualized form of the ACLC were derived from a population of 311 nursery and elementary school children, primarily from Tallahassee, Florida, and from families representing middle socioeconomic and educational backgrounds. Only about one-third of the normative population was of lower socioeconomic level or represented racial variation. Results were divided into 6-month age intervals from 3 years to 6 years, 5 months.

Normative data from a study by Darley (1979) suggest that most "normal" children, upon entering kindergarten, have developed the language comprehension skills probed by the ACLC. This study also reported that there were no statistically significant differences in sex or race. However, these normative data are not conclusive, due to the restricted geographic and racial sampling and the paucity of scores at certain age levels. No normative data exist on the screening form.

The authors disclose no tests of reliability or validity. However, odd-even reliability coefficients were determined to assess item consistency in measuring the same skills. After correction for attenuation, the results imply adequately high interval consistency.

Administration and Scoring

The ACLC consists of 41 spiral-bound picture plates, a pad of score sheets, and a test manual. The test takes approximately 15–20 minutes to administer and score. The first test plate contains five simple training items. For each item, the examiner reads the stimulus, prefacing it with, "point to ———" or "show me ———."

Part A, a vocabulary test of single critical elements, consists of ten plates, each with five stimulus items. If the child misses a large number of items, the authors suggest training in error items prior to continuing with the test. Since Part A contains most of the single critical elements that make up Parts B, C, and D, correct responses in Part A guarantee that errors in subsequent sections do not signify a vocabulary problem.

In Part B, the child must indicate comprehension of two critical elements by choosing one of the four pictures in each of the ten test plates. These pictures contain syntactic combinations of agent, attribute, action, and object.

Part C test items consist of three critical elements among which various relations exist. One element is varied in each of the four pictures on each of 10 plates. The child must comprehend every element in order to choose the correct item.

Part D displays five pictures on each of the 10 test plates. Four critical elements make up the items. Stimuli express agent-action relations, for example, "boy standing in the house."

Part A is scored by combining the number of accurate responses. Parts B, C, and D allow for an analysis of the pattern of errors in each section, according to the first, second, or third critical element. Word-order errors can be easily detected. In addition to this pattern description, the last three sections yield a percent-correct score.

Summary

The ACLC is a practical test in terms of length of administration and scoring. It is relatively unique in assessing auditory comprehension and word memory in noncomplex grammatical constructions arranged in an order of increasing difficulty. However, the ACLC lacks comprehensive statistical data. Broader normative groups would improve test standardization. More explicit instructions on score- and error-pattern analyses would improve interpretation of results.

The ACLC has been criticized on other counts. For example, the black-shadow test pictures have been criticized for their lack of detail. Also, pictures representative of objects are not always consistent throughout the test. A final cautionary word should be noted regarding the attempt to evaluate language out of social context.

Auditory Discrimination Test

Description

The Auditory Discrimination Test (ADT) (Joseph Wepman, Language Research Association, 1973) is designed to assess the ability of children, ages 5 to 8, to recognize the five differences that exist between the phonemes used in English speech.

Technical Information

The author does not specify in the manual the number of children in the normative group or their characteristics. Wepman does report two test-retest reliability coefficients greater than .90, but the sample used to obtain these measures is not described.

Validity claims are based on eight studies reported in the ADT manual. One cross-sectional and two longitudinal studies indicate that mean raw scores increased slightly, but significantly, with age. However, Locke (1979) argues that there are serious problems with the test's validity. By demonstrating the lack of voicing and manner-of-articulation contrasts on the ADT, he counters Wepman's claim that auditory discrimination ability is relevant to articulation. Using Snow's (1963) common phoneme substitutions, Locke points out that the ADT lacks the voicing and manner-of-articulation contrasts that constitute the majority of Snow's phoneme confusions.

Administration and Scoring

The ADT is available in two equatable forms, each containing 40 word pairs. Of the 40 word pairs, 30 differ from each other by one phoneme; 10 consist of identical words. The examiner reads each word pair and the child must indicate verbally, by gesturing, if the two words are the same or different. Through a table in the test manual, the child's raw score is converted to a five-point rating scale based on percentile ranks. The scores of the bottom 15 percent of the normative group are designated as indicating inadequate discrimination. If a child responds correctly to 10 items or less or responds incorrectly to four or more same-word pairs, the test is considered invalid.

Summary

Salvia and Ysseldyke (1978) state that the content of the ADT represents a sufficient sample of behavior for a screening device. However, the test has limited relevance to articulation, reading, or language. In addition, the normative data are inadequately described.

Bankson Language Screening Test

Description

The Bankson Language Screening Test (BLST) (Nicholas W. Bankson, University Park Press, 1977) was designed to indicate children in need of language remediation and to determine expressive and perceptual skill areas that require further testing. The BLST assesses language skills in 17 subtests that are organized into five general categories: semantic knowledge, morphological rules, syntactic rules, visual perception, and auditory perception.

Technical Information

Normative data were obtained from a sample of 637 children, aged 4 years, 1 month to 8 years, living in semirural counties bordering the Washington, D.C., metropolitan area. Of the sample children, 80 percent were white, and the remainder represented various minority groups. Socioeconomic status ranged from lower-middle class to upper-middle levels. Subjects were grouped in 6-month age levels, with reported means and standard deviations for raw scores on each subtest. Percentile ranks were included only for the total test score in the 6-month categories. The normative sample indicates that the BLST is responsive only to developmental variations at the lower age levels, between 4 and 6 years of age.

To determine reliability, the BLST was administered to 70 children on two occasions with a 1-week interval. Point-to-point reliability for all items reached the .94 level. However, interpretation is limited because age and selection criteria were not provided.

Internal consistency within subtests is not reported, nor are interitem or intersubject correlations. Though Bankson presents the finding that 38 out of the 153 items were most discriminating between age levels, those specific age levels are not listed. There are also no data on the use of this screening test with children who exhibit language problems.

Administration and Scoring

The BLST takes approximately 25 minutes to administer. Test items are scored as correct or incorrect. Raw scores on each subtest can be compared to means reported for each 6-month category. Percentile ranks are provided for each age level.

Cutoff-score guidelines for those children who need further language testing are suggested, but are not backed with evidence. The examiner is urged to observe the type of errors that the child makes. Bankson provides instructions for the use of several of the basic vocabulary and semantic knowledge subtests as receptive tasks so that expressive item errors can be tested receptively.

Summary

The BLST is effective as a broad screening instrument for children from ages 4 to 6. Darley (1979) states that this test "does not yield extensive information about the language skills commonly impaired in children within the upper preschool and early elementary school years suspected or known to have language problems." (p. 8). The BLST also lacks comprehensive normative data.

Basic Concept Inventory

Description

According to the author, the Basic Concept Inventory (BCI) (Siegfried Englemann, Follett Educational Corporation, Field Research Edition, 1967) furnishes "a broad checklist of basic concepts that are involved in new learning situations in the first grade" (Englemann, 1967, p. 1). He indicates that the BCI can also serve to evaluate the individual or group instruction of elementary academically related concepts. He notes that the test is designed for use with special groups of children, including mentally retarded, culturally disadvantaged, and emotionally disturbed children.

Technical Information

Since the present version of the BCI is an experimental edition, statistical evaluation of its adequacy is limited. Predictive reliability and construct validity for the BCI have not been established. No age norms are provided; the author states that age norms are inappropriate, that they are actually "achievement norms."'

Administration and Scoring

According to the author, if the purpose of the evaluation is diagnosis or special placement of a subject, the BCI should be administered by a trained examiner. However, if remedial instruction is the intended purpose, the classroom teacher would be the most appropriate administrator. Much of the BCI manual is devoted to teaching young children specific linguistic forms. The author directs the reader to the more comprehensive guide to the content of instruction, Bereiter and Englemann's *Teaching Disadvantaged Children in the Preschool* (1966).

The BCI consists of 90 test items divided into three sections. Part 1 requires the child to point to pictures and to utter a verbal response to demonstrate comprehension of target words. Part 2 assesses a child's ability to imitate sentences and to answer questions that relate to specific information. Part 3, Pattern Awareness, evaluates the child's auditory sequential memory and sound-blending abilities. The child is required to repeat sequences of clapping or digits and also to blend syllables into words.

A low score indicates a high performance level. Although the author states that a child who fails 40 or more items will probably experience difficulty in new learning situations, the interpretation of results is mostly qualitative. The manual provides six cases, with indications of the possible use of the performance scores on the three levels.

Summary

The BCI evaluates an important aspect of language and cognition, namely the comprehension of concepts relating to the academic setting. It is however, reliant on verbal expressive ability and is therefore limited for use with the population addressed in the BCI text.

Boehm Test of Basic Concepts

Description

The Boehm Test of Basic Concepts (BTBC) (Ann E. Boehm, Psychological Corporation, 1971) is designed to evaluate children's understanding concepts that are considered necessary for achievement in the primary levels of school. Its purpose is to pinpoint individual concepts that a child does not comprehend.

Technical Information

The test standardization sample consists of children from five cities in the United States. A southeastern city school system contributed a disproportionate number of low socioeconomic-class children, thus producing an unrepresentative normative sample (McCandless, 1972). Mean scores are exceedingly high for second graders of low, middle, and high socioeconomic groups. A study by Noll (1970) suggests that the BTBC is easily mastered by first graders of upper-income levels. Therefore, the test may be most appropriate for kindergarteners and children in the first grade from lower socioeconomic levels.

Content validity appears to be adequate, since test items were selected on the basis of relevance to primary-grade curriculum materials. However, no data on construct, predictive, or concurrent validity are available.

Administration and Scoring

The BTBC consists of two forms, each comprised of two booklets containing 25 test pictorial items arranged in order of increasing difficulty. The test can be administered to a class or to an individual child. The subjects are verbally instructed by the examiner to mark an X on the picture that is described. The manual provides tables of means and percentile equivalents for raw scores by grade and socioeconomic level. The tables may be used either with separate raw scores from each booklet or with combined raw scores from both booklets. The tables also show percentages of those passing each item by grade and socioeconomic level. A class record form enables the teacher readily to identify problem areas for each child.

Summary

The BTBC can be a valuable instrument in identifying deficits in knowledge of basic concepts. However the author provides no explanation to support the premise that knowledge of basic concepts affects achievement in the primary school grades. The test's validity is questionable. When supplemented with informal measures of concept development, however, results on the BTBC have value as pretest and posttest indexes.

Carrow Elicited Language Inventory

Description

The Carrow Elicited Language Inventory (CELI) (Elizabeth Carrow, Teaching Resources Corporation, 1974) is a diagnostic test of children's productive use of selected features of language structure. It permits identification of specific grammatical forms on which a child may be in error.

Technical Information

Even though Carrow reports little information on the subject, the content validity of the CELI is high. An adequate number of representative grammatical features are included in the test. Criterion-related validity has not been definitively assessed. Carrow (1974) reports a study by Cornelius that found a significant correlation between Lee and Canter's Developmental Sentence Scoring (DSS) (1971) and the CELI. However, a study by Sinclair, Khan, and Saxman (1977) found that subjects' performances on the DSS and CELI did not correlate closely.

Carrow reports a high correlation coefficient for test-retest and interexaminer reliability. However, she does not elaborate on how these coefficients were obtained, and reliability is therefore difficult to interpret. The normative population was composed of white middle-class children from an urban community. The test does not allow for children whose grammatical systems differ from standard English because of social or ethnic dialects.

Administration and Scoring

The CELI consists of 52 sentences ranging from 2 to 10 words which the child is asked to imitate. The grammatical constructions include articles, adjectives, nouns, pronouns, verbs, negatives, adverbs, prepositions, demonstratives, conjunctions, plurals, and contractions. The child's repetitions of test stimuli are recorded on audiotape and transcribed onto the test form. Each utterance is classified on the test form according to grammatical categories. The total score consists of the total number of errors; subscores represent the number of errors within each grammatical category. A verb protocol sheet affords more detailed analysis of the child's verb usage. According to the manual, the mean time required for administration, transcription, and scoring is 45 minutes. This may be an underestimation for the inexperienced examiner.

Summary

The CELI offers efficiency in the number of grammatical constructions that can be assessed using relatively few items. However, the scoring of the CELI is time consuming, especially for those with limited experience with grammatical references. In addition, there are limitations in the test's construction. In terms of a child's grammatical performance, the CELI may not give a representative sampling. Even though findings by Menyuk (1963) and Ervin (1964) suggest that a child's imitations of adult sentences will closely approximate the child's productions of these sentences in spontaneous speech, these imitations may be more grammatically complex than the spontaneous utterances. Also, children who exhibit auditory processing deficits may have difficulty with repetition tasks. With these cautions in mind, the CELI is still a useful test of expressive language.

Deep Test of Articulation: Picture Form

Description

According to the author of the Deep Test of Articulation (Eugene T. McDonald, Stanwix House, 1964), speech sounds are the result of a series of overlapping, ballistic movements or coarticulation. The Deep Test of Articulation evaluates speech sounds as such and samples representatively the possible phonetic contexts of the sound, including those contexts in which they are parts of phoneme blends. The length of the test permits observation of the degree of variability in the subject's production of a sound.

Technical Information

McDonald's text, *Articulation Testing and Treatment: A Sensory-Motor Approach,* provides standardization, validity, and reliability information for the test. The validity of overlapping motor movements during connected speech is well established in the research literature (Daniloff, 1973). The author provides data indicating significant correlations between results of four different forms of the test. This lends support to the validity of deep testing as an approach.

Administration and Scoring

The picture form of the Deep Test of Articulation was designed for use with subjects whose reading ability is below the third grade level. The format consists of two sets of adjacent, spiral-bound pictures. The subject is told that pictures can be turned to make "funny big words out of two little words." Each sound is tested in several contexts by keeping one card stationary and turning the adjacent card.

A record sheet is provided for recording the type of misarticulations and correct and incorrect articulations of the sounds tested. To score the test, a percentage of correct articulations of each sound is calculated. Therapy can be based on phonetic contexts in which a child can correctly articulate an error sound. Analyses of these contexts reveal the distinctive features related to the successful production. The author provides a progression continuum for sounds from "almost never correct" to "almost always correct," which allows for evaluation of the therapy.

Summary

Though lengthy in administration, the Deep Test of Articulation can yield information directly applicable to therapy. Like other articulation instruments, it measures pronunciation proficiency. Contexts in which an error sound is correctly articulated can serve as a therapeutic foundation. The test also provides a means of gauging therapy progress. However, as an articulation test, it requires a language base and verbal ability at least equivalent to late preschool age.

Del Rio Language Screening Test, English/Spanish

Description

The Del Rio Language Screening Test (DRLST) (Allen S. Toronto, D. Leverman, Cornelia Hanna, Peggy Rosengweis, and Antoneta Maldonado; National Educational Laboratory Publishers, 1975) is designed to detect language disorders in children of ages 3 to 6 years, 11 months, from the following groups: Anglo-English-speaking; Mexican-American, English-speaking; and Mexican-American, Spanish-speaking. The content of the test items is congruous with the linguistic and cultural backgrounds of the southwest United States. The test can be administered in English or Spanish.

Technical Information

Items for each subtest were selected on the basis of their representativeness of the language and culture of Del Rio, Texas. The normative group consisted of 384 normal children, equally distributed among the three groups: Anglo-English-speaking; Mexican-American, English-speaking; and Mexican-American, Spanish-speaking. Each cultural group had the same sex and age distribution and was divided into age groups of 1-year intervals from 3 years to 6 years, 11 months. Each age group was comprised of 32 children.

The authors used 32 subjects from each cultural group to establish test-retest reliability. The reliability coefficients were significant at the .01 level of confidence for all subtests in each cultural group. The authors established internal validity by the test-item ability to discriminate differences between language and age groups, as revealed by statistical analysis.

Administration and Scoring

The DRLST consists of five subtests that assess (1) receptive, single-word, noun and verb vocabulary; (2) repetition of sentences of increasing length; (3) repetition of sentences of increasing grammatical complexity; (4) memory for oral directions of increasing length; and (5) story comprehension. Each subtest has an English and Spanish version. Administration of the DRLST is simple and brief (about 15 minutes), with specific instructions for administration and scoring provided in the manual. The number of correct responses on each subtest constitutes the raw score.

The manual provides separate norms for each of the three cultural groups. Norms for each subtest are reported as age ranges in yearly intervals, as percentile ranks, and as positions relative to the mean on a standard curve. A score below the 10th percentile is indicative of the need for further evaluation, while a score of −2 standard deviations below the mean signals the necessity of intervention.

Summary

Because the DRLST was standardized on three separate language groups, it permits evaluation of deviancy in terms of children's performances in their own language. Since it was developed specifically for the intended subjects, the DRLST has high content validity. The language measure taps a variety of language behaviors and is easy to administer and score. Test use is flexible because of the separate scoring and discriminative aspect of each subtest. However, until the effectiveness of the test with other Spanish-speaking cultural groups has been demonstrated, application to other populations not representative of the normative group should be avoided.

Denver Articulation Screening Examination

Description

The Denver Articulation Screening Examination (DASE) (Amelia F. Drumwright, University of Colorado Medical Center, Ladoca Project and Publishing Foundation, 1971) purports to detect articulation disorder in culturally disadvantaged children between the ages of 2 years, 6 months, and 6 years. The test assumes that these children not be judged according to the standards of more "advantaged children."

Technical Information

The sounds tested represent those correctly articulated by 85 percent of 6-year-old children in Templin's experimental population (1957). The author standardized these sounds on 1,455 black, Anglo, and Hispanic preschoolers in Denver, Colorado. This population was equally divided by sex and cultural group.

Test-retest reliability determined on 110 children by the same examiner with a 4- to 8-day interval was found to be .95. A longer interval between testing and different examiners may have increased the usefulness of these data. Validity of the instrument is questionable. The DASE scores were compared to performance on the Hejna Articulation Test (1968) to yield copositivity and conegativity scores. Although these values were fairly high, the use of a criterion test without published validity or reliability studies does not provide an adequate measure of validity.

Administration and Scoring

Test administration is direct and simple. The child is asked to imitate the examiner's words. The author provides coordinated line drawings to help elicit responses in hard-to-test children. To score the DASE, the correct sounds are totaled to produce a low score. In addition, the examiner judges intelligibility of articulation on a four-point scale. The raw score is compared with percentile ranks by age provided on the test form. The author assigns the 15th percentile as the cutoff score for normal articulation. A rank of "normal" is given to those children who score above the 15th percentile on articulation and normal on intelligibility. A score below the 15th percentile is abnormal and indicates need of therapy.

Summary

The DASE is an easily administered test. While it may be as reliable as other single-phoneme measures, further validity studies are needed before it can be confirmed that the DASE is able to detect normal versus abnormal articulation in culturally and economically disadvantaged children.

Detroit Tests of Learning Aptitude

Description

The Detroit Tests of Learning Aptitude, (DTLA) (Harry J. Baker and Bernice Leland, Bobbs-Merrill, 1967) according to the authors, can serve as an aid to psychologists in solving children's learning difficulties. The authors indicate that the three tests—the Auditory Attention Span for Unrelated Words Test, the Auditory Attention Span for Related Syllables Test, and the Oral Commissions Test—all evaluate a child's auditory attentive ability. The tests reveal also strengths and weaknesses in the psychological composition of the subject. In addition, the Oral Commissions Test purports to assess "practical judgment, "motor ability," and "number ability."

Technical Information

The normative sample for the DTLA consisted of 150 students who were tested at 3-month intervals from the ages of 3 to 19 years. The students were drawn from the Detroit public school system, were in the appropriate grade for their age, and had IQs from 90 to 110. Only the norms for the tests are presented in the DTLA manual. Therefore, the distribution of scores by percentile rank or standard scores is not available.

Test-retest reliability estimates were high for 48 normal subjects with a 5-month interval between testing. A coefficient of .675 was obtained for 792 mentally retarded, delinquent, and emotionally unstable subjects with a testing interval of 2 to 3 years. The reliability samples and measures are not outlined adequately, nor do the three tests have separate reliability measures.

The authors report no statistical analysis or research findings to support test-score interpretation in terms of school performance. The rationale for possible interpretations is not presented. Baker and Leland indicate a study of over 4,000 cases which found the DTLA appropriate for evaluation of mentally retarded subjects as well as average students. Unfortunately, this study's research design and statistical analysis are not sufficiently described.

Administration and Scoring

To administer the Auditory Attention Span for Unrelated Words Test, the examiner instructs the child to repeat groups of unrelated words in the exact order of presentation. The number of words varies from two to eight. A score is obtained by assigning one point to each word recalled in any order. A weighted score is the product of the number of correct words in each group and the number of words in the span. The Auditory Attention Span for Related Syllables Test requires the child to repeat 43 sentences ranging in length from 5 words (6 syllables) to 22 words (27 syllables). Each sentence receives a score of 0 to 3, depending upon the number of omitted, added, and substituted words. The Oral Commissions Test requires the child to perform a sequence of commands that increase in number from one to four. Each correctly performed command receives one point.

Scores from each test are converted to a mental age (MA) by means of a normative table. Mental ages can then be recorded on a profile. The DTLA manual provides straightforward administration and scoring procedures. The authors interpret test scores with regard to their relationship to performance in school subjects and present six exemplary cases to assist in test-score interpretation.

Summary

The three tests in the DTLA may provide some valuable information about short-term auditory memory skills in children. Administrative and scoring procedures are clearly described. Though normative data include mental ages, no comparative measure within each age level is provided. Reliability studies are not adequately described, and validity measures are practically nonexistent. However, it seems logical that these tests can help to assess aspects of auditory attentive ability. They may provide one aspect to clinical evaluation related to auditory processing and language, albeit with children beyond the scope of the present text in regard to age.

Developmental Articulation Test

Description

At the time of its publication, the Developmental Articulation Test (Robert F. Hejna, Speech Materials, 1968) offered the novel feature of a developmentally arranged articulation scoring sheet. According to the author, the developmental age level represents the age at which 90 percent or more of children have mastered a particular sound.

Technical Information

No data on validity or reliability are available. Moreover, no information on standardization procedures for the instrument are reported.

Administration and Scoring

The Developmental Articulation Test consists of picture plates containing three to five pen and ink drawings. All consonant sounds except /hw/ and /ʒ/ are tested in initial, medial, and final positions; 14 blends are also included. Test procedures require the child to name the pictures. The examiner notes the type of misarticulation (substitution, omission, or distortion) in the appropriate phoneme position for an indication of whether or not a child can produce a sound in isolation.

Summary

The Developmental Articulation Test is criterion-based, not a standardized instrument. Much criticism is focused on this issue. However, the concept of the test is unique and can provide helpful information for those working with very young children in early stages of phoneme production.

Environmental Language Inventory

Description

The Environmental Language Inventory (ELI) (James D. MacDonald and Judith P. Blott, Charles E. Merrill, 1978) is designed to assess expressive language through rules, context, and generalization. It is based on an analysis of semantic-grammatical rules that describe the early constructions of normally developing children (Darley, 1979). The ELI approximates the environmental context of the "language units" by eliciting them with parallel linguistic and nonlinguistic cues. The assessment samples the child's language in three production modes—imitation, conversation, and play—to allow for generalization. The diagnostic model serves as the basis for the therapeutic scheme. The semantic-grammatical rules shown to be absent by ELI evaluation are targeted for therapy.

Technical Information

In the test manual, the authors report reliability and validity data drawn from the 1974 ELI and the revised semantic-grammatical rules and procedures of the current edition. Reliability was determined by the administration of the ELI to 10 mentally retarded children whose mean length of utterance (MLU) ranged from one to four words. The interexaminer reliability coefficient for semantic-grammatical rule content and utterance length was reported to be .93. The authors mention several experimental language programs that applied the ELI model to teach semantic complexity and encourage "expressive spontaneity" with positive results. The subjects (age 2 years to adult) were drawn from autistic, visually impaired hearing-impaired, and mentally retarded populations. The ELI is also effective for subjects with good receptive language skills but delayed expressive skills and with utterances from one to four words in length.

Administration and Scoring

To evaluate a child's production of phrases according to semantic intent, the examiner must be familiar with the eight semantic-grammatical rules included in the ELI. The examiner must also gather the array of nonlinguistic stimuli (objects, toys, etc.). Although the authors designate specific items to evoke each rule, items can be altered to suit the particular child. Administration proceeds with the child seated with the examiner or in a play setting. Total time for the test averages about 30 minutes.

The examiner presents 24 stimulus sets, testing each rule three times. Each stimulus set contains one nonlinguistic cue (environmental enactment of the rule) and two linguistic cues. All eight rules are assessed in conversation, imitation, and play, with each linguistic cue preceded by a nonlinguistic cue.

To assess language in free play, it is suggested that the examiner obtain 50 responses during a play session. Contextual cues should be noted, and, to facilitate analysis, responses should be catalogued as imitation, question, or spontaneous.

Details of the scoring procedure are provided in the manual. Measures of expressive language that can be derived include the proportion, frequency, and rank order of each rule; the mean length of utterance for total words and intelligible words; and the frequency of intelligible and unintelligible words. Analysis of test scores indicates which rules the child is producing in the various production modes. Distribution of the semantic-grammatical rules in free speech can be compared to the distributions provided in the manual for normal and delayed speakers.

Summary

The ELI provides a viable alternative to traditional language measures. Since the model concentrates on expressive skills, receptive skills are assumed, as in language-sample analyses. Based on a diagnostic model, the program provides consistent coordination between assessment and programming. The flexibility of the ELI is also a favorable point, in that it may be used with a variety of clients. Further research will indicate its ultimate value as a language evaluation instrument.

Environmental Pre-Language Battery

Description

The Environmental Pre-Language Battery (EPB) (De Anna Horstmeier and James D. MacDonald, Charles E. Merrill, 1978) is a diagnostic procedure designed to assess preliminary skills necessary for the development of social language. The test aims toward prescriptive intervention.

Technical Information

The EPB is not a standardized instrument, therefore, no normative data are available. The authors justify inclusion of skills as part of an intervention program that the assessment tool facilitates.

The EPB has been used extensively with mentally retarded and language-delayed individuals at the Nisonger Center for Mental Retardation and Developmental Delay in Columbus, Ohio. The battery has been effectively adapted for use with young or difficult-to-test children, in addition to children with auditory, visual, or physical impairments.

The intent of the EPB is to derive a behavioral description of the child's prelanguage skills that will aid in appropriate intervention planning. By incorporating teaching strategies into the assessment, applicable information about the value of these strategies is obtained.

Administration and Scoring

The EPB consists of two components. The nonverbal portion includes a history of early sound productions (obtained from the parent), observation of preliminary skills, observation of functional play and motor imitation, and assessment of receptive language. The verbal section evaluates sound imitation, single-word imitation and production, and two-word phrase imitation and production. As with the ELI, the examiner uses a variety of toys and pictures as test stimuli, and the child may be seated in a somewhat formal setting or in a play situation. For each skill, four test items are presented by the examiner. If a child fails an item, the child is immediately trained on that item. The manual details specific instructions on skill training. If a child responds correctly during training, the test item is readministered.

Each correct test item receives three points; a readministered correct item receives one point. A test level is passed if the child obtains at least 75 percent of the total possible score; 50 percent or more of the possible score denotes emerging level. The assessment continues until two skill levels are failed. The behavioral description of a child's mastery of prelanguage skills yielded by the EPB helps in determining appropriate therapy planning and goal-setting.

Summary

The EPB is recommended for use with very young or severely language-delayed individuals. It has been shown to be effective with maladaptive children with hyperactivity or short attention span, as well as with individuals who do not respond to formalized testing procedures. The close alliance and incorporation of teaching techniques in the EPB is a unique and valuable asset.

Fisher-Logemann Test of Articulation Competence

Description

The Fisher-Logemann Test of Articulation Competence (Hilda A. Fisher and Jerilyn A. Logemann, Houghton Mifflin, 1971) is designed to evaluate a client's phonological system, analyze phonetic notations of articulation, and aid in complete and accurate analysis and categorization of articulatory errors. The test stresses analysis of misarticulations within the framework of the individual's native dialect.

Technical Information

As a pilot study, 30 speech pathologists in the greater Chicago area tested 500 children representing various dialectal backgrounds. The population also included cleft-palate and mentally retarded subjects. All of the therapists in the study expressed favorable views of the test. No norms by sociologic background or age are presented in the manual. Examiners must make interpretations on the basis of individual discretion.

No quantitative measures of reliability are reported, nor are criterion-related or construct validities noted. However, the Fisher-Logemann test contains such an adequate sampling of phonological behavior that construct validity is fairly certain.

Administration and Scoring

The Fisher-Logemann picture test consists of 109 colored picture cards designed to elicit spontaneous one-word responses. A selected portion of the picture form can be used as a screening test. The sentence test form, used with children beginning at the third grade, is read by the subject. Both test forms assess all English phonemes in systematic occurrence according to syllabic function in initial, medial, and final positions.

The record sheet for each form groups articulation errors according to the nature of the articulatory deficiency. Errors are analyzed and summarized according to the distinctive features involved. Consonant phonemes are analyzed on the basis of a three-parameter system: (1) place of articulation, (2) manner of articulation, and (3) voicing. Vowel phonemes are interpreted on the basis of (1) place of articulation, (2) tongue height, (3) tension, and (4) lip rounding. The manual provides more detailed instructions for administration, recording, and distinctive-feature analysis of articulation errors. Tables of native dialect patterns provide data for distinguishing between misarticulations and dialectal variations. Total test time is estimated at 20 to 45 minutes.

Summary

The Fisher-Logemann test's recording of a subject's error responses with phonetic symbols and subsequent distinctive-feature analysis yields more precise and meaningful information than other available articulation tests. The inclusion of dialect tables allows for selective interpretation of results. Because of these complexities, however, a higher level of examiner skill is necessary, and testing requires more time. Reliability and validity information is sketchy, although face validity is high. The picture-identification approach requires that the picture label be part of a child's expressive repertoire. Children with limited vocabulary would therefore be at a disadvantage.

Goldman-Fristoe-Woodcock Auditory Memory Tests

Description

The Goldman-Fristoe-Woodcock (G-F-W) Auditory Memory Tests (Ronald Goldman, Macalyne Fristoe, and Richard W. Woodcock; American Guidance Service, 1974) are concerned with one of the four categories of auditory perception in the total G-F-W Auditory Skills Test Battery (1974). (The other three categories are covered in subsequent test descriptions.) The purpose of the G-F-W Auditory Memory Tests is to assess the individual's ability to recall items presented orally via short-term memory and to describe any deficiencies in this area. The tests include recognition memory, memory for content, and memory for sequence.

Technical Information

The technical manual for the G-F-W Auditory Skills Test Battery contains descriptive information on standardization, validity, and reliability. The normative population for the three tests consisted of approximately 300 normal subjects and approximately 120 mildly-to-severely dysfunctional subjects for each test. The manual describes age, race, and geographical distribution of the sample. The normative group was approximately 87 percent white, 8 percent black, and 5 percent representing "other" races. The majority of the subjects were from Minnesota. The age norms ranged from 3 to 85 years, but the majority of the sample consisted of subjects under 18 years of age.

Internal consistency reliability data are reported for age groups 3–8, 9–18, and 19+. Values are consistently high for the memory-for-sequence test, while the recognition-memory test has significant coefficients only for the 3–8 and 19+ age groups. It is therefore not recommended that the examiner estimate total raw scores on subjects for whom administration of the entire test is discontinued because of poor performance. Test-retest reliability is not reported for any age group.

Justified claims of content validity are weakened by the fact that the recognition-memory and memory-for-content tests involve negation. This construction complicates the instruction for all subjects, especially young children who have not mastered the form. The authors provide data to support their inference that each of the three tests measures a distinct short-term auditory memory ability that is independent of other auditory skills measured in other tests of the G-F-W Auditory Skills Test Battery. In addition, the authors cite references that support the notion that auditory memory is related to language, articulation, reading, writing, learning disabilities, and mental retardation.

Administration and Scoring

Three separate tests, presented in serial order, constitute the G-F-W Auditory Memory Tests. The examiner administers each test via recorded auditory test stimuli. Preteaching is provided for each test to ensure task familiarity and to lessen the effects of prior vocabulary.

Test 1, recognition memory, assesses the subject's ability to recognize a word over a short time lapse. The subject is instructed to respond "yes" or "no" to each word heard, depending on whether or not the subject has heard it earlier. There are five lists of 22 words each; 11 words in each list are repeated at least once.

Test 2, memory for content, measures the ability to recognize an auditory message regardless of the sequence of elements. The subject listens to a list of recorded words and is then shown a set of pictures containing all the recorded words and two additional ones. The subject must point to the two unnamed pictures, each with one score point. The test begins with two stimulus words and increases to seven by the end of the test.

Test 3, memory for sequence, involves recall of an auditory sequence. The examiner presents a set of stimulus pictures for the subject to arrange in the sequence specified on the taped list of words. The subject receives one point for correct placement of the first or last card and for any correct sequencing of two cards. Word lists progress in length from two to eight words.

The number of correct responses constitutes a subject's raw score, which can be converted to percentile rank, age equivalent, or standard score by means of tables in the test manual. These values are then plotted on a profile provided in the test booklet.

Summary

The G-F-W Auditory Memory Tests are intended for use with children who experience reading, spelling, writing, language, articulation, or listening problems in an attempt to identify related-term, auditory memory deficits. The G-F-W battery of tests constitutes one of the most comprehensive attempts to achieve this goal. In conjunction with other measures of auditory ability, these tests may yield valuable information, within the constraints of observed statistical support, for children of prekindergarten age or older. The taped format is not particularly conducive for use with hearing-impaired subjects.

Goldman-Fristoe-Woodcock Auditory Selective Attention Test

Description

The Goldman-Fristoe-Woodcock (G-F-W) Auditory Selective Attention Test (Ronald Goldman, Macalyne Fristoe, and Richard W. Woodcock; American Guidance Service, 1974) is designed to assess an individual's ability to attend to a listening task within the context of background noise, based on three distortion factors: intensity (shift of signal-to-noise ratio), variability, and meaningfulness.

Technical Information

The test's normative population is made up of subjects between age 3 and 80 years (the majority between 3 and 12) from locations in California, Florida, Maine, and Minnesota. The population represents both normal and pathological subjects. The authors present internal consistency reliability coefficients for both groups by age range and by the G-F-W Auditory Skills Test Battery.

Administration and Scoring

The G-F-W Auditory Selective Attention Test consists of 110 items divided into four subtests with 15 training items for adequate subject preparation. All auditory stimuli are prerecorded on cassette tape and presented via earphones. The subject is asked to respond to a set of four pictures, one of which relates to the auditory stimulus.

The first 11 items constitute the quiet subtest (no background noise). The remaining 99 items are divided equally into the fan-like noise subtest, the cafeteria noise subtest, and the voice subtest. The number of correct items on each subtest and the total number of correct items for the entire test yield raw scores that are converted into age equivalency and percentile ranks. These results are combined with those of the other battery tests to form a profile for each subject. Total administration time is approximately 20 minutes.

Summary

The G-F-W Auditory Selective Attention Test attempts to measure auditory skills that are believed to be vital to the educational process. It is designed to be used independently if a time constraint prohibits administration of the total G-F-W battery.

Test validity and reliability remain questionable. Further research is necessary to establish sensitivity to auditory processing problems. Also, the test provides no guidelines for sequencing of remedial tasks and therefore limits the applicability of results.

Goldman-Fristoe-Woodcock Sound Symbol Tests

Description

The purpose of the Goldman-Fristoe-Woodcock (G-F-W) Sound Symbol Tests (Ronald Goldman, Macalyne Fristoe, and Richard W. Woodcock; American Guidance Service, 1974) is to measure specific attributes of oral-written language skills.

Technical Information

The technical manual for the G-F-W Auditory Skills Test Battery (Goldman et al., 1974) presents information on the construction of the G-F-W Sound Symbol Test. The normative sample was drawn from schools and institutions in California, Florida, Maine, and Minnesota. The authors attempted to obtain representative data from ages 3 to 80 with an emphasis on the 3- to 12-year-old interval. The population size for all tests except the Reading of Symbols Test appears to be adequate; however, approximately 88 percent of the subjects were white. Separate normative data for the Reading of Symbols Test were obtained from results from 4,790 subjects on the Word Attack Test of the Woodcock Reading Mastery Tests (1973). Norms for this test encompass only school-aged subjects.

Data are reported for two additional populations: subjects with mild speech and learning problems, and those with severe learning problems. The mild clinical group was best represented in the 7- to 12-year-old interval, while the severe-learning-problem group was best represented in the 11- to 16-year-old category. The number of subjects for each test and clinical group ranged from 48 to 60.

The range of test reliability coefficients for normal subjects on each test by age group is as follows: 3–8 years, .81 to .97; 9–19 years, .73 to .96; and 19 years and over, .87 to .97. For five of the tests, coefficients for the mild clinical group ranged from .74 to .98, while those for the severe clinical group ranged from .93 to .97.

Inferential interpretation of intercorrelations among the tests indicated that each test measured a different skill. Further correlations between test scores and age became progressively less with age increase. Goldman et al., (1974) interpreted these data as evidence of "age-related growth and decline of auditory skills" (p. 27). A comparison of mean score variance for normal subjects and mild and severe clinical groups indicated a significant distinction between normal subjects and those with severe problems.

The majority of the normal-to-mild clinical group comparisons were significant; the age-within-group comparison was often a more substantial source of variance than subject grouping.

Administration and Scoring

The G-F-W Sound Symbol Tests consist of seven separate measures of auditory comprehension skills:

1. sound mimicry: the ability to repeat a nonsense syllable immediately after it is presented
2. sound recognition: the ability to synthesize isolated sounds comprising a word
3. sound analysis: the ability to identify phonemic component sounds of nonsense syllables
4. sound blending: the ability to synthesize isolated sounds into meaningful words
5. sound symbol association: the ability to learn associations between unfamiliar visual and auditory symbols
6. reading of symbols: the ability to translate graphemes to phonemes
7. spelling of sounds: the ability to translate phonemes to graphemes

The easel-kit provides test instructions and training procedures for each test, as well as test stimuli for the sound recognition and association tests. A prerecorded tape provides stimuli for the sound-mimicry, recognition, analysis, blending, and spelling tests. Administration time is approximately 20 minutes.

Information on scoring and interpretation of test results are included in the test manual section of the easel-kit. Percentile ranks, age equivalents, standard scores, and stanines are also provided for each test.

Summary

The test format and materials for the G-F-W Sound Symbol Tests are easily employed, and instructions for administration and scoring are clearly specified. Reliability and validity measures are considered sufficiently adequate to meet clinical application of the tests within the best standardized age group, 3 to 12 years. As with the other G-F-W battery tests, difficulty arises in the use of an auditory-only stimulus with many hearing-impaired individuals, especially very young children and clients with poorly developed listening ability. Perhaps if interpretation were based on criteria reference, helpful information could be derived that could be used in aural habilitation and rehabilitation programming.

Goldman-Fristoe-Woodcock Test of Auditory Discrimination

Description

The Goldman-Fristoe-Woodcock Test of Auditory Discrimination (Ronald Goldman, Macalyne Fristoe, Richard Woodcock; American Guidance Service, 1974) attempts to assess speech-sound discrimination under conditions relatively free from the subject's level of vocabulary and relative familiarity with test materials, the difficulty of the memory tasks, interexaminer variability, and the contrived situation of "ideal" conditions. As a comparative measure of auditory discrimination, this instrument also tests in the presence of controlled background noise.

Technical Information

The normative group consisted of 745 subjects from 3 to 84 years of age. Kindergarten and school-aged children were drawn from schools, while preschool and adult subjects were selected by personal contact. There is no mention in the test manual of geographical or racial distribution.

Reported split-half reliabilities and test-retest reliabilities are relatively low. The subtests of the G-F-W Test of Auditory Discrimination have face validity based on test construction. However, there are no correlations reported between the test and other measures of auditory discrimination. Additional validity data are needed.

Administration and Scoring

The test is comprised of three parts: the training procedure, the quiet subtest, and the noise subtest. The latter two parts are presented on audiotape.

The purpose of the training procedure is to familiarize the subject with the word-picture associations presented in the two subtests. The examiner asks the subject to point to specific pictures. If the response is incorrect, the examiner may use verbal or gestural cues to help in word-picture association.

Before the recorded quiet subtest, the examiner reads instructions to the subject. The tape presents the 30 stimulus items while the examiner manipulates the test plates and records the subjects responses.

The recorded noise subtest presents three training plates with increasing levels of background noise to adjust the listener to the "masked" portion. These plates are not counted in the score. The background noise is 9 dB less intense than the speech signal on the tape. This decibel figure represents the intensity level differences at which normal subjects showed a marked decrease in discrimination.

The authors present two levels of scoring for the test. A total error score can be translated into a percentile score and a standard score, for comparison with normative tables. Another level of scoring, which sorts errors into a speech-sound matrix, is recommended only for research and clinical inquiry.

Summary

The G-F-W Test of Auditory Discrimination is recommended as a screening test for auditory discrimination. In its administration, the test attempts to eliminate many factors that interfere with accurate assessment of discrimination. The training procedure ensures that errors are due to problems in auditory discrimination and not in word-picture association. However, though the test has some face validity based on test construction, no correlations between the G-F-W Test of Auditory Discrimination and other measures of auditory discrimination are presented. Validity data are incomplete, and reliability measures are low. Before further evaluation can be made of this test, more clinical data would be helpful.

Houston Test for Language Development

Description

The Houston Test for Language Development (HTLD) (Margaret Crabtree, Houston Test Company, Part I, 1958, Part II, 1963) was designed to measure language development in children from 6 months to 6 years of age.

Technical Information

Data on reliability and validity available in the test manual are scant. The author provides a rationale for item selection in support of validity. For Part I, an interexaminer reliability correlation of .84 is presented. However, sampling procedures and sample size are not specified. Parts I and II were both developed on insufficient sample groups of 113 and 215, respectively, taken from the white community of Houston, Texas. Interpretation of test results, therefore, should be cautious.

Administration and Scoring

Part I of the HTLD, for use with children from 6 months to 3 years of age, is essentially an observational device modeled on normal maturational charts. Part II examines language in children through age 6. Test items measure both expressive and receptive language skills in such categories as vocabulary, articulation, rhythm, identification of body parts, gestures, geometric drawings and designs, counting, and a language sample of 10 responses. The test items are grouped in 6-month age intervals to 3 years and in 1-year intervals to 6 years. The weight of each test item is determined by the total number of items at that age level. A basal age, ceiling age, and language age are obtained from the raw score. Children who score 2 or more years below their chronological age are considered to have a language problem. The test takes approximately 30 minutes to administer.

Summary

The HTLD represents an early attempt at language testing but is now of limited use when compared to more recent and sophisticated measures. The inadequacy of statistical data curtails diagnostic or remedial interpretation of test results. Item selection reflects a general theory of language that is not in accordance with language acquisition knowledge (Smith and Miller, 1966). The HTLD manual lacks specific stimuli for test items, and subjective judgments on scoring may contaminate responses. Finally, the full-year age levels are not sensitive enough to differentiate normal and language-delayed children.

Illinois Test of Psycholinguistic Abilities

Description

The Illinois Test of Psycholinguistic Abilities (ITPA) (Samuel A. Kirk, James J. McCarthy, and Winifred D. Kirk; University of Illinois Press, rev. ed., 1968) was designed as a diagnostic device to tap and differentiate various aspects of cognitive ability in children between the ages of 2 years, 4 months, and 10 years, 3 months. The test is based on Osgood's theoretical model of psycholinguistic communication, which consists of three dimensions of cognitive ability: channels of communication, psycholinguistic processes, and organizational levels. By delineating specific abilities and disabilities in children with different sensory modalities, the ITPA purports to facilitate selection for remedial programming.

Technical Information

The statistical information on the ITPA is extensive. The test was standardized on 962 "average," middle-class children between the ages of 2 years, 7 months, and 10 years, 1 month, from cities in Illinois and Wisconsin. However, according to Paraskeropoulous and Kirk (1969), the ITPA was designed "for use with children encountering learning difficulties" (p. 51), and the normative population is not representative of this group.

The discussion of reliability presented in the ITPA manual is most adequate. Internal consistency coefficients for each of the eight age groups are reported by age and subtest. These coefficients fall below .90 for the 12 subtests only between the ages of 5 years, 7 months, and 6 years, 1 month. Test-retest reliability was computed for the three age levels of 4, 6, and 8 years. No subtest estimate exceeded .86.

Test validity on the ITPA is, at present, a debatable issue. No validity estimates with other language measures are presented. The assumption that psycholinguistic abilities, as defined by the authors, can be separated and measured is questionable.

Content validity of various subtests is another area of concern. According to developmental research on the complexity of psycholinguistic behaviors, the ordering of numerous items in the subtests is in need of revision. Hammill and Larsen (1974) reviewed 38 studies that attempted to train children in psycholinguistic skills, using the ITPA as a guideline. Only verbal expression and manual expression appeared to be amenable to training.

Administration and Scoring

The ITPA consists of 12 subtests, 6 of which assess abilities at the representational level while the remainder assess abilities at the automatic level. The subtests tap auditory and visual modalities (auditory-vocal, auditory-motor, visual-motor, visual-vocal) and psycholinguistic processes (expressive and receptive) within their respective levels. Each subtest has specific administration and scoring procedures. The order of subtest presentation is specified in the manual. For each separate subtest, a scaled score or an age score can be derived. The total raw score can be converted to an overall "psycholinguistic age." Kirk and Kirk (1971) have provided a book on interpretation and remediation based on the ITPA results. They suggest comparison of intraindividual differences within a child's performance on the ITPA subtests and encourage supplementary testing and observation for a more valid diagnosis.

Summary

The ITPA can assist in providing information pertaining to auditory and visual skills, but it must be used with cognizance of existing limitations. The norms appear inadequate for stringent use. The validity of the test is questionable. The theoretical model emphasizes abilities that, although related to language, are not language per se. One also runs the risk of attending to a discrete-skill orientation when applying the test to processing ability. Perhaps the best use of the ITPA at this point in time is as a supplement to additional testing and observation. It is not recommended for very young children or children with language development levels below late preschool age.

Language Facility Test

Description

The Language Facility Test (LFT) (John T. Darley, Allington Corporation, 1977) employs pictures to elicit verbal responses in persons with "mental ages" from 3 to 15. The test was devised as a short measure that could be administered by teachers or aides with little training in test administration. The author suggests that the LFT be used in programs for the mentally retarded or physically handicapped, bilingual educational programs, foreign language programs, and other groups where language is not standard English.

Technical Information

Normative data were collected on a sample of 4,000 subjects from ages 3 to 20 years in 10 U.S. cities. Of the 10 cities, 8 were located in the southern United States, which limits the representativeness of the sample. The LFT manual does not report the number of subjects in each age group, the sex distribution, or the socioeconomic spread. These omitted factors would appear to be crucial to language facility. Norms are reported by age-equivalents and percentile scores.

Examiner reliability was determined in several studies. Pearson product-moment correlations (between .88 and .94) were obtained for poorly identified samples. Test-retest correlations for five groups range from .46 to .90. However, interval length was quite prolonged, 15 weeks and 12 weeks, respectively.

The LFT manual does not discuss validity, except to present two tables that give correlations of the LFT with other tests. The author reports a correlation of .20 with the Science Research Associates (SRA) achievement tests and .18 with the Stanford Binet. These low correlations do not support concurrent validity.

Administration and Scoring

The LFT consists of 12 pictures, grouped into sets of three; with three extra plates for alternate use. The first set contains simple drawings; the second consists of photographs of children of migrant workers interacting with a teacher; and the third contains reproductions of detailed, shaded Spanish paintings. The examiner selects the set of pictures that is most meaningful to the particular child. The subject is directed to tell a complete story about each picture in a set. Directions for administration are clear and specific, indicating the number of prompts that are appropriate for each picture before its withdrawal.

Responses to each picture are scored on a scale of 0 to 9, according to complexity and organization. The LFT manual provides a detailed description for each scale value as well as response examples. However, very few examples of nonstandard English responses are given. This factor contradicts the notion that the test scores are independent of the subject's facility for standard English.

Summary

In light of the inadequate data on standardization, reliability, and validity, the LFT, in its current form, has little utility as a standardized instrument. The LFT offers the advantage of short administration and scoring time. And the idea of a language assessment instrument independent of dialect, specifically standard English, is appealing. However, much developmental work on the LFT is still needed.

Michigan Picture Language Inventory

Description

The Michigan Picture Language Inventory (MPLI) (William Wolski and Louis Lerea, University of Michigan, Department of Communication Disorders, 1962) was devised as a measure of vocabulary and grammatical structures. Both structures are evaluated in terms of verbal expression and receptive comprehension. The MPLI was initially developed by Lerea (1958) and revised by Wolski (1962).

Technical Information

The MPLI was standardized on 180 children, 30 boys and 30 girls in each age group of 4-, 5-, and 6-year-olds. The normative subjects were Caucasian singletons from the Flint, Michigan, area, which limits the applicability of the derived norms. The authors present questionable reliability and validity data in the test manual. They assert content validity on the basis of test-item selection and the fact that older groups of children in the normative population performed better than the younger children on both the vocabulary and language-structure subtests. However, the linguistic model upon which the test is based (Fries, 1952) is based on a rather shallow perception of language. It does not consider the importance of more recent views of language, such as transformational grammar (Chomsky, 1965), generative semantics (Fillmore, 1968), or pragmatics (Bates, 1976). Evaluation of language with a focus on superficial grammatical structure will produce a biased, deceptive, and incomplete picture of language behavior.

Administration and Scoring

The MPLI consists of a vocabulary subtest and a language-structure subtest. The vocabulary subtest contains 35 vocabulary items, all nouns, selected from the Buckingham and Dolch word count for children. The language-structure subtest employs 50 stimulus plates to assess 69 examples of such syntactic forms as singular and plural noun forms, personal pronouns, adjectives, demonstratives, possessives, articles, adverbs, verbs, and prepositions.

The examiner first administers the expressive portion of the vocabulary subtest. Each test plate contains one stimulus picture and two items. The examiner points to the test picture, and the child is required to name it. To administer the expressive portion, the examiner asks the child to indicate by pointing to a specific picture in each test plate.

The language-structure subtest is divided into three sections. Nine structures are tested separately in three stages. The stimulus cards are described by the examiner to familiarize the child with the significant structures. In the expressive portion, the examiner models the test structure, as with the vocabulary subtest, and then requests that the child respond on a subsequent example. Only those items failed in the expressive portion of the language-structure subtest are tested receptively. The child receives credit for receptive ability for all correct items on the expressive portion of the subtest. Correct items receive one point in scoring. Receptive and expressive scores on each of the subtests are compared to norms in the test appendix to evaluate a subject's performance.

Summary

The MPLI fails to use new knowledge related to language acquisition. The linguistic model upon which it is based does not reflect contemporary views of language. The information obtained from administration of this lengthy test has little relevance to a child's expressive and receptive language abilities.

Northwestern Syntax Screening Test

Description

The Northwestern Syntax Screening Test (NSST) (Laura L. Lee, Northwestern University Press, 1969, 1971) was designed to identify children between 3 and 8 years of age whose syntactic development diverges enough to warrant further evaluation. It does not provide a comprehensive analysis of a child's syntax but rather a quick estimate of his level of development.

Technical Information

Test norms for the NSST are based on scores collected from 344 children. However Arndt (1977) countered that these norms were not generalizable because of the homogeneity of the standardization population in terms of socioeconomic level and geographic location.

A study by Prutting, Gallagher, and Mulac (1975) suggests that results on the expressive portion of the NSST are not reflected in spontaneous speech. Test validity is questionable. No statistical analysis indicating item-selection criteria is included in the manual. Also, a study by Larson and Summers (1976) found no significant differences between subjects' means in age groups of 5 years, 6 months; 6 years; and 6 years, 6 months. Test norms differed little in the 7 year to 7 year, 11 month range.

Test reliability coefficients, derived in a study by Ratusnik and Koenigknecht (1975) were poor (.55 and .67) for the receptive portion of the NSST and only moderate (.81 and .78) for the expressive portion.

Administration and Scoring

The NSST contains a receptive and expressive portion, each with 20 items of increasing difficulty. Both portions test the same grammatical structures but use different contrasting sentence pairs. No specific subject training is required, but demonstration items are included. Each test stimulus on the receptive portion contains four pictures. The child must match with the proper picture a sentence spoken by the examiner.

In the expressive portion, the examiner identifies the two pictures on each test plate with sentences and asks the child to repeat the sentences. Expressive items are scored incorrect if the child changes the linguistic form being tested or does not produce a grammatically and semantically correct sentence.

The scores on each test portion can be compared with norms for 6-month intervals from 3 years to 7 years, 11 months. The author suggests that children who score less than 2 standard deviations below the mean on either section are probably candidates for language therapy. The time required for test administration is approximately 15 minutes.

Summary

The NSST should not be used beyond its stated intent as a screening tool. It can be quickly and simply administered. However, limitations in its construction and in its validity, reliability, and normative data prevent its use in qualitative analysis.

Photo Articulation Test

Description

The Photo Articulation Test (PAT) (Kathleen Pendergast, Stanley E. Dickey, John W. Selmac, and Anton L. Soder; Interstate Printers and Publishers, 1969) is designed as a means of rapidly evaluating the articulation skills of children of ages 3 to 12. The test stimuli consist of color photographs of objects. Separate scores may be obtained for tongue, lip, and vowel sounds.

Technical Information

The authors provide normative data for 684 white, middle-class children on the tongue, lip, and vowel subscales. Mean and standard deviations are reported for boys and girls in 6-month age groups from 3 to 12 years of age. At least 25 children of each sex were tested at each age group. It should be noted that children with very different phoneme error patterns could obtain the same test score. In this case, norms would provide little valuable information.

Validity and reliability tests were carried out on 100 children. Test-retest reliability was reported to be .99. A concurrent validity coefficient of .975 was obtained by comparing results on PAT to results on the Templin-Darley Tests of Articulation. Given the subscale norms and test rationale, validity coefficients at the subscale level would have been more meaningful.

Administration and Scoring

The PAT contains 72 color photographs of objects that were considered familiar to most young children. The examiner evaluates the adequacy of the target sound uttered by the child and records the response on the score sheet. Altogether, 23 consonants are tested in all positions, and 18 vowels are assessed. Three levels of distortions, omissions, and substitutions, as well as of imitative ability, are recorded. Connected speech is observed through the use of three story-making pictures. In scoring, the number of errors on each subscale are totaled and compared to the age norms.

Summary

The PAT can provide a quick survey of a child's articulation ability. It offers the advantage of utilizing photographs rather than line drawings. However, the PAT does not appear to be as fully developed an articulation test as the Goldman-Fristoe-Woodcock, Templin-Darley, or Fisher-Logemann articulation measures, all of which present more relevant information on phonological development and use. Another shortcoming is the limited spontaneous sample that can be obtained during the test. The user of the PAT should keep in mind that the instrument touches only the surface of a child's phonological system.

Porch Index of Communicative Ability in Children

Description

The Porch Index of Communicative Ability in Children (PICAC) (Bruce E. Porch, Consulting Psychologists Press, 1975) measures selected verbal, gestural, and graphic abilities in children. Ultimately, according to the author, the test results will provide differential diagnostic, prognostic, and therapeutic information.

Technical Information

No validity, normative, or reliability data are available at this time, since the PICAC is available only in a research edition. However, the author emphasizes tester reliability, requiring 40 hours of preparation, to ensure test adequacy.

Administration and Scoring

The PICAC contains two batteries. The basic battery, to be used with preschool children, consists of 15 subtests. The advanced battery, to be used with children aged 6 to 12 years, has 20 subtests. Subtests are grouped according to the response modality (verbal, reading, gestural, auditory, visual, graphic). The test objects, 10 items considered common to children, are set before the child in a predetermined order. The examiner administers each subtest in a fixed sequence. The child is instructed to respond according to the requirements of each subtest. The average testing time is 1 hour, but the child may be given more time, as needed.

The administration and scoring procedures are elaborate. The scoring system provides 16 categories to score subject responses and five dimensions of "rightness" (accuracy, responsiveness, completeness, promptness, and efficiency) that help determine the point value of a response. Mean scores for individual modalities, as well as a total mean score, can be derived from the subtest scores.

Summary

Since no clinical research on the PICAC is available to date, its worth as an evaluation tool and aid for diagnostic, prognostic, and remedial conclusions has yet to be established. The obvious strength of this instrument is the in-depth detail of its administration and scoring procedures.

Preschool Language Scale

Description

The Preschool Language Scale (PLS) (Irla L. Zimmerman, Violette G. Steiner, and Roberta L. Evatt; Charles E. Merrill, 1969, 1979) was designed to pinpoint areas of strength and weakness in auditory comprehension and verbal expression. It provides "language ages" for these aspects as well as a total language age from 1 year, 6 months, to 7 years.

Technical Information

No validity or reliability data are presented for the PLS. Only previously obtained normative data for each item are given. The authors stress that the scale is not a test but rather an evaluation instrument still in experimental form.

Reliability data for a revised edition of the PLS, are reported in a new manual (Zimmerman, Steiner, & Evatt, 1979). Coefficients ranging from .75 to .92 are presented as derived from test presentations to students enrolled in two Head Start programs. No further reliability data are included. Content validity is based on the rationale provided for test items. Concurrent validity is reported for comparisons with several other tests (the Illinois Test of Psycholinguistic Abilities, the Utah Test of Language Development, the Peabody Picture Vocabulary Test (PPVT), etc.). Correlations ranged from .26 to .99, depending on the test and sample of children.

Administration and Scoring

Items on both the auditory-comprehension and verbal-ability sections are sequenced in an order that reflects normative data obtained from the developmental literature. There are four items at each age level with 6-month intervals from 1 year, 6 months, to 5 years and yearly age intervals from 5 to 7 years. Administration of each section begins at an age level that is slightly below the child's estimated ability. Basals and ceilings are determined by success and failure on all four items at each age level. Each item is scored by a plus or minus, but each response should be recorded in full to allow for more comprehensive evaluation. Scoring procedures, which are clearly outlined in the manual, yield an auditory comprehension age, a verbal ability age, and an overall language age. These can be compared by converting each to a quotient.

Summary

The PLS features a dichotomy of test items between auditory comprehension and verbal expressive abilities, but this differentiation is a gross one. Neither scale assesses a discrete ability, and the verbal tasks, in particular, reflect an interaction between receptive and expressive skills.

Receptive-Expressive Emergent Language Scale

Description

The Receptive-Expressive Emergent Language (REEL) Scale for the measurement of language skills in infancy (Kenneth R. Bzoch and Richard League, Tree of Life Press, 1971) attempts to assess graded language behaviors in terms of both expressive and receptive skills from birth to 36 months of age.

Technical Information

The standardization population consists of only 50 linguistically competent infants. No information is provided on the geographical distribution on age. Test-retest reliability on 28 normal infants was .71, a reasonable coefficient. However, such a small number of subjects, coupled with the 3-week interval, makes interpretation of this reliability coefficient difficult. No validity data have been reported, although the authors claim a high degree of validity when the Stanford Binet and Vineland Test of Social Maturity are used as criteria.

Administration and Scoring

The REEL Scale is administered through an informant interview. The manual suggests general questioning to elicit information on each item before direct questioning. Direct observation of the child is recommended to confirm ambiguous parent responses. Each item is scored as "plus," "minus," or "emergent." The results yield two scores: a developmental age score and a combined language age. A total language quotient can be derived, which assumes that receptive and expressive ability are parallel in development.

Summary

The REEL Scale should be used with caution and only as a rough screening device. While the scale is rich in detail, the items and age equivalents are not sufficiently founded empirically or theoretically. No data on effectiveness in diagnosing deafness, infantile autism, or mental retardation have been reported. In addition, the authors provide no variation in the phrasing of items to communicate them effectively to parents of varying degrees of sophistication.

Scales of Early Communication Skills for Hearing Impaired Children

Description

The Scales of Early Communication Skills for Hearing Impaired Children (Jean S. Moog and Ann V. Geers, Central Institute for the Deaf, 1975) assess the speech and language development of hearing-impaired children from age 2 to 8 years. It is designed to be given by the child's teacher, since the teacher has a great deal of contact with the child and is familiar with the child's behavior.

Technical Information

The standardization sample consisted of 372 children enrolled in 14 oral programs for the hearing impaired in Georgia, Tennessee, Missouri, Ohio, California, and Colorado. Normative tables were constructed with mean hearing levels and standard deviations at yearly intervals for seven age groups from 2 years to 8 years, 11 months.

Reliability coefficients were derived from correlation of test scores and teacher ratings of speech and language abilities of 31 students, aged 4 through 8 years, enrolled in the Central Institute for the Deaf. Reliability coefficients were lowest for receptive A items (.76) and highest for expressive A items (.91). Children under 4 years of age were not included in the reliability data, nor were reliability measures for separate age groups reported.

No statistical measures of validity are provided by the test authors. Items were selected on the basis of experience in teaching deaf children.

Rationales for inclusion of each item and criteria for rating are the only attempts to demonstrate face or criterion-related validity.

Administration and Scoring

The test is designed around four separate scales: receptive language skills, expressive language skills, nonverbal receptive skills, and nonverbal expressive skills. In the sections on receptive language skills and expressive language skills, the child is rated in two situations: a highly structured context (A) and a natural spontaneous context (B). Many of the items in each scale can be scored by the teacher on the basis of a knowledge of the child. The ratings on the nonverbal scales, which test understanding and use of gestures, are not added to the raw scores for these sections.

The scoring procedure is as follows:

- + (1 point)—frequently demonstrated skill
- ±(1/2 point)—emerging skill, demonstrated on occasion
- – (0 point)—unacquired skill, not demonstrated by child

A criterion for acceptable performance is listed under each skill. Since the items in each scale are listed hierarchically, testing stops in a particular section once the child receives a – rating. Three receptive and three expressive raw scores are computed and entered onto tables for comparison with deaf children in the normative sample at the appropriate age level.

Summary

The Scales of Early Communication Skills for Hearing-Impaired Children may be helpful to teachers of hearing-impaired children as a general screening instrument, but the scales fail to evaluate language ability in any depth. Many items are language-related but do not truly reflect language function. Administration of the test is easy and requires no examiner training.

However, the application of test results is limited because the scales are standardized only on hearing-impaired children in selected oral programs and thus afford no further comparisons. Additional evaluation is necessary to compare these children to normal-hearing peers. The reliability coefficient for the receptive scales is only moderate, compared with the high reliability coefficient for the expressive scales. There is a need for more comprehensive reliability data. Also the validity of the test items as legitimate indexes of language development is disputable.

Sequenced Inventory of Communication Development

Description

The Sequenced Inventory of Communication Development (SICD) (Dona Lea Hedrick, Elizabeth Prather, and Annette R. Tobin; University of Washington Press, 1975) was designed to assess discretely the expressive and receptive factors of communication development in children between the ages of 4 months and 4 years. The inventory is in a kit format with accompanying score and summary forms.

Technical Information

Proposed test items—drawn from the Denver Development Scale, the Illinois Test of Psycholinguistic Abilities, and the authors' research—were administered to 82 children in the 1969 experimental edition of the SICD. The test was then standardized on 252 Caucasian children in the Seattle, Washington, area. Three age levels per year, from 4 to 48 months, were included. Equal numbers of children from each social class—low, middle, and high—were represented at every age level. The numbers of male and female subjects were approximately equal. Only children with "normal" development were included in the sample.

Interexaminer reliability was estimated through simultaneous administration by two examiners on 16 subjects. The mean percentage of agreement was 96. The mean test-retest reliability coefficient was 92.8 for 10 subjects, with a testing interval of 1 week.

The authors contend that high correlation between the receptive communication age (RCA) and expressive communication age (ECA) and the proximity of a subject's chronological age to the means of RCAs and ECAs lend support to test validity. In addition, they report the rigid controls on test administration and scoring as another validity index. Test items are drawn from well-established measures of prelinguistic communicative behavior.

According to the authors, the SICD does seem to be effective in assisting remedial programming for deviant children at the University of Washington clinic. McLean (1979) claims that the SICD can be most useful in identifying brand areas in communication development that require "intensive clinical prescriptive development" (p. 69). Further studies are underway to determine the measure's clinical usefulness.

Administration and Scoring

The two major parts of the SICD are the receptive scale and the expressive scale. Responses include informant reports of a child's behavior at home and elicited items in the testing situation. Receptively, the SICD samples motor responses to environmental sounds and speech. Behavior responses are classified by test items on awareness, discrimination, and understanding of verbal directives.

Expressive items sample such behaviors as imitation of a motor or speech activity, imitation of a motor or speech behavior, and spontaneous response (any nonimitative vocal and verbal behavior). In addition, a 50-response language sample is obtained for all children 2 years old and over, and structural complexity and mean length of utterance are determined. The SICD also provides for an inventory of articulation skills and scoring along a developmental continuum.

There are 32 items on the receptive scale and 67 items on the expressive scale, excluding the articulation inventory. Test items are scored "yes" or "no." Test items can be compared to a norm-referenced scale to provide a score or age for both the receptive and expressive scales. The receptive communication age (RCA) and the expressive communication age (ECA) can be contrasted with the subject's chronological or mental age, as determined by another measure, to determine deficiencies.

Summary

The SICD presents an eclectic approach to quantifying young children's positions on a developmental continuum of communication behavior. As such, it may be helpful in directing the examiner to areas that should be further evaluated to determine specific deficits. In this way, language programming can result. Rieke, Lynch, and Soltmon (1977) have demonstrated that the SICD meets this goal.

In addition, high interrater and test-retest reliability has been reported. Testing procedures are standardized and clearly defined. The inclusion of parent-report items reduces the artificiality of results.

Unfortunately the language sample for the SICD does not extend downward to children at single-word or preverbal stages. Also, the standardization population needs to be enlarged. Hopefully, this will occur with extended use of the instrument. Like many other language tests, the SICD does not address pragmatics as an integral part of language behavior. However, it does give a more representative sample of context than most currently available instruments.

Templin-Darley Tests of Articulation

Description

The Templin-Darley Tests of Articulation (Mildred D. Templin and Frederic L. Darley, University of Iowa Bureau of Educational Research and Service, 2nd ed., 1969), a revision of the 1960 Templin-Darley Screening and Diagnostic Tests of Articulation, are designed to assess a subject's habitual and optimum phoneme production in a shorter, more flexible format than was available in the original version. The test purpose is to describe a pattern of misarticulations and to prescribe a phoneme sequence to be followed in therapy. To meet these aims, the 141-item Diagnostic Test has been organized into nine overlapping test areas. The 50-item Screening Test measures general articulation adequacy, while the 43-item Iowa Pressure Test of Articulation assesses the adequacy of a palatopharyngeal closure through production of oral pressure consonants. The other seven tests include a 42-item grouping of initial and final consonants and groupings of various consonant clusters, vowels, and diphthongs.

Technical Information

The present version of the Templin-Darley test manual presents an updated review of relevant literature and more detailed instructions for interpretation of results. Test validity was established in a study by Jordan (1960). Raw scores obtained by 5- to 10-year-olds on several item categories were significantly related to adult judges' ratings of the subjects' articulation characteristics during contextual speech. Recent critics of the measure claim that it provides a quantitative measure of errors but no information about phonological rules, such as that obtained with a distinctive feature-analysis approach.

Templin's normative sample consisted of white children of normal intelligence and hearing enrolled in 35 public schools and nursery schools in Minneapolis and St. Paul. Norms are presented by mean scores at ages of 3, 3½, 4, 4½, 5, 6, 7, and 8 years for both sexes together and separately and for upper and lower socioeconomic levels.

Reliability data are available only for the screening test. The Iowa Pressure Test of Articulation was determined to be a reliable predictor of palatopharyngeal competence by Van Demark, Kuehn, and Thorp (1975).

Administration and Scoring

The examiner evokes responses from nonreaders with picture stimuli. Prompts are provided to elicit these responses. The author suggests that misarticulated phonemes be imitated by the subject in isolation, in syllables, and in words. In addition, intelligibility of conversational speech should be assessed. For older children who can read, two test words containing the target phoneme are provided in each test sentence. Imitation and spontaneous speech evaluation follow. Responses are recorded on a test form on which each subtest has an overlay to facilitate scoring. The child's scores are compared with appropriate test norms.

The author recommends that errors on the Diagnostic Test be analyzed according to the type of error, consistency, and stimulability. Differential diagnosis, interpretation of inconsistency patterns, therapy planning, and so forth, are discussed in the manual. Unfortunately, norms for the scores on the Iowa Pressure Test of Articulation were derived from Templin's normal subjects. Therefore, interpretation of results must take this into consideration.

Summary

The Templin-Darley Tests of Articulation represent a practical, albeit traditional, measure that enjoys wide use by speech-language pathologists. The various subtests, especially the Iowa Pressure Test of Articulation, allow for the description of a child's misarticulation patterns. The test manual provides detailed guidance for administration, scoring, and interpretation of results. Advocates of articulation as expressions of phonological rules question the validity of the tests' rationale. However, keeping in mind the normative group description and the limitations relating to inattention to distinctive-feature analysis or phonotactic processes of early phonological development, the teacher/clinician may find these tests helpful in support of other evaluation and observation.

Test for Auditory Comprehension of Language

Description

The Test for Auditory Comprehension of Language (TACL) (Elizabeth Carrow, Teaching Resources Corporation, 5th ed., 1973) has the objective of providing a developmental level to describe a child's understanding of spoken language. Test items are derived from language categories that are divided into the following subscales: (1) form class and function words, (2) morphological constructions, (3) grammatical categories, and (4) syntactic structure. A screening version of the TACL, the Screening Test for Auditory Comprehension of Language (STACL) (Carrow, 1973a), is also available. Both the abridged and unabridged test forms are published in English and Spanish.

Technical Information

The standardization sample for the TACL was comprised of 200 middle-class Anglo-American, Mexican-American, and black children, aged 3 to

6. The age levels 3, 4, 5, and 6 years each contained 50 children. Given this limited population size and vaguely reported geographical distribution, the application of the normative data is restricted. The author also failed to report separate norms for boys and girls. Reliability data are available only for the 1971 and prior versions of the TACL. Test-retest reliability coefficients and intercorrelations were all deemed insignificant.

Test validities for the TACL are difficult to determine. Darley (1979) lists several studies that suggest that the TACL does distinguish between normal and language-deficient children. But item-selection criteria and the rationale for selection of specific syntactic constructions are deficient.

Administration and Scoring

The TACL consists of 101 plates, each displaying three line drawings. One drawing represents the referent for the linguistic form being tested, and the other two pictures denote referents for contrasting forms. Score sheets are separate. Stimulus items are administered orally by the examiner, and the child responds by pointing to the corresponding picture. Test items are arranged in order of grammatical levels.

Each response is scored as correct or incorrect. The total raw score can be converted into an age-score equivalent and a percentile rank. There is a section for the analysis of performance on specific item classes. However, no scoring device is provided to distinguish between lexical and grammatical errors in individual responses. The author does provide ages at which 75 and 90 percent of children pass each item.

Summary

Due to the numerous limitations of the TACL, it should be utilized only as an initial probe in assessment. The deficiencies that children exhibit on the test must be further explored in varied contexts, modes of presentation, meanings, and sentence length.

As with many tests of language comprehension, the construct validity of the TACL is questionable because of incomplete association of comprehension to production and the restrictions that the test format places on item selection. Many grammatical forms cannot be symbolized in pictures.

The TACL lacks broadly applicable normative data in terms of size of population, and it fails to include norms by sex. Interpretation of individual responses is complicated by variables, such as guessing rate, order effects, stimulus length, and method of stimulus presentation.

Utah Test of Language Development

Description

The Utah Test of Language Development (UTLD) (Merlin J. Mecham, J. Lorin Jex, and J. Dean Jones; Communication Research Associates, 1967) is designed to measure the expressive and receptive language skills of children between the ages of 1½ and 14½ years. It contains 51 items arranged in increasing difficulty by age levels. Each age level presents several "language" behaviors characteristic of that particular age in relation to normal development.

Technical Information

The normative data for the UTLD are questionable, due to the small size and limited geographical distribution of the sample. Split-half correlations and correlations of UTLD scores with scores on the informant interview edition of the test, the Verbal Language Development Scale, were used to establish an adequate reliability. The authors claim face validity for the instrument, since all items were selected from standardized sources. Other measures, however, are needed to support assumptions of validity.

Administration and Scoring

The 51 items on the UTLD are divided approximately equally into those that measure "sequential language ability" and "selective language ability." To administer the test, the examiner gives the child verbal instructions, involving the use of paper and pencil and six objects and various picture plates provided in the test kit. The examiner scores the child's responses as correct (+) or incorrect (−) on the score sheet. Ceilings and basals are outlined in the manual. The total raw score can be converted to language-age scores from 9 months to 16 years and to a language quotient. Standard scores and percentile equivalents are not possible to calculate, due to the small normative sample. The test administration is untimed and may vary with each child.

Summary

The examiner should be wary of using the UTLD as anything more than a general screening device. It is questionable whether many of its items actually test language abilities. Many of the items pertain to visual motor ability. Therefore, any child suspected of having visual or motor impairments should not be evaluated with this instrument, since limitations in these areas will be designated as language deficiency. Also, maximum interpretation of item responses is restricted because of the paucity of directions and insufficient space for verbatim responses on the score sheet.

Vane Evaluation of Language Scale

Description

The Vane Evaluation of Language Scale (Vane-L) (Julia R. Vane, Clinical Psychology Publishing Company, 1975) is a screening device for assessing the receptive language, expressive language, memory, and handedness of children aged 2½ to 6½ years.

Technical Information

The standardization population for the Vane-L consists of 470 children from New Jersey, New York, and Vermont. The sample adheres closely to the 1970 U.S. Census data in terms of age, sex, race, and parental occupation. There is a somewhat disproportionate number of urban children, however.

No reliability or validity measures are available to give the scale further credibility. According to Rosenbaum (1978), the Vane-L does not differentiate between children with respect to developmental rate, form, and content of language behavior.

Administration and Scoring

The Vane-L test is intended for administration by preschool and kindergarten teachers. It contains a receptive language scale and an expressive language scale, as well as a test of auditory and visual memory. The test items, chosen from a wide range of language constructions, were field-tested over a 4-year period in nursery schools, Head Start, day-care centers, kindergartens, and first grades. The author designed the stimulus sentences so that all elements, except the concepts being tested, are known to the child.

The receptive language scale, which is administered first, requires nonverbal responses. On the expressive language scale, the child must repeat sentences of increasing length and complexity and define vocabulary items. The child's speech is assessed as "good," "fair," or "poor"; and misarticulations are scored as "initial" and "other" sound substitutions. Auditory-memory items require the child to repeat a tapping sequence, while visual-memory items call for motor responses (block arrangements) and the designation of relative quantity (beans in transparent containers).

Scores on the three subtests have equivalent percentile ranks. If 75 percent of the time the child uses one hand to point to and manipulate objects in the test, the child is either "predominantly" right- or left-handed (75 to 95 percent) or "consistently" right- or left-handed (100 percent).

Summary

The Vane-L is an easily administered scale with fairly well-designed receptive items. Estimates of speech intelligibility according to the vague severity levels are likely to be subjective. Though items were field-tested, the scale lacks sufficient statistical data. Even as a screening device, the Vane-L may attempt to evaluate across too many categories. Caution should also be exercised with respect to examiner sophistication regarding language.

Verbal Language Development Scale

Description

The Verbal Language Development Scale (VLDS) (Merlin J. Mecham, American Guidance Service, 1971) utilizes an interview format to assess indirectly a child's language through an informant's knowledge of the child's language performance. The VLDS is suggested for use with children who are not responsive to direct testing methods.

Technical Information

The normative population consisted of 237 white, normal-speaking children from central and midnorthern Utah. The number of children in any age group was below 27. Ages ranged from 2 through 12 years. While 10 or fewer children were tested at ages 1, 13, and 14, no information on characteristics—that is, age, sex, socioeconomic status, or relationship of informant to the subject—was reported.

Reliability and validity studies on the VLDS are incomplete. Two studies of test-retest reliability are reported in the manual. In these studies, a "spot check" on 15 of the children from the original sample and on 28 mentally retarded children, correlation coefficients of .96 were derived. The author claims item and content validity for the instrument based on relatively small standard deviations in a study involving mentally retarded children.

Administration and Scoring

The VLDS consists of 50 items ranked in developmental order from infancy to 14 years of age. The examiner questions an individual who is familiar with the child regarding the extent to which the child exhibits each age-level communication skill. Items are scored as passed, emerging, or failed according to the informant's response to an item description. The majority of items are oriented toward speech skills; the remainder pertain to reading, writing, and listening abilities. No examiner training is necessary, and the test is not timed. The test manual provides a table for converting raw scores into language-age equivalent scores.

Summary

One of the major criticisms of the VLDS concerns the ambiguity of informant reporting and the three-level ranking system. Only a gross estimate of language development can be obtained with such variation in interviews and informant interpretation. As noted with some other instruments, it is also questionable whether items that address visual and/or auditory "skills" in the test measure language at all.

Washington Speech-Sound Discrimination Test

Description

The Washington Speech-Sound Discrimination Test (WSSDT) (Elizabeth M. Prather, Adah Miner, Margaret Anne Addicott, and Linda Sunderland; Interstate Printers and Publishers, 1971) was developed to assist in acquiring quick baseline appraisal of phoneme discrimination ability in children from ages 3 to "Kindergarten." It also aids in discernment of specific error types that are present. Additionally, the authors suggest the test can be used as a research tool.

Technical Information

Neither the validity nor the reliability of the WSSDT has been established. Validity is based on children's performances on the original 66 items. Of these items, 13 were discarded because three or fewer children made errors on them. The WSSDT was not compared to other speech sound discrimination tests for validity purposes. No data on test reliability are presented in the manual.

A description of the standardization population is not included in the test manual. Norms for each age group are based on small sample groups: 20 children for age 3½, 23 for age 4, 21 for age 4½, and 75 for kindergarteners for whom ages are not given. Norms are further limited by the overlapping of scores in the youngest three age groups.

Administration and Scoring

The WSSDT consists of 53 test items (18 presentations of five key words and 35 foils). The five key words (cup, fish, sun, crackers, toothbrush) are depicted on picture plates. The foils represent incorrect productions of the key words, varying in manner or place of articulation, voicing, or substitutions. The key words, randomly distributed among the foils, are separated by no more than three foils.

Before actual test administration, a teaching-testing procedure is followed to ensure that the child understands the listening task and that all five key words are in the child's receptive vocabulary. To administer the test, the examiner reads the key words and foils, having the child point to the picture only when the examiner says the key word. Neither same-different discrimination nor a verbal response is required of the child. The total number of correct responses is the raw score, which is compared to mean and standard deviations for age levels of 3½, 4, 4½, and kindergarten.

Summary

The WSSDT is not recommended for general use because of its serious limitations in standardization, validity, and reliability. While the pointing response may permit assessment of auditory discrimination of isolated words in nonverbal and language-limited children, it does not provide clues or the parameters that a child uses to judge the examiner's utterances. Haller (1972) indicates that some of the foil items represent dialectal pronunciations that may be identified as correct by the child.

REFERENCES

Anderson, R., Miles, M., & Matheny, P. *Communication evaluation chart from infancy to five years*. Cambridge, Mass.: Educators Publishing Service, 1963.

Arlt, P. E. *Illinois Children's Language Assessment Test*. Danville, Ill.: Interstate Printers and Publishers, 1977.

Arndt, W. B. A psychometric evaluation of the Northwestern Syntax Screening Test. *Journal of Speech and Hearing Disorders*, 1977, *42*, 316–319.

Baker, H. J., & Leland, B. *Detroit Tests of Learning Aptitude*. Indianapolis, Ind.: Bobbs-Merrill, 1967.

Bangs, T. E. *Language and learning disorders of the preacademic child*. New York: Appleton-Century-Croft, 1968.

Bankson, N. W. *Bankson Language Screening Test*. Baltimore, Md.: University Park Press, 1977.

Bates, E. *Languages and context: The acquisition of pragmatics*. New York: Academic Press, 1976.

Bayley, N. *The Bayley Scales of Infant Development*. New York: Psychological Corporation, 1969.

Berko, J. The child's learning of English morphology. *Ward*, 1958, *14*, 150–177.

Bloom, L. *Language development: Form and function in emerging grammars*. Cambridge, Mass.: MIT Press, 1970.

Bloom, L., & Lahey, M. *Language development and language disorders*. New York: John Wiley & Sons, 1978.

Boehm, A. *Boehm Test of Basic Concepts*. New York: Psychological Corporation, 1971.

Brown, R. *A first language*. Cambridge, Mass.: Harvard University Press, 1973.

Brown, R., & Bellugi, U. Three processes in the children's acquisition of syntax. *Harvard Educational Review*, 1964, *34*, 133–151.

Bruner, J. The ontogenesis of speech acts. *Journal of Child Language*, 1975, *2*, 1–19.

Bzoch, K. R., & League, R. *Receptive Expressive Emergent Language Scale*. Gainesville, Fla.: Tree of Life Press, 1971.

Carrow, E. *Screening Test for Auditory Comprehension of Language*. Boston, Mass.: Teaching Resources Corporation, 1973. (a)

Carrow, E. *Test for Auditory Comprehension of Language* (5th ed.). Boston, Mass.: Teaching Resources Corporation, 1973. (b)

Carrow, E. *Carrow Elicited Language Inventory*. Boston, Mass.: Teaching Resources Corporation, 1974.

Chomsky, N. *Syntactic structures*. The Hague: Mouton, 1957.

Chomsky, N. *Aspects of the theory of syntax*. Cambridge, Mass.: MIT Press, 1965.

Chomsky, N., & Halle, M. *The sound pattern of English*. New York: Harper & Row, 1968.

Crabtree, M. *Houston Test for Language Development* (Part I). Houston, Tex.: Houston Test Company, 1958.

Crabtree, M. *Houston Test for Language Development* (Part II). Houston, Tex.: Houston Test Company, 1963.

Daniloff, R. G. Normal articulation process. In F. D. Minifie, T. J. Nixon, & F. Williams (Eds.), *Normal aspects of speech, hearing, and language*, 1973.

Darley, F. L. *Evaluation of appraisal techniques in speech and language pathology*. Reading, Mass.: Addison-Wesley, 1979.

Darley, J. *Language Facility Test*. Alexandria, Va.: Allington Corporation, 1977.

Doll, E. A. *Preschool attainment record*. Minneapolis, Minn.: American Guidance Service, 1966.

Dore, J. A pragmatic description of early language development. *Journal of Psycholinguistic Research*, 1974, *3*, 343–350.

Drumwright, A. F. *Denver Articulation Screening Examination*. Denver: University of Colorado Medical Center, Ladoca Project and Publishing Foundation, 1971.

Englemann, S. *Basic Concept Inventory* (Field research ed.). Chicago, Ill.: Follett Educational Corporation, 1967.

Ervin, S. Imitation and structural change in children's language. In E. Lenneberg (Ed.), *New direction in the study of language*. Cambridge, Mass.: MIT Press, 1964.

Fillmore, C. The case for case. In E. Bach & R. Horms (Eds.), *Universals in linguistic theory*. New York: Holt, Rinehart, and Winston, 1968.

Fisher, H. A., & Logemann, J. A. *Fisher-Logemann Test of Articulation Competence*. Boston: Houghton Mifflin, 1971.

Foster, R., Gidden, J. J., & Stark, J. *Assessment of children's language comprehension.* Palo Alto, Calif.: Consulting Psychologists Press, 1973.

Fraser, E., Bellugi, U., & Brown, R. Control of grammar in imitation, comprehension, and production. *Journal of Verbal Learning and Verbal Behavior,* 1963, *2,* 121–135.

Fries, C. C. *The structure of English.* New York: Harcourt Brace, 1952.

Gesell, A. *The first five years of life.* New York: Harper & Row, 1940.

Gesell, A. *Developmental Schedules.* New York: Psychological Corporation, 1956.

Goldman, R., Fristoe, M., & Woodcock, R. W. *Technical manual for Goldman-Fristoe-Woodcock Auditory Skills Test Battery.* Circle Pines, Minn.: American Guidance Service, 1974.

Greenfield, E., & Smith, H. *The structure of communication in early language development.* New York: Academic Press, 1976.

Haller, R. M. A review of the Washington Speech Sound Discrimination Test. In O. K. Buros (Ed.), *The eighth mental measurements yearbook* (Vol. 2). Highland Park, N.J.: Gryphon Press, 1972.

Halliday, M. *Learning how to mean.* New York: Elsevier, 1977.

Hammill, D., & Larsen, S. The effectiveness of psycholinguistic training. *Exceptional Children,* 1974, *41,* 5–14.

Hannah, E. *Applied Linguistic Analysis II.* Pacific Palisades, Calif.: Sencom, 1979.

Hannah, E., & Gardner, M. *Preschool Language Screening Test.* Northridge, Calif.: Joyce Publications, 1974.

Hargis, C. *English syntax.* Springfield, Ill.: Charles C Thomas, 1977.

Hedrick, D., Prather, E., & Tobin, A. *Sequenced Inventory of Communication Development (SICD).* Seattle: University of Washington Press, 1975.

Hejna, R. F. *Developmental Articulation Test.* Ann Arbor, Mich.: Speech Materials, 1968.

Horstmeier, D., & MacDonald, J. D. *Environmental Pre-Language Battery.* Columbus, Ohio: Charles E. Merrill, 1978.

Jordan, E. P. Articulation test measures and listener ratings of articulation defectiveness. *Journal of Speech and Hearing Research,* 1960, *3,* 303–313.

Kirk, S. A., & Kirk, W. D. *Psycholinguistic learning disabilities: Diagnosis and remediation.* Urbana: University of Illinois Press, 1971.

Kirk, S., McCarthy, J., & Kirk, W. *Illinois Test of Psycholinguistic Abilities* (Rev. ed.). Urbana: University of Illinois Press, 1968.

Kretschmer, R., & Kretschmer, L. *Language development and intervention with the hearing impaired.* Baltimore, Md.: University Park Press, 1978.

Larson, G. W., & Summers, P. A. Response patterns of pre-school age children to the Northwestern Syntax Screening Test. *Journal of Speech and Hearing Disorders,* 1976, *40,* 486–497.

Lee, L. *Northwestern Syntax Screening Test.* Evanston, Ill.: Northwestern University Press, 1969.

Lee, L. *Northwestern Syntax Screening Test.* Evanston, Ill.: Northwestern University Press, 1971.

Lee, L. *Developmental Sentence Analyses.* Evanston, Ill.: Northwestern University Press, 1974.

Lee, L., & Canter, S. Developmental sentence scoring: A clinical procedure for estimating syntactic development in children's spontaneous speech. *Journal of Speech and Hearing Disorders,* 1971, *36,* 315–340.

Lerea, L. Assessing language development. *Journal of Speech and Hearing Research,* 1958, *1,* 75–85.

Ling, D. *Speech and the hearing impaired.* Washington, D.C.: A. G. Bell Association for the Deaf, 1976.

Locke, J. L. Review of Auditory Discrimination Test. In F. L. Darley (Ed.), *Evaluation of appraisal techniques in speech and language pathology.* Reading, Mass.: Addison-Wesley, 1979.

MacDonald, J. D., & Blott, J. P. *Environmental Language Inventory.* Columbus, Ohio: Charles E. Merrill, 1978.

McCandless, G. A review of the Boehm Test of Basic Concepts. In O. K. Buros (Ed.), *The seventh mental measurements yearbook.* Highland Park, N.J.: Gryphon Press, 1972.

McCarthy, D. *The McCarthy Scales of Children's Abilities.* New York: Psychological Corporation, 1972.

McDonald, E. T. *Deep Test of Articulation: Picture Form.* Pittsburgh, Pa.: Stanwix House, 1964.

McLean, J. E. Review of the Sequenced Inventory of Communication Development. In F. L. Darley (Ed.), *Evaluation of appraisal techniques in speech and language pathology.* Reading, Mass.: Addison-Wesley, 1979.

Mecham, M. J. *Verbal Language Development Scale.* Circle Pines, Minn.: American Guidance Service, 1958.

Mecham, M. J. *Verbal Language Development Scale, Revised Edition.* Circle Pines, Minn.: American Guidance Service, 1971.

Mecham, M. J., Jex, J. L., & Jones, J. D. *The Utah Test of Language Development.* Salt Lake City, Utah: Communication Research Associates, 1967.

Menyuk, P. Comparison of grammar of children with functionally deviant and normal speech. *Journal of Speech and Hearing Research,* 1964, *7,* 109–121.

Menyuk, P. A preliminary evaluation of grammatical complexity in children. *Journal of Verbal Learning Behavior,* 1963, *2,* 429–439.

Menyuk, P. *Sentences children use.* Cambridge, Mass.: MIT Press, 1969.

Moog, J. S., & Geers, A. V. *Scales of Early Communication Skills for Hearing Impaired Children.* St. Louis, Mo.: Central Institute for the Deaf, 1975.

Muma, J. R. *Language handbook, concepts, assessment, intervention.* Englewood Cliffs, N.J.: Prentice Hall, 1978.

Newcomer, P. L., & Hammill, D. D. *The Test of Language Development.* Austin, Tex.: Empiric Press, 1977.

Noll, V. H. A review of the Boehm Test of Basic Concepts. *Journal of Educational Measurement,* 1970, *7,* 139–140.

Paraskeropoulous, J. N., & Kirk, S. A. *The development and psychometric characteristics of the revised Illinois Test of Psycholinguistic Abilities.* Urbana: University of Illinois Press, 1969.

Pendergast, K., Dickey, S. E., Selmac, J. W., & Soder, A. L. *Photo Articulation Test.* Danville, Ill.: Interstate Printers and Publishers, 1969.

Piaget, J. *The language and thought of the child.* New York: Harcourt, Brace, Jovanovich, 1926.

Piaget, J. *The origin of intelligence in children.* New York: Norton & Company, 1952.

Porch, B. E. *Porch Index of Communicative Ability in Children.* Palo Alto, Calif.: Consulting Psychologists Press, 1975.

Prather, E. M., Miner, A., Addicott, M. A., & Sunderland, L. *Washington Speech Sound Discrimination Test.* Danville, Ill.: Interstate Printers and Publishers, 1971.

Prutting, C. A., Gallagher, T. M., & Mulac, A. The expressive portion of the NSST compared to a spontaneous language sample. *Journal of Speech and Hearing Disorders,* 1975, *40,* 40–48.

Reynell, J., & Huntley, R. New scales for the assessment of language development in young children. *Journal of Learning Disabilities,* 1979, *4,* 10–18.

Rieke, J., Lynch, L., & Soltmon, S. *Teaching strategies for language development.* New York: Grune and Stratton, 1977.

Rosenbaum, R. L. A review of the Vane Evaluation of Language Scale. In O. K. Buros (Ed.), *The eighth mental measurements yearbook* (Vol. 2). Highland Park, N.J.: Gryphon Press, 1978.

Russell, W., Quigley, S., & Power, D. *Linguistics and deaf children.* Washington, D.C.: A. G. Bell Association for the Deaf, 1976.

Salvia, J., & Ysseldyke, J. E. *Assessment in special and remedial education.* Boston, Mass.: Houghton Mifflin, 1978.

Scroggs, C. Analyzing the language of hearing impaired children with severe language acquisition problems. *American Annals of the Deaf,* 1977, *122,* 403–406.

Sheridan, M. D. *Stycar Language Test.* Windsor Berks, England: NFER Publishing Company, 1976.

Sinclair, S., Khan, L., & Saxman, J. *Do differing test conditions predict equivalent language ages?* Paper presented at Boston University Conference on Language Development, Boston, Mass., 1977.

Skarakis, E., & Prutting, C. Early communication: Semantic functions and communicative intentions in the communication of preschool children with impaired hearing. *American Annals of the Deaf,* 1977, *122,* 382–391.

Smith, F., & Miller, G. A. (Eds.). *The genesis of language: A psycholinguistic approach.* Cambridge, Mass.: MIT Press, 1966.

Snow, K. A detailed analysis of articulation responses of "normal" first grade children. *Journal of Speech and Hearing Research,* 1963, *6,* 277–290.

Templin, M. D., & Darley, F. L. *Templin-Darley Tests of Articulation* (2nd ed.) Iowa City, Iowa: University of Iowa Bureau of Educational Research and Service, 1969.

Terman, L., & Merrill, M. *Stanford Binet Intelligence Scale* (1972 norms ed.). Boston, Mass.: Houghton Mifflin, 1973.

Toronto, A. S., Leverman, C., Hanna, C., Rosengweis, P., & Maldonado, A. *Del Rio Language Screening Test, English/Spanish.* Austin, Tex.: National Educational Laboratory Publishers, 1975.

Tyack, D., & Gottsleben, R. *Language sampling, analysis and training: A handbook for teachers and clinicians.* Palo Alto, Calif.: Consulting Psychologists Press, 1974.

Van Demark, D. R., Kuehn, D. P., & Thorp, R. F. Prediction of velopharyngeal competence. *Cleft Palate Journal,* 1975, *12,* 5–11.

Vane, J. R. *Vane Evaluation of Language Scale.* Brunelon, Vt.: Clinical Psychology Publishing Company, 1975.

Vygotsky, L. *Thought and language,* Cambridge, Mass.: MIT Press, 1962.

Wechsler, D. *Wechsler Preschool and Primary Scale of Intelligence.* New York: Psychological Corporation, 1967.

Wepman, J. *Auditory Discrimination Test.* Chicago: Language Research Association, 1973.

Wolski, W. *Language development of normal children, four, five and six years of age, as measured by the Michigan Picture Language Inventory*. Doctoral dissertation, University of Michigan, 1962.

Wolski, W., & Lerea, L. *Michigan Picture Language Inventory*. Ann Arbor: University of Michigan, Department of Communication Disorders, 1962.

Zachman, L., Huisingh, R., Jorgensen, C., & Barrett, M. *The Oral Language Sentence Imitation Screening Test*. Moline, Ill.: Lingui Systems, 1976.

Zachman, L., Huisingh, R., Jorgensen, C., & Barrett, M. *The Oral Language Sentence Imitation Diagnostic Inventory*. Moline, Ill.: Lingui Systems, 1977.

Zimmerman, I. L., Steiner, V. G., & Evatt, R. *Preschool Language Scale*. Columbus, Ohio: Charles E. Merrill, 1969.

Zimmerman, I. L., Steiner, V. G., & Evatt, R. *Preschool Language Scale* (Rev. ed.). Columbus, Ohio: Charles E. Merrill, 1979.

SUGGESTED READINGS

Darley, F. L. *Evaluation of appraisal techniques in speech and language pathology*. Reading, Mass.: Addison-Wesley, 1979.

Schiefelbusch, R. L., & Lloyd, L. L. *Language perspectives—acquisition, retardation, and intervention* (4th ed.). Baltimore, Md.: University Park Press, 1978.

Chapter 6

Bare Essentials in Assessing Really Little Kids (BEAR): An Approach

M. Suzanne Hasenstab and Joan Laughton

In Chapter 5, various evaluative instruments were presented and briefly described as to their use with young hearing-impaired and language-delayed children. The purpose of the present chapter is to present an approach or process that is used in the Comprehensive Services Program. This process is comprised of two primary components: a testing kit for the purpose of evaluating conceptual understanding and a language sample analysis technique that examines the child's linguistic behavior.

The evaluation of language in the very young child requires an alternative to traditional standardized instruments. Bear Essentials in Assessing Really Little Kids (BEAR) represents such an attempt. The purpose of the BEAR process of evaluating language in young children is to allow for in-depth determination of a child's language problem once a delay has been noted. The need for this is obvious, based on the growing awareness and identification of infants and preschool children who exhibit language delay. Identification represents the first step in the intervention chain. This must be followed by accurate and appropriate assessment that will provide a foundation for educational programming.

GENERAL DESCRIPTION OF BEAR

BEAR in its entirety represents the core of the third component of assessment, language evaluation. It contains four individual language evaluation processes that may be used either singularly or in support of one another:

1. concept analysis profile summary (BEAR CAPS)
2. syntactic/morphological analysis profile summary
3. phonological analysis profile summary
4. semantic/pragmatic analysis profile summary

The last three aspects make up BEAR. The first is referred to as BEAR-CAPS.

CONCEPT ANALYSIS PROFILE SUMMARY

The first component, CAPS, does not require verbalization on the part of the child. It is designed to evaluate conceptual understanding of relationships that usually appear in language development between the ages of 18 months and 5 years. CAPS is the "kit" part of the language package. It contains simple and attractive materials that are manipulated by the child according to instructions of the examiner. A score/summary sheet is used to record the child's performance on each item. The information that CAPS yields is used to develop instructional objectives in program planning for the child.

Concepts represent commonality among groups of symbols that stand for objects or events within our experience. They represent the content of language or what is understood about the world about us. Concepts allow us to handle large amounts of information efficiently.

Language and cognition, although not synonymous, are based in concept development. Concepts are coded in language, and language can provide a measure of a child's understanding of concepts. Words, which are symbols, represent a concept's meanings which develop and elaborate over a child's infancy and preschool years.

Concept acquisition is necessary because conceptual relationships must be mastered before the child can use these relationships in language (Ault, 1977). Bloom and Lahey (1978) indicate that conceptual development is needed in order for form, the dictionary of sounds and words and their corresponding governing rules, and use, the function of language, also to develop. If concept development is weak, there is an effect on all components of language. If a child demonstrates language delay, a logical starting point in evaluation is to determine what concepts are understood. Concept growth is developmental. In other words, children normally comprehend certain relationships and their representative words at certain ages, as understanding matures toward adult meaning. Therefore, based on normal age ranges of concept development, we can determine delay in concept understanding of children with language problems. Language programming based on concept development can then be implemented.

Although most of the tests described in Chapter 5 contain items that are related to the understanding of particular concepts, this aspect is part of an overall language investigation. The items do not examine concepts in depth, nor do they provide a basis for program development. There are tests designed to evaluate specifically conceptual understanding, for example, the Vocabulary Comprehension Scale (Bangs, 1975), the Boehm Test of Basic Concepts (Boehm, 1971), the Conceptual Sorting Test (Kagan, Rosman, Day, Albert, & Phillips, 1964), and the Basic Concept Inventory (Englemann, 1967). However, these tests are designed to be used with children with normal or minimal language delay or with children of school age (5 years and older) and are therefore not appropriate for the population addressed in this text.

Indeed, it would be impossible to design an instrument to evaluate all of the possible concepts a child could develop during the preschool years. Exact repertoires will vary with each child depending on a multitude of variables in environmental experiences. Therefore, while CAPS cannot evaluate all possible concepts, it does present a select group of concepts that are within the range of common experiences of preschool children, both normal and with language and hearing impairment.

Concepts can be divided into categories: position/location, quantity, quality, size, pronouns, and body parts. Concepts in each category, the normal age range of comprehension, and the relevant materials in CAPS are shown in Table 6–1.

The general procedure in administering CAPS is indicated by the following seven points:

1. In each category of concepts, the examiner presents only those items that are to be used for the particular concept being evaluated.
2. Unless otherwise designated by the directions, the materials are placed in front of the child in a neutral position.
3. The examiner directs the child to perform the appropriate manipulation for the specific concept, for example, "Put the button in the box." The verbal instructions are precise and simple.
4. The child receives three trials, directions for each one becoming more simple. The directions may be given in sign language or cued speech. For example, "Put the button in the box." The examiner points to the button. "Put in." The examiner holds up the button and hands it to the child. "In."
5. The child performs the activity. (The tasks do not require that the child interact verbally; there are no verbal response requirements, but rather nonverbal solutions.)
6. The examiner scores appropriately on the score sheet.
7. The examiner proceeds to the next concept until all are completed or the child misses three out of five concepts (concept-tasks).

The score sheet/summary profile is arranged in developmental sequence for each concept area evaluated. The age norms for concept comprehen-

Table 6–1 CAPS Concepts

Concept	*Normal Age Range of Comprehension*	*Materials*
Position/Location		
in	2 to 2½	one round button and one plastic box (1″ × 3″)
off	2 to 2½	same
on	2½ to 3	same
under	2½ to 3	same
out	2½ to 3	same
together	2½ to 3	plastic egg
away	2½ to 3	plastic box and small car (approx. 3″)
up	3 to 3½	any item in this category
top	3 to 3½	plastic box with lid
apart	3 to 3½	two small cars
open	3 to 3½	plastic egg plastic box with lid
toward	3 to 3½	small car
around	3½ to 4	small car and plastic box
in front	3½ to 4	small stuffed animal
high	3½ to 4	any item in this category
beside	4 to 4½	small stuffed animal
bottom	4 to 4½	plastic box
backward	4 to 4½	small car
forward	4 to 4½	small car
down	4½ to 5	any item in this category
low	4½ to 5	any item in this category
through	4 to 4½	plastic ring and string
behind	5 to 5½	small stuffed animal
first	5 to 5½	three small cars
last	5 to 5½	three small cars
between	5 to 5½	small cars and stuffed animal
over	5 to 5½	small stuffed animal and plastic box
Quantity		
one	2 to 2½	The materials for this category are wooden beads and two plastic boxes (4″ × 4″)
more	2½ to 3	
all	2½ to 3	
empty	3 to 3½	
full	3½ to 4	

Note: Quantity concepts 2 through 5 are normally comprehended at one quantitative set below age, i.e., a 3-year-old normally understands the quantitative concepts indicated for up to 2 years of age.

Table 6–1 continued

Concept	*Normal Age Range of Comprehension*	*Materials*
less	3 to 4½	
each	4 to 4½	
some	3 to 3½	
Quality		
soft	2½ to 3	a foam rubber ball
heavy	2½ to 3	a 3″ square beanbag stuffed with dry beans
same	3 to 3½	2 identical stuffed animals; 1 different stuffed animal
different	4½ to 5	2 identical stuffed animals; 1 different stuffed animal
light	3½ to 4	a 3″ square beanbag stuffed with foam
rough	4 to 4½	4″ circle, sandpaper
smooth	4 to 4½	4″ circle, smooth paper
Size		
big	2½ to 3½	two identical stuffed animals, one measuring 4″ × 4″, the other 2½″ × 2½″
tall	2½ to 3	mounted photograph of a tall animal standing beside a short animal
little	3½ to 4	same as for big
long	3½ to 4	30″ ribbon
short	4 to 4½	same as for tall
fat	4 to 4½	dowel rods 4″ in length, ⅜″ diameter and 1½″ diameter
thin	4½ to 5	same as for fat
Pronouns		
Subjective pronouns:		Materials for this category consist of a four-piece picnic set with four cups, four dishes, four forks, four spoons, and four
I	2 to 2½	
you (sing.)	3 to 3½	
he	2½ to 3	
she	2½ to 3	
it	3 to 3½	

Table 6–1 continued

Concept	*Normal Age Range of Comprehension*	*Materials*
they	3 to 3½	knives; a boy doll and a girl doll appropriate to the color/race of the child; a stuffed puppy; and a large napkin. The examiner and child set up a picnic.
we	4½ to 5	
Objective pronouns:		
me	2½ to 3	
him	2½ to 3	
her	2½ to 3	
you	3 to 3½	
us	3½ to 4	
them	3½ to 4	
Possessive pronouns:		
my	2 to 2½	
mine	2 to 2½	
your	2 to 2½	
Body Parts		
eyes	18 mos. to 2 years	A mirror is the only material needed for this category.
nose	18 mos. to 2 years	
hair	2 to 2½	
mouth	2 to 2½	
ears	2 to 2½	
hands	2 to 2½	
feet	2 to 2½	
stomach or tummy	2 to 2½	
head	3 to 3½	
arm	3 to 3½	
leg	3 to 3½	
knee	3½ to 4	
elbow	3½ to 4	
chin	4½ to 5	
eyebrow	4½ to 5	

sion were taken from various references. The test itself has not been normed. The developmental ages are to serve as a reference point both for the usual sequence in which children comprehend various concepts and for the extent of delay in the language growth of an individual child with respect to various concept areas.

Since one major purpose of the test is to develop a base for appropriate programming, scoring and summaries are criterion- or communication-referenced descriptions. Bloom and Lahey (1978) suggest that, although norm-referenced descriptions can assist in the determination of a concept (or content) problem in language, criterion- or communication-referenced descriptions in content assessment are best for programming or remediation. The purpose of criterion- or communication-referenced measures is to provide information about behaviors relative to certain goals or tasks. These measures are especially helpful in reassessing progress and determining program effectiveness.

The CAPS score sheet presents the concepts by categories, beginning with those that are comprehended earliest and progressing through the more difficult ones. The examiner checks as to whether the child completes the required task on the first, second, or third trial or indicates no response. The first trial presents the concept within the context of a meaningful sentence. The second trial simplifies the sentence to a short two- or three-word phrase and adds a visual clue. The third trial presents the concept word in isolation accompanied by a more concrete visual clue. The complete CAPS score/summary form is presented in Exhibit 6–1.

LANGUAGE SAMPLE ANALYSIS

Rather than observe language acquisition by expectations based on chronological age, it is more meaningful to look at where an individual child falls on a continuum of language development. Children acquiring language typically develop through a sequence beginning with preverbal behaviors and moving on through one-word, two-word, three-word, and finally four-word utterances. The final stages of language development involve the refinement and expansion of earlier stages, adding length and complexity to linguistic ability. In assessing this progression of language development, observation becomes the primary source of evaluative information. The observation includes both spontaneous and elicited utterances that a child produces in various settings.

This process of observing, recording, and analyzing language behaviors of young children constitutes the approach of BEAR. At whatever point along the continuum a child demonstrates the behaviors, valuable information can be derived through language samples to facilitate programming.

Exhibit 6–1 BEAR-CAPS Scoring/Summary Form

BARE ESSENTIALS IN ASSESSING REALLY LITTLE KIDS (BEAR)

CONCEPT ANALYSIS PROFILE SUMMARY (CAPS)

Name: ________ D.O.B. ________ Date Eval: ________

Address: ________ Age: ________ Sex: ________

________ Phone: ________ Disability: ________

Parents: ________ Examiner: ________ ________

Referred by: ________ Informant: ________ Communication Mode: ________

POSITION/LOCATION

Materials	Concept	Verbal Directive	Response Level	Comment
button/box—set button next to box	in	1. Put the button in the box.	____	
		2. Put in. (Touch button)	____	
		3. In. (Give button to child)	____	
box with top in place	off	1. Take the top off the box.	____	
		2. Take off. (Touch top)	____	
		3. Off. (Give box to child)	____	
box with top removed and set next to box	on	1. Put the top on the box.	____	
		2. Put on. (Touch top)	____	
		3. On. (Give top to child)	____	
button/box—set button next to box	under	1. Put the button under the box.	____	
		2. Put under. (Touch button)	____	
		3. Under. (Give button to child)	____	
button/box—button inside box	out	1. Take the button out of the box.	____	
		2. Take out. (Touch box)	____	
		3. Out. (Point to button inside)	____	
egg halves—next to each other	together	1. Put the egg together.	____	
		2. Put together. (Point to halves)	____	
		3. Together. (Give halves to child)	____	
car-near child—in front position	away	1. Push the car away from you.	____	
		2. Push away. (Push car slightly)		
		3. Away. (Put child's hand on car)	____	
puppy (or any item)	up	1. Put the puppy up.	____	
		2. Put up. (Touch the puppy)	____	
		3. Up. (Give puppy to child)	____	

Exhibit 6–1 continued

Materials	Concept	Verbal Directive	Response Level	Comment
box with top in place	top	1. Show me the top of the box. 2. Show top. (Touch box) 3. Top. (Give box to child)	_____ _____ _____	
egg halves together	apart	1. Take the egg apart. 2. Take apart. (Touch egg) 3. Apart. (Give egg to child)	_____ _____ _____	
box with top in place	open	1. Open the box. 2. Open. (Touch box) 3. Open. (Give box to child)	_____ _____ _____	
car at one end of table—puppy at other	toward	1. Push the car toward the puppy. 2. Push toward. (Point to the car and puppy) 3. Toward (Place child's hand on car)	_____ _____ _____	
box with top removed	close	1. Close the box. 2. Close (Touch box and top) 3. Close. (Give child top of box)	_____ _____ _____	
car next to box	around	1. Push the car around the box. 2. Push around. (Touch the car) 3. Around. (Put child's hand on the car)	_____ _____ _____	
puppy (or any item) off to side from child	in front	1. Put the puppy in front of you. 2. Put in front. (Touch puppy) 3. In front (Give puppy to child)	_____ _____ _____	
puppy (or any item)	high	1. Put the puppy high. 2. Put high.)touch puppy) 3. High. (Give puppy to child)	_____ _____ _____	
puppy (or any item)	beside	1. Put the puppy beside*you.* 2. Put beside (Touch puppy) 3. Beside. (Give puppy to child)	_____ _____ _____	
box with top in place	bottom	1. Show me the bottom of the box. 2. Show bottom. (Touch box) 3. Bottom. (Give box to child)	_____ _____ _____	
car facing left/right	backward	1. Push the car backward. 2. Push backward. (Touch car) 3. Backward. (Put child's hand on car)	_____ _____ _____	
puppy (or any item)	down	1. Put the puppy down. 2. Put down. (Touch puppy) 3. Down. (Give puppy to child)	_____ _____ _____	
car facing left/right	forward	1. Push the car forward. 2. Push forward. (Touch car) 3. Forward. (Put child's hand on car)	_____ _____ _____	
puppy (or any item)	low	1. Put the puppy low. 2. Put low. (Touch puppy) 3. Low. (Give puppy to child)	_____ _____ _____	
large bead and string	through	1. Put the string through the hole/bead. 2. Put through. (Touch string) 3. Through. (Give string to child)	_____ _____ _____	
puppy (or any item)	behind	1. Put the puppy behind you. 2. Put behind. (Touch puppy) 3. Behind. (Give puppy to child)	_____ _____ _____	
3 cars all facing same direction left/right	first	1. Show me the first car. 2. The first car. 3. First.	_____ _____ _____	

Exhibit 6–1 continued

Materials	Concept	Verbal Directive	Response Level	Comment
3 cars all facing same direction left/right	last	1. Show me the last car. 2. The last car. 3. Last.	_____ _____ _____	
2 cars/ 1 puppy	between	1. Put the puppy between the cars. 2. Put between. (Touch puppy) 3. Between. (Give puppy to child)	_____ _____ _____	
puppy/box	over	1. Put the puppy over the box. 2. Put over. (Touch puppy) 3. Over. (Give puppy to child)	_____ _____ _____	
QUANTITY				
box of beads	one	1. Give me one bead. 2. Give one. (Point to beads in box) 3. One. (Hold out hand)	_____ _____ _____	
2 boxes of beads—one with noticeably more than the other	more	1. Show me more beads. 2. More beads. (Point to beads in boxes) 3. More. (Point to beads in boxes)	_____ _____ _____	
beads on table beside box	all	1. Put all the beads in the box. 2. Put all in. (Touch beads) 3. All. (Point to all beads and box)	_____ _____ _____	
1 full box of beads	empty	1. Show me the empty box. 2. The empty box. (Touch boxes) 3. Empty. (Touch boxes)	_____ _____ _____	
2 boxes of beads—one with noticeably less than the other	less	1. Show me less beads. 2. Less beads. (Point to beads in boxes) 3. Less. (Point to beads in boxes)	_____ _____ _____	
1 full box of beads 1 empty box	full	1. Show me the full box. 2. The full box. (Touch boxes) 3. Full. (Touch boxes)	_____ _____ _____	
2 boxes and 2 beads set away from boxes	each	1. Put a bead in each box. 2. Put in each box. (Touch the beads) 3. Each. (Give beads to the child, point to boxes)	_____ _____ _____	
Box of beads	some	1. Give me some beads. 2. Give me some. (Hold out hand) 3. Some. (Hold out hand)	_____ _____ _____	

Note: Number concepts 2 through 5 are normally comprehended one quantitative set above chronological age. (A three-year-old normally understands the quantitative concepts up to 4)

Materials	Concept	Verbal Directive	Response Level	Comment
beads in box	two	1. Give me 2 beads. 2. Give 2. (Point to beads in box) 3. 2. (Hold out hand)	_____ _____ _____	
beads in box	three	1. Give me 3 beads. 2. Give 3. (Point to beads) 3. 2. (Hold out hand)	_____ _____ _____	
beads in box	four	1. Give me 4 beads. 2. Give 4. (Point to beads) 3. 4 (Hold out hand)	_____ _____ _____	
beads in box	five	1. Give me 5 beads. 2. Give 5. (Point to beads) 3. 5. (Hold out hand)	_____ _____ _____	

Exhibit 6–1 continued

QUALITY:

Materials	Concept	Verbal Directive	Response Level	Comment
2 balls (soft/hard)	soft	1. Give me the soft ball	______	
		2. The soft ball. (Place one in each of child's hands)	______	
		3. Soft. (Hold out hand)	______	
2 beanbags (heavy/light)	heavy	1. Give me the heavy bag.	______	
		2. The heavy bag. (Place one in each of child's hands)	______	
		3. Heavy. (Hold out hand)	______	
2 like animals 1 different animal	same	1. Show me the same animals.	______	
		2. The same animals. (Touch each animal)	______	
		3. Same. (Hold out hand)	______	
2 balls (hard/soft)	hard	1. Give me the hard ball.	______	
		2. The hard ball. (Place one in each of child's hands)	______	
		3. Hard. (Hold out hand)	______	
2 beanbags (heavy/light)	light	1. Give me the light bag.	______	
		2. The light bag. (Place one in each of child's hands)	______	
		3. Light. (hold out hand)	______	
2 dowel rods (fat/thin)	fat	1. Show me the fat one.	______	
		2. Show me fat. (Touch each dowel)	______	
		3. Fat. (Hold out hand)	______	
2 circles (smooth/rough)	smooth	1. Show me the smooth one.	______	
		2. Show me smooth. (Place one in each of child's hands)	______	
		3. Smooth. (Hold out hand)	______	
2 like animals 1 different animal	different	1. Show me the different animal.	______	
		2. Show me different. (Touch each animal)	______	
		3. Different. (Hold out hand)	______	
2 circles (smooth/rough)	rough	1. Show me the rough one.	______	
		2. Show me rough. (Place one in each of child's hands)	______	
		3. Rough. (Hold out hand)	______	
2 dowel rods (fat/thin)	thin	1. Show me the thin one.	______	
		2. Show me thin. (Touch each dowel)	______	
		3. Thin. (Hold out hand)	______	

SIZE:

Materials	Concept	Verbal Directive	Response Level	Comment
2 animals (big/little)	big	1. Show me the big dog.	______	
		2. Show me big. (Touch each dog)	______	
		3. Big. (Trace circumference of each dog)	______	
picture— tall and short people	tall	1. Show me the tall person.	______	
		2. Show me tall. (Point to people in picture)	______	
		3. Tall. (Trace height of each person)	______	
2 ribbons (long/short)	long	1. Show me the long ribbon.	______	
		2. Show me long. (Touch each ribbon)	______	
		3. Long. (Trace length of each ribbon)	______	

Exhibit 6–1 continued

Materials	Concept	Verbal Directive	Response Level	Comment
2 animals (big/little)	little	1. Show me the little dog.	______	
		2. Show me little. (Touch each dog)	______	
		3. Little. (Trace circumference of each dog)	______	
2 ribbons (long/short)	short	1. Show me the short ribbon.	______	
		2. Show me short. (Touch each ribbon)	______	
		3. Short. (Trace length of each ribbon)	______	

PRONOUNS: The words *milk* or *juice* may substitute for *tea*

Materials	Concept	Verbal Directive	Response Level	Comment
cups	me	1. Give me a cup.	______	
		2. Give me a cup. (Point to cups)	______	
		3. Give me a cup. (Give cup to child)	______	
cups	him	1. Give him a cup.	______	
		2. Give him a cup. (Point to cups)	______	
		3. Give him a cup. (Give cup to child)	______	
cups	her	1. Give her a cup.	______	
		2. Give her a cup. (Point to cups)	______	
		3. Give her a cup. (Give cup to child)	______	
teapot	my	1. Put tea in my cup.	______	
		2. Put tea in my cup. (Point to teapot)	______	
		3. Put tea in my cup. (Give child teapot)	______	
spoons	mine	1. Put a spoon in mine.	______	
		2. Put a spoon in mine. (Point to spoon)	______	
		3. Put a spoon in mine. (Give spoon to child)	______	
teapot Give child a cup	your	1. Put tea in your cup.	______	
		2. Put tea in your cup. (Point to teapot)	______	
		3. Put tea in your cup. (Give teapot to child)	______	
dishes	I	1. I want a dish.	______	
		2. I want a dish. (Point to dish)	______	
		3. I want a dish. (Give dish to child)	______	
dishes	he	1. He wants a dish.	______	
		2. He wants a dish. (Point to dish)	______	
		3. He wants a dish. (Give dish to child)	______	
dishes	she	1. She wants a dish.	______	
		2. She wants a dish. Point to dish)	______	
		3. She wants a dish. (Give dish to child)	______	
dishes	you (subj.)	1. You want a dish.	______	
		2. You want a dish. (Point to dish)	______	
		3. You want a dish. (Give dish to child)	______	
spoon	you (obj)	1. Give you a spoon.	______	
		2. Give you a spoon. (Point to spoon)	______	
		3. Give you a spoon. (Give spoon to child)	______	
dog dish	it	1. It wants a dish.	______	
		2. It wants a dish. (Point to dish)	______	
		3. It wants a dish. (Give dish to child)	______	
spoons	they	1. They want spoons.	______	
		2. They want spoons. (Point to spoons)	______	
		3. They want spoons. (Give spoons to child)	______	
teapot	them	1. Give them tea.	______	
		2. Give them tea. (Point to teapot)	______	
		3. Give them tea. (Give teapot to child)	______	

Exhibit 6–1 continued

Materials	Concept	Verbal Directive	Response Level	Comment
napkins	us	1. Give us napkins.	______	
		2. Give us napkins. (Point to napkins)	______	
		3. Give us napkins. (Give napkins to child)	______	
forks	we	1. We want forks.	______	
		2. We want forks. (Point to forks)	______	
		3. We want forks. (Give forks to child)	______	
you- obj pl you- sub pl	These forms are not usually mastered by preschool children and are therefore not included.			

BODY PARTS:

A large mirror may be used.

* If child responds at level 2 by pointing to Examiner indicate you want him to point to his eyes.

Concept	Verbal Directive	Response Level	Comment
eyes	1. Show me your eyes.	______	
	2. Show me eyes. (Point to your eyes)	______	
	3. Eyes. (Point to your eyes)	______	
nose	1. Show me your nose.	______	
	2. Show me nose. (Point to your nose)	______	
	3. Nose. (Point to your nose)	______	
hair	1. Show me your hair.	______	
	2. Show me hair. (Point to your hair)	______	
	3. Hair. (Point to your hair)	______	
mouth	1.Show me your mouth.	______	
	2. Show me mouth. (Point to your mouth)	______	
	3. Mouth. (Point to your mouth)	______	
ears	1. Show me your ears.	______	
	2. Show me ears. (Point to your ears)	______	
	3. Ears. (Point to your ears)	______	
hands	1. Show me your hands.	______	
	2. Show me hands. (Point to your hands)	______	
	3. Hands. (Point to your hands)	______	
feet	1. Show me your feet.	______	
	2. Show me feet. (Point to your feet)	______	
	3. Feet. (Point to your feet)	______	
head	1. Show me your head.	______	
	2. Show me head. (Point to your head)	______	
	3. Head. (Point to your head)	______	
arm	1. Show me your arm.	______	
	2. Show me arm. (Point to your arm)	______	
	3. Arm. (Point to your arm)	______	
leg	1. Show me your leg.	______	
	2. Show me leg. (Point to your leg)	______	
	3. Leg. (Point to your leg)	______	
knee	1. Show me your knee.	______	
	2. Show me knee. (Point to your knee)	______	
	3. Knee. (Point to your knee)	______	

Exhibit 6–1 continued

Concept	Verbal Directive	Response Level	Comment
elbow	1. Show me your elbow.	_____	
	2. Show me elbow. (Point to your elbow)	_____	
	3. Elbow. (Point to your elbow)	_____	
chin	1. Show me your chin.	_____	
	2. Show me chin. (Point to your chin)	_____	
	3. Chin. (Point to your chin)	_____	
eyebrow	1. Show me your eyebrow.	_____	
	2. Show me eyebrow. (Point to your eyebrow)	_____	
	3. Eyebrow. (Point to your eyebrow)	_____	

For example, the case of an 8-month old baby who is just presenting mid- and low vowels suggests an intervention objective for the stimulation for mid- and mid-high vowel production based on the results of an utterance sample analysis.

Kretschmer and Kretschmer (1978) note two advantages in using the language-sample approach with spontaneous utterances. First, since much of the research on language of normals has been analyzed via this approach, there is in existence a large amount of normative data. Second, formal testing situations are too often unnatural estimates of performance, while the setting for a collection of spontaneous utterances may be representative of how a child actually uses language. The latter approach thus appears feasible for young children. In addition to its use in the Kretschmer spontaneous language analysis procedure, the language-sample approach has been used by Lee (1966, 1974), Tyack and Gottsleben (1974), Hannah (1979), Hannah and Gardner (1974), and Bloom and Lahey (1978), as described in Chapter 5.

Procedure

The language sample may be recorded either on a portable cassette recorder or, preferably, via a narrative approach, using the form shown in Exhibit 6–2. The sample is then analyzed after the observation session has been completed.

There are three general ways in which a language sample may be recorded, depending on finances, the context in which the sample is taken, and the language level of the child to be evaluated. The first method, videotaping, is ideal because it provides the truest record of context, facial expression, and body movement as well as the utterances produced. The second method, the audiotape or cassette recording, is less expensive and less obtrusive but more portable. However, only vocalizations can be

Exhibit 6–2 Language Sample Analysis: Narrative Recording Sheet

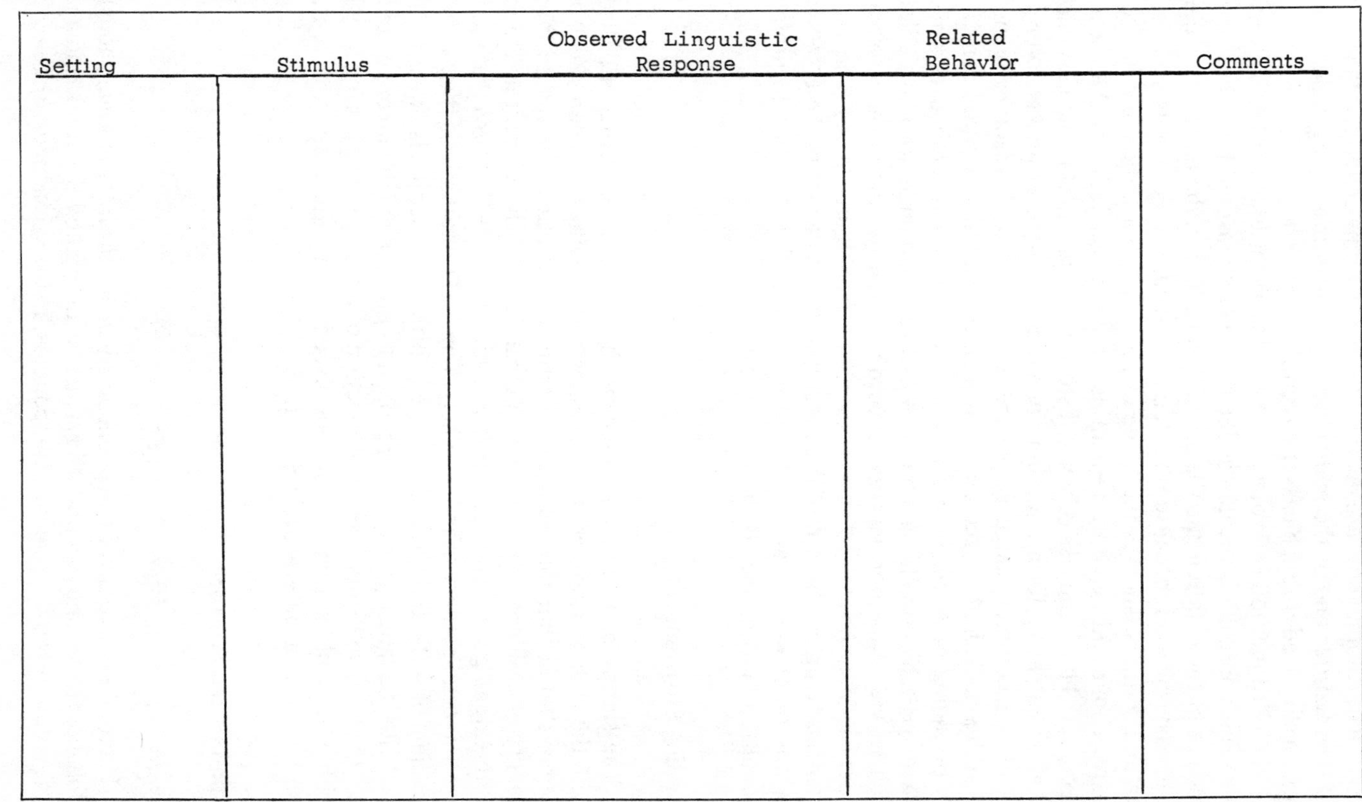

Setting	Stimulus	Observed Linguistic Response	Related Behavior	Comments

recorded. Another concern in taping voices of young children is the quality of the recorder and of the audiotape. The voice of a young child is often lost or distorted through cassette recordings.

The third method is through the narrative recording of a language sample. This approach is recommended for several reasons. First, because of the age of the children and the low language levels, the narrative is quick and easy. Second, because we attempt to secure spontaneous samples in natural settings, such as the home or nursery school, the child is free to move about and need not remain in the close proximity of the cassette recorder. Third, the risk of voice distortion on tape is eliminated. Fourth, a good narrative form and some minimum training of an observer can produce a complete language picture second only to a videotape record.

Although videotape recordings would undoubtedly be more beneficial in providing both visual and auditory information regarding the child's language behavior, this method is not always available nor affordable. If neither videotape nor narrative recording are used, the examiner should note pertinent behaviors relating to responses and utterances. The examiner may employ the use of the parent(s), the materials in the CAPS kit, or any other items that might appeal to the individual child to promote vocalization using the language-sample approach.

Testing Environment

The setting or testing environment should be a free situation, ideally with the child performing daily routines and activities. Cazden (1970) has demonstrated that the testing environment will affect the quantity and quality of children's utterances to a great degree. Therefore, relaxed and unthreatening surroundings are desirable. Axline (1947) states that play is the universal activity of infants and young children, that it is their natural medium of self-expression. Thus, the informal play setting is suggested for use with the language-sample approach to provide maximum opportunity for a natural and spontaneous production of language. The setting may be within the child's home, preschool placement, or the evaluation center, but it should be natural and relaxed.

Analysis and Scoring

Syntactic/Morphological Analysis

Utterances are transcribed phonetically, using the international phonetic alphabet (IPA), and in standard English as uttered by the child, and analysis is completed via language components. In the syntactic/morphological analysis, descriptions are made and based primarily on those presented by Hannah (1979), Hargis (1977), and Kretschmer and Kretschmer (1978), as shown in Table 6–2.

In this table, expansion level III represents sentence patterns and transformations that are employed by children who are closely approximating or actually employing adult grammar. This normally occurs as a perfection process at about age 5 and continues through the elementary school years. Since the purpose of the language evaluation process is centered on the preschool child with language delay, we would not expect the child to demonstrate proficiency at this level. Therefore, a few commonly used transformations are presented at expansion level III to provide the examiner with a point of reference for normal language. There is also the possibility that a child with a slight language delay may produce some of these syntactic examples while the bulk of the child's productions are still being perfected at the earlier levels.

Table 6–2 Categories and Descriptions in Syntactic/Morphological Analysis

One-Word Utterances		
N	(nouns)	Mama
V	(verbs)	go
Desc	(description)	pretty
Two-Word Utterances		
N + V	(noun + verb)	Mommy go
N + N	(noun + noun)	Patty girl
N + Adj	(noun + adjective)	Mommy pretty
N + Adv pl	(noun + adverb of place)	Daddy bye-bye
V + N	(verb + noun)	Take Patty
V + Adj	(verb + adjective)	See pretty
V + Adv pl	(verb + adverb of place)	Go bye-bye
Adj + N	(adjective + noun)	Pretty Patty
Yes/no quest		Mommy go?
Wh-quest + X		Where Mommy?
Expansion Level I		
Structural Elements		
N pl reg	(noun plural, regular form)	girl/girls, dress/dresses
Def Art	(definite article)	the
Indef Art	(indefinite article)	a/an, some
NCN	(noncount noun)	courage

Table 6-2 continued

Pron	(pronouns)	Subjective: Singular Plural 1. I we 2. you you 3. he, she, it they Objective: Singular Plural 1. me us 2. you you 3. him, her, it them
D1	(demonstrative)	this, these
D2		that, those
D1 or D2 del	(deletion of noun following demonstrative)	I see that (boy)
Tense reg	(verb tense, regular form)	walk(s)/walked
M	(modal)	will/would, shall/should, can/could, may/might, must
QM	(quasimodal)	*I am going* to tell Mommy. (*I'm gonna* tell Mommy.)
Be + NP	(Be verb form + noun phrase)	Patty *is a baby.*
Be + Adj	(Be verb form + adjective)	Patty *is little.*
Be + Adv pl	(Be verb form + adverb of place)	Patty *is in bed.*
V + ing	(Verb + ing, participial ending without *be* in aux)	Stop *running.*
V + Adv pl	(Verb + adverb of place)	Daddy *went to work.*
V + Adv t	(Verb + adverb of time)	Patty *naps after lunch.*
V + Adv m	(Verb + adverb of manner)	Patty *runs awkwardly.*
V + Adv f	(Verb + adverb of frequency)	Mommy *bathes Patty daily.*
Transformations		
T neg	(Use of not, contracted form *n't,* or *no* to indicate Negative)	Patty is *not* here. Patty *isn't* here. Patty is *no* help.
T do	(Addition of *do* to verb phrase, obligatory in formation of negative or question form when only tense is present in aux followed by a verbal)	Patty *does* not live here. *Does* Patty live here?
T contr	(Any contracted form)	Is not = is*n't*

Table 6–2 continued

T conj	(Conjunction *and*)	Patty *and* Mommy . . . . Patty cried *and* cried. Patty is a cute *and* chubby baby.
T poss	(Possessive—pronoun or noun form with 's/s')	Pronouns: Singular — Plural 1. my — our 2. your — your 3. his, her, its — their Noun possessive form: Patty'*s* book The boy'*s* bikes
T pos/del	(Possessive form of pronoun or noun with modified noun deleted)	Pronoun-possessive-deleted form: Singular — Plural 1. mine — ours 2. yours — yours 3. his, hers, its — theirs Noun-possessive-deleted form: That book is Patty'*s* (book). Those are the boys' (bikes).
T there	(Not adverb of place as in *The doll is there.* Can be used only when noun is preceded by indefinite article)	There is (there's) *a* doll for Patty.
T imp	(Imperative sentence)	Go away. Stop running.
T got	(Use of *got* in child language, usually substituted for *have*)	Patty *gots* new boots.
T yes/no	(Yes-no question form)	Is Daddy home now? Did Patty eat dinner?
T wh quest	(Question forms using Wh-introductory forms)	
	Who	*Who* is your mother?
	What	*What* is that animal?
	What-do	*What* did Patty *do?*
	Where	*Where* is Patty?
	When	*When* is her mother coming?
	How	*How* do you make cookies?

Table 6–2 continued

	How +	*How many* cookies do you want? *How much* will the cookies cost? *How come* Mommy is at the store?
T Inv	(Inversion of adverb position to precede verb)	*Sometimes* Patty is naughty. Patty *usually* is a pleasant child.
T Adj	(Adjective modifier—*not* adjective form following "be ")	Patty is a *happy, pleasant* child.
T Adv mod	(Adverb modifying an adjective, adverb, or verb *not* classified as time, place, frequency, or manner)	Patty is *very* tired.
Expansion Level II		
Structural Elements		
Tense irreg	(Verb tense irregular)	run/ran, come/came
V + prt	(Verb + particle-phrasal verbs)	Patty *fell down.* Patty *picked* her toys *up.*
V + prt move	(Movement of participle immediately to follow verb or precede N.P. acting as the direct object)	Patty *picked up* her toys.
Be + ing (aux)	(Be + verb + ing)	Patty *is running.*
Have + en (aux)	(Have + verb + en)	Patty *has fallen.*
VI + comp	(Intransitive verb followed by a prepositional phrase or other modifier not classified as one of the four adverbial forms)	Patty cried *for one whole hour.*
N pl irreg	(Noun plural, irregular)	Child/children, goose/geese
Indef Pron	(Indefinite pronouns)	Everyone, somebody, etc.
Number or #	(In determiner, either cardinal or ordinal)	Cardinal: one, four, ninety-seven Ordinal: first, third, seventy-second (indicates position in a series)

Table 6–2 continued

Transformations		
T Conj II	(Conjunctions other than *and*)	Patty *or* me . . . . Patty is asleep *but* . . . .
T Conj del or series	(Deletion of *and* between items listed in a series)	Mommy, Daddy, Patty, and Grandma . . . . Patty walks, runs, and jumps well.
T pronom	(Pronominalization—substitution of *one* for noun referent *not* used as cardinal number)	Patty wants *one* too.
T VT to + comp	(Transitive verb followed by infinitive marker and complement)	Mommy *asked* Patty *to close the door.*
T VT to comp del	(Transitive verb followed by infinitive marker with complement deleted)	from: Patty *asked* Mommy *to read her a story.* to: Patty *asked* Mommy *to read.*
T VT ing + comp	(Transitive verb followed by participial and complement)	Patty *heard* Daddy *singing a song.*
V VT ing comp del	(Transitive verb followed by participial with complement deleted)	from: Patty *heard* Daddy *singing a song.* to: Patty *heard* Daddy *singing.*
TV T_3 + comp	(Transitive verb followed by a be deletion complement)	from: Patty's new mittens keep. . . . Her hands are warm. to: Patty's new mittens keep *her hands warm.*
Trel	(Relative clauses)	
Trel/subj	(Relative clause that functions as a subject of a sentence)	*Whoever did this* is in serious trouble. *Whatever you do,* don't tell Paul.
Trel/obj	(Relative clause that functions as the object of a transitive verb)	Patty eats *what(ever) you feed her.* I will call *who(ever) you want.*
Trel/pos		The mothers *whose children attend the nursery session* will have conferences next week.

Table 6–2 continued

Trel/N Mod subj	(Relative clause that functions as a noun modifier for the subject or object of a sentence)	Patty, *who is my baby sister,* is a pest. The puppy *that we got last week* is all black and furry. Mommy read us a story *that was funny.*
Trel/del	(A case in which the relative pronoun when the clause is acting as a noun modifier can be deleted from the sentence)	from: Patty, *who is my sister,* is 2 years old. to: Patty, *my sister,* is 2 years old.
T ind obj	(Indirect object)	Mommy read a story *to/for* me.
T ind obj/del	(*To* or *for* is deleted and the indirect object immediately follows the verb)	Mommy read *me* a story.
T adv cl	(Adverbial clauses of time, place, frequency, and manner)	
	Place:	Patty stays *where the other children play.*
	Time:	Mommy will come home *when she finishes grocery shopping.*
	Manner:	He ran *like a monster was chasing him.*

Expansion Level III

(In normal language development, all elements are in use at this level.)

Transformations		
T comp	(Comparative form)	My daddy's *bigger than your daddy.*
T reflex	(Reflexive form of the pronoun)	Singular Plural 1. myself ourselves 2. yourself yourselves 3. himself, herself, itself themselves
T tag	(Tag question)	Daddy isn't outside, *is he?* Patty is two years old, *isn't she?*
T sub	(Subordinate clauses)	I will go *if you go.*

Table 6–2 continued

T elp	(Ellipsis)	from: Paul can run fast but Patty can't run fast. to: Paul can run fast but Patty can't.
T corel conj	(Correlative conjunctions—either/or neither/nor)	*Either* my mommy is sleeping *or* she is fooling me.
T conj III	(Conjunctions such as however, although, nevertheless, etc.)	

Source: Summary of information from Hargis, 1977; Kretschmer & Kretschmer, 1978; and Hannah, 1979.

Phonological Analysis

Phonologically, the utterance sample is analyzed through the productive development of stages of speech growth, through distinctive-feature analysis (Hannah & Gardner, 1974; McReynolds & Engmann, 1975), and through phonotactic processes (Ingram, 1976; Menn, 1971; Muma, 1978). The general stages of phonological development are shown in Table 6–3.

These are not isolated stages; they rather blend and overlap into one another. They are gross demarcations of where the child is functioning at the one-word-utterance level or earlier. The child's utterances are then further analyzed to determine which vowels and consonants are being produced and which distinctive features are present.

Although they are not presently included in the BEAR language sample analysis, Hasenstab (in press) strongly suggests that the stages of phonation, which Oller (1975, 1980) proposes occur during the first 12 months of infancy, be used for more specific evaluation in this component. (See Chapter 7.)

Speech production for the child at the one-word-utterance level or beyond is first examined to determine which consonants and vowels are present. Table 6–4 summarizes generally the production of consonants and consonant blends. Following this examination, a more intensive evaluation is undertaken through a distinctive-feature analysis and the examination of phonotactic processes.

Distinctive-feature analysis is based on the original theory advanced by Jakobson, Fant, and Halle (1952) and expanded by Chomsky and Halle (1968) and on the analytical processes developed by Hannah and Gardner (1974) and McReynolds and Engmann (1975). (See Table 6–5.)

Table 6–3 General Stages in Phonological Development

Vocalization		Age Range of Usual Production
Crying:		At birth
Variations in cry—"Mewing" changes in frequency and timing patterns		By 2 months
Vocal Play:		
Production of neutral vowel /ʌ/		Between 2 and 4 months
Production of back vowels /u/ /ʊ/ /o/ /ɔ/ /a/	Vowel production begins at the neutral position and moves out to include front and back vowels from low to high tongue position	Between 2 and 4 months
Production of front vowels /i/ /I/ /e/ /ae/		Between 4 and 6 months
Babbling and Consonant Production (consonant production begins, with back consonants moving forward):		
Addition of consonants to vowels with intonation.	Includes stops, then nasals and some fricatives	10 months
Babbling sets—random		About 6 months
Babbling sets—imitative		About 8 months
Words		
First words		Between 9 and 12 months

Table 6–4 Summary of Production of Consonants and Consonant Blends

Consonant Production	*Median Age of Usage*	*Age of 90% Competency in Production*
Consonants		
/p/ /m/ /h/ /n/ /w/	1 year, 6 months	3 years
/b/	1 year, 6 months	4 years
/k/ /g/ /d/	2 years	4 years
/t/ /ŋ/	2 years	6 years
/f/	2 years, 6 months	4 years
/r/ /l/	3 years	6 years
/s/	3 years	8 years
/z/ /j/	4 years	7 years
/v/	4 years	8 years
Blends		
/ʃ/ /tʃ/	3 years, 6 months	7 years
/θ/ /dʒ/	4 years, 6 months	7 years
/ð/	5 years	8 years
/ð/ /ʍ/	6 years	8 years, 6 months
thr	7 years	8 years, 6 months
sk, st, sl, sn, etc.	5 years	8 years, 6 months
Others (f plus, b plus, g plus, etc.)	5 years	8 years, 6 months

Source: Summation of information based on Poole, 1934; McCarthy, 1954; Templin & Darley, 1957; and Winitz, 1969 .

Within a given utterance sample of 50 to 100 items, children will use repetitions of the vocalizations and phonemes in their repertoires. Therefore, distinctive-feature analysis procedures may be used to determine the presence of correct feature production. The feature-analysis approach used in the present context differs from the usual feature analysis in that phonemes need not be analyzed with respect to target phoneme and various substitutions (see the Exhibit 6–1 scoring summary sheets). The phonemes may be analyzed as the child produces them. Since young children are expected to produce misarticulations due to age or, in our cases, to language difficulty, the purpose is to examine the features the child has mastered at this level, not correct phoneme production. This should be noted in the general analysis section of the phonological summary.

Confining the analysis of a child's speech beyond word utterances to a general description and feature analysis still leaves unanswered the types

Table 6–5 Distinctive-Feature Descriptions

Features	*Vowels*	*Consonants*	*Definitions*
Voiced	All vowels	/r/ /l/ /b/ /d/ /g/ /m/ /n/ /ŋ/ /ð/ /v/ /z/ /ʒ/ /dʒ/ /j/ /w/	Vocal cord function present.
Vocalic	All vowels	/r/ /l/	Airstream passes through the vocal tract unobstructed Voicing is present
Low	/ɛ/ /ae/ /ɔ/ /ɑ/	/h/	Tongue position low
High	/i/ /u/ /I/ /u/	/w/ /j/ /k/ /g/ /ŋ/ /ʃ/ /ʒ/ /tʃ/ /dʒ/	Tongue position high
Back	/u/ /ʊ/ /o/ /ɔ/ /ɑ/	/k/ /g/ /ŋ/ /w/	Tongue position back from neutral
Anterior/front*	/i/ /I/ /ae/ /e/ /ɛ/	/l/ /p/ /b/ /t/ /d/ /m/ /n/ θ/ /ð/ /f/ /v/ /s/ /z/	Tongue position or sound near front of mouth
Round	/u/ /ʊ/ /o/ /ɔ/ /ɑ/	/w/	Rounded lips
Tense	/i/ /u/ /e/ /o/ /ɑ/ /ae/ /ɝ/		Tension of musculature over relatively long time
Consonantal		All consonants except /h/	Airstream meets narrow obstruction at some point in vocal tract
Nasal		/m/ /n/ /ŋ/	Airstream passes through nasal port
Continuant		/r/ /l/ /θ/ /ð/ /f/ /v/ /s/ /z/ /ʃ/ /ʒ/ /h/	Obstruction minimal to allow continuous flow of airstream
Strident		/f/ /v/ /s/ /z/ /ʃ/ /ʒ/ /tʃ/ /dʒ/	Airstream affected by elongated vocal tract, rapid speed, and small obstruction
Coronal		/r/ /l/ /t/ /d/ /n/ /θ/ /ð/ /s/ /z/ /ʃ/ /ʒ/ /tʃ/ /dʒ/	Blade and anterior part of tongue raised

Source: These descriptions are based on categories proposed by Chomsky and Halle (1968). The order has been changed, however, to more closely approximate the developmental sequence.

*The anterior/front category has been expanded to include front vowels.

of variations exhibited in the child's spoken language. There is more to the description of early speech than substitutions, omissions, and distortions in various phoneme positions.

Further analysis of vocalizations by examination of phonotactic processes helps to account for child variations in phonology (Bloom & Lahey, 1978; Muma, 1978). The eight phonotactic processes described in Table 6–6 are based on definitions and descriptions proposed by Ingram (1976).

In addition to these eight processes, the phonotactic aspect of the phonological analysis includes two additional characteristic productions sug-

Table 6–6 Phonotactic Processes

Phonological Variation	*Definition*	*Example*
Reduplication	Repetition of syllable	mama, dada, byebye
Simplification	Reduction of closed syllable (CVC) to open syllable (CV) by deletion of final consonant	boat: - bo cat: - ca
Consonant cluster reduction	Cluster features deleted, produces reduced cluster	stop: top fast: fas
Voicing	Voiced initial consonant; unvoiced final consonant	soup: zup cookie: doti
Deletion of weak syllable	Omission of unaccented syllable	elephant: phant potato: tato
Diminutive	Addition of high front vowel (i or I) to end of proper noun	Mommy, Daddy
Assimilation (coarticulation):	The influence of one consonant on another when one phonetic activity replaces another:	
(1) Forward assimilation	Final or forthcoming consonant features replaced initial or earlier ones	coat: tot
(2) Backward assimilation	Initial or earlier consonant features replace final or forthcoming ones	soup: sos
Fronting	Usual phonetic activity is replaced by anterior movement of the tongue	sit: thit

Source: Summarized from Ingram, 1976, and Muma, 1978.

gested by Ingram (1976) and illustrated by deVilliers and deVilliers (1978). These are shown in Table 6–7. (Phonological development, including phonotactic processes, is discussed in detail in the following chapters on intervention.)

The development of the phonological component, involving both perception and production, is extremely complex. In the utterance analysis, on the theory that perception precludes production (although there are exceptions), only production is examined. It must be remembered that a simple listing of phonemes present in a child's vocalization repertoire cannot fully explain the child's speech development. Distinctive-feature analysis can provide information regarding feature rules the child has mastered and can also provide the basis for prespeech and early speech development in programming, such as breath and tongue control, voicing, and so forth. Further, examination of phonotactic processes can evaluate the vocalizations of the child based on variations of child phonology rather than on a model of adult pronunciation, as in the traditional articulation approach where phonemes are isolated entities and misarticulations consist of sound omission, distortion, or substitution in various positions (initial, medial, final). Phonemic production is a result of coarticulation in spoken language and must be viewed as such. The production of a phoneme in isolated context is no guarantee of correct use in connected speech.

Semantic/Pragmatic Analysis

We must be aware of the structure of language. There is much to be learned about a child's command of the structure of language to give us clues to underlying linguistic competence. It is, however, the functional use of that language structure in a language-using world that becomes a major concern in language assessment, since the main objective of assess-

Table 6–7 Additional Phonotactic Productions

Phonological Variation	*Definition*	*Example*	
Glide/liquid substitution	Substitutions between the consonant glides (h, w, y) and the consonant liquids (r, l).	run: yellow:	wun lellow
Stop/fricative substitution	Substitutions between the consonant stops (p, b, t, etc.) and the consonant fricatives (f, v, s, etc.)	that:	dat

Source: Summarized from deVilliers and deVilliers, 1978, and Ingram, 1976.

ment is always to propose instructional, acquisition, or facilitative procedures when the assessment indicates deficiency.

Effective language users must have both linguistic competence and communicative competence (Kretschmer & Kretschmer, 1978). Earlier in this chapter, we examined strategies for assessing the syntactic and phonologic aspects of a young child's language. In the present section, we will deal with semantic/pragmatic assessment, or meaning in context. The semantic description of the child's utterances is based on the studies and work of Brown (1973), Leonard (1976), Bloom and Lahey (1978), Kretschmer and Kretschmer (1978), and Muma (1978). A list of semantic descriptions is presented in Table 6–8.

Table 6–8 Descriptions in Semantic Assessment

	Definition	*Example*
Noun Cases:		
Agent	(the performer or initiator of an action)	*Patty* hit Tom.
Object	(that which receives the action or is acted upon)	Patty tore *the papers.* Patty kicked *Tom.*
Complement	(that which occurs *because* of the action)	Mommy baked *a cake.*
Recipient	(the receiver of an object)	Mommy gave *Patty* a cookie.
Possessor	(used to indicate ownership)	*Patty* has a bunny. *Patty's* bunny.
Entity	(an object or person in existence)	That's a *ball.*
Vocative	(call for attention)	*Mommy,* look!
Experiencer	(person/object involved with process or internal feeling)	*Patty* slept.
Verb Cases:		
Action/causative	(transitive verb)	Patty *hit* Tom.
Action/affect	(intransitive verb)	Patty *cried.*
Process/causative	(transitive verb)	Patty *wants* two cookies.
Process/affect	(intransitive verb)	Patty *thinks.*
Stative	(verb indicating state, i.e., existence, condition)	Patty *is* cute.
Modifier Cases:		
Specification	(indicates a particular person or object)	I see *that* bird.

Table 6–8 continued

Noun Cases:	*Definition*	*Example*
Existence	(indicates notice of a person or object)	See *the* puppy.
Nonexistence	(indicates a person or object is not present)	There is *no* bird here.
Recurrence	(indicates repetition)	Patty wants *more* milk.
Disappearance	(indicates absence of a person or object previously present)	Patty's milk is *all gone.*
Condition/quality	(indicates a state or attribute of a person or object)	Patty's doll is *broken.* The bunny is *fuzzy.*
Size	(indicates size description)	Patty is *little.*
Shape	(indicates form description)	The ball is *round.*
Color	(indicates color description)	The sweater is *yellow.*
Age	(indicates age description)	Mommy is *old.*
Quantity	(indicates amount)	Patty has *two* cookies.
Position:ordinal number	(indicates location relationship of a person or object)	Mommy is *second* in line.
Adverbial Cases:		
Location/position	(indicates where)	Daddy is *at work.* Patty is *next to me.*
Time	(indicates when)	Daddy went to work *this morning.*
Manner	(indicates how an action occurred)	Patty hits *hard.*
Frequency	(indicates how often, how many, etc.)	Mommy plays with Patty *every day.*

Other cases should be specifically stated. For example, an adverbial depicting "reason," as "in Mommy made soup *for lunch.*"

Question Forms:		
yes/no	(a question that is either true or false)	Is that Patty?
Who	(indicates a person)	*Who* is here?
What	(indicates an object)	*What* is this?
What - did	(indicates action)	*What* did you do?
When	(indicates time)	*When* is Daddy coming home?
Where	(indicates location)	*Where* is Patty?
How	(indicates manner)	*How* did you fall?

Table 6–8 continued

Noun Cases:	*Definition*	*Example*
Why	(indicates reason)	*Why* do bunnies hop? (How come?)
Other:		
Rejection	(indicates refusal)	*No more* cookies for me.
Denial	(indicates falsity)	I *didn't do it.*

Source: Summarized from Bloom and Lahey, 1978; Brown, 1973; Kretschmer and Kretschmer, 1978; Leonard, 1976; and Muma, 1978.

It must be noted that, as in the case of syntactic descriptions, not all possible semantic rules are represented in Table 6–8; only those that occur most often in early language are included. For example, when the verb *be*, is used, there may be such variations expressed as the following, noted by Kretschmer and Kretschmer (1978):

Stative-static	Something exists	Patty's dress *is* blue.
Stative-dynamic	A result of a process of time	Patty *is* tired.
Ambient-stative	A condition	It *was* a pleasant time.
Ambient-action	A natural phenomenon (pronoun has no referent)	It *is* snowing.

Descriptions of other elaborated semantic cases are presented in Appendix A.

Stages in Semantic/Pragmatic Acquisition

Preverbal Level

At the preverbal level, nonlinguistic prerequisites to language that signal the beginning phrases of the communicative process are observed. These prerequisites can be differentiated as cognitive and communicative behaviors. Cognitive behaviors that are prerequisite to expressive single-word use relate to the language acquirer's ability to represent, symbolize, focus attention, organize information, solve problems, and test hypotheses at a level prior to the use of language to accomplish these functions (Bloom

& Lahey, 1978). These skills can be considered as a type of cognitive/motor readiness for language. These cognitive behaviors may be categorized as:

- *motor imitation*—making a reasonable attempt to copy the gross movements of another person
- *body image*—perceiving one's body as separate from others and capable of performing tasks
- *eye contact*—visually focusing on another person with whom the child is interacting
- *object permanence*—knowing objects exist in space and time even when the child no longer sees or acts on them
- *ordering*—putting things into a specific, intentional arrangement
- *embedding*—inserting something into a previously established arrangement
- *categorizing*—grouping things according to characteristics they have in common
- *relational concepts*—making some association between or among things based on function or ownership
- *causality*—noting that one event or action will regularly cause another event or action to take place

Characteristic of emerging pragmatic use of language at a preverbal level are communicative behaviors related to early speech or elocutionary acts (Searle, 1969). In these cases, the child has specific intents for communicative behavior or for perlocutionary acts, in which the acts may not be present but adults interpret the behaviors as intentional. Communicative behaviors may be categorized as:

- *pointing/gesturing*—conveying information or making known wants or needs by gesturing/pointing at persons or objects in the environment; may be used to refer to objects or actions or to show relationships between objects and actions
- *crying*—differentiated to indicate need for attention, food, or removal of discomfort
- *gazing*—an early form of eye contact used for communication with child and adult maintaining eye contact; may be accompanied by smiling, touching, and vocalizing
- *facial expression*—emotions that can be easily observed in facial expressions; for example, fear, surprise, contentment, pleasure
- *posturing*—turning body or head toward or away from adult in a social/communicative fashion

- *babbling/jargon/vocal play*—series of vocalizations with or without intonation; short sentence-like utterances with no meaning; gurgles and chuckles
- *turn-taking*—an interaction in which the adult/child speaks or acts, waits to allow the child/adult a response (turn), with the adult permitted to take the child's turn if the child declines a turn
- *touching/holding/tugging*—social behavior that establishes a bond between the child and adult, for example, pulling the adult to or away from a task to indicate wishes or needs
- *showing*—taking the object to the adult or the adult to the object to indicate requests, wishes, or action
- *requesting/questioning*—bringing the object to the adult and questioning or requesting by facial expression and/or vocalization
- *negating/nodding*—shaking head to indicate nonexistence, denial, or rejection, or covering or throwing an object to remove it from the immediate environment

One-Word Level

The one-word level of utterances marks the use of true words or the referential use of language. Receptive or comprehension abilities at the one-word-utterance level may be difficult to assess, since contextual cueing probably has more influence than vocabulary (Huttenlocher, 1974). Early comprehension of language appears to be basically semantic, consisting largely of proper nouns with some common nouns and action words. Expressively, basic semantic relationships appear to begin emerging at the one-word-utterance level. These have been described by Muma (1978) as substantive functions—such as comments, vocatives, agents, objects, actions, and possession—and as relational functions—such as recurrence, nonexistence, disappearance, rejection, cessation, and existence.

Production at this level consists usually of function words that express existence, nonexistence, and recurrence (Bloom, 1973). These are followed by expressions of causality or location, possession or attribution, and internal experience. Language may be basically performative, that is, communication is primarily an aspect of the child's actions. There may be some continued, incomplete separation of word and referent, as in greetings or responses in which the child acts to a request from someone other than the language user. During this phase, it is assumed that the child is acquiring semantic categories that will be combined at the two- and three-word levels into semantic propositions. As they are combined into semantic relationships, these semantic categories are defined in the two-word level. The communicative intents described in the present section are the focus of the one-word-utterance level. Communicative intents described by several authors (Dore, 1974; Greenfield & Smith, 1976; Skarakis & Prutting, 1977) provide the basis for the following descriptive categories at the one-word-utterance level:

- *imitation*—repeating one word of someone else's utterance
- *comment*—any comment, remark, or observation about an obvious or visible topic (run, pretty)
- *response*—any single-word answer to a question or any stimulus in the environment ("yes" to "do you want a cookie?" or "hot" after touching the stove)
- *initiation*—using any single-word attempt to begin a dialogue rather than responding to it ("water?" looking toward mother)
- *labeling*—giving names to people, objects, and actions (bathroom, Ted, girl)
- *turn maintaining*—using a word to hold one's place (signing "wait" to hold a turn)
- *requesting*—any single word plus rising intonation, facial expression, or body movement to form a question, later the use of question words (car? walk? where?)
- *demanding*—any single word plus intonation, facial expression, or body movement (cookie! come!)
- *description (attribution)*—using one of several types of one-word utterances to add information about a person, object, event, or situations (big, my, funny)
- *location*—using one word to give the position of an object (here, under, chair)
- *protest/denial/nonexistence/rejection*—opposing the stimulus word or situation (no, not, gone, don't, can't)
- *greeting/attention/vocative*—using one word to attract the attention of the desired person to self, object, or event (Hi! Tom! Uh, oh!)

The one-word level usually includes some semantic categories that combine at the two-word level into basic semantic relationships that form the meaning base for language. At the one-word level, many children will use single words for a variety of purposes, such as responding, protesting, questioning, or describing. The single-word vocabulary may consist of several classes of words—nouns, verbs, prepositions, adjectives, adverbs, and negatives. The verb is perhaps the most significant of these, since it serves as the basis for coding into language the action-based life of the young child and for later grammatical development.

There is an intermediate stage between one-word utterances and two-word utterances that occurs in some children's language systems. This is the stage of successive utterances (Bloom, 1973), which can probably be best described as several concepts presented in a linear fashion by the child without expressing more well-defined, two-word semantic relationships. Examples would be utterances like "hit, fall" or "boy, girl" or "blue, red."

Two-Word Level

The two-word-utterance level is marked by the acquisition of semantic relationships. These semantic relationships consist mainly of (1) functional or linear relationships, such as existence, nonexistence, or recurrence, and (2) grammatical or hierarchical relationships, such as agent-action. The verb determines the semantic role of the noun. Some authors have indicated that the order of early two-word utterances is based on the old-new information theory (Bates, 1976; Greenfield & Smith, 1976), in which the first word is a comment and the second word is a topic. Developmentally, it appears that, when they are functioning at a one-word level, children make a comment about a topic supplied by the environment. Later, they presuppose somewhat less shared information with the listener or receiver and offer the topic with the comment following the topic, that is, their syntax and semantic development emerges (Bates, 1976; Bates & Johnston, 1977). Some authors have suggested the existence of an intermediate phase in which babbling and jargon are used in a communicative, expressive, game-like way, along with some pat phrases that extend the mean length of utterance (MLU) prior to the actual use of the two-word semantic relationship (Feagans, 1979).

The semantic relationships relevant to the present context are based on information presented by case grammarians (Chafe, 1970; Fillmore, 1978) who describe sentences as consisting of underlying semantic intents or propositions that determine what syntactic form the sentences will ultimately take. The verb has the major influence on how the base relationships will occur. The major types of verb cases in English are action, process, and state. Combinations can also occur, such as action-process or stative-process. The following semantic relationships typically occur at the two-word level:

agent + action	(boy hit)
experiencer + process/ state	(me like)
action + object	(watch monkey)
process + object	(like cookie)
state + modifier	(is hot)
action + complement	(paint picture)

agent + object	(dentist tooth)
x + location	(go home)
modifier + x	(new clothes)
x + modifier	(fire yellow)
possessive/recipient + x	(my boat; daddy car; give [ball] Mommy)
negative + x	(no cookie)
x + time	(go yesterday)
introducer + x	(hi, Mark)

In the modifier + x relationship in the above list, the variation of x + modifier also occurs frequently. This variation can be expanded to a sentence with the words remaining in the same order. For example, "Mother strong" becomes "Mother is strong." However, not all modifier + x relationships can be rewritten as x + modifier and then expanded. An utterance such as "Mother my" would be considered an inappropriate reversal of modifier + x rather than a variation.

Three-Word Level

Three-word utterances are combinations and expansions of two-word utterances and thus, in effect, become basic sentences. Basic relationships are expanded across categories such as agent + action + object, which is developed from agent + action in combination with action + object.

Two important processes emerge at the three-word-utterance level: conjoining and embedding. Conjoining occurs when two *grammatical* relationships sharing a common term join (e.g., me eat + eat cookie = me eat cookie). Embedding occurs with the insertion of a *functional* relationship (nonexistence, recurrence, existence) into a grammatical relationship (e.g., no cookie + eat cookie = eat no cookie). A greater variety of relationships become functional and approximate sentences. It is not uncommon for these emerging sentences to lack morphological markers (past tense, plural), conjunctions, or modifiers, although they usually develop in conjunction with such relationships in normally hearing children.

The major combined relationships that occur at the three-word level are:

- agent + action + object
- agent + location + x
- action + location + x
- agent + action + location

- agent + object + location
- agent + be + location
- agent + modifier + x
- action + modifier + x
- agent + modifier + object
- agent + be + modifier/agent
- agent + negative + x
- action + negative + x

Examples of other three-word utterances in which young children may combine some of the above would be such utterances as agent + negative + location (Mommy not outside) and location + negative + modifier (outside not pretty). The four-word level is included in the model to demonstrate the progression from semantic relationships expressed in two- to three-word-utterance levels to the more complete syntactic use of sentences that is characteristic of utterances beyond these levels. The language structure used by the children at this later level may be in the form of complete, short sentences or nearly complete short sentences with some omissions. At this level, a definite sentence sense is demonstrated.

Four-Word Level

Children at the four-word level may use some syntactically correct sentences, but the majority of their utterances will be three-word-level relationships. The additional word may be in the form of modification or location, agents and actions, or emerging transformational or morphological use. This phase is a transition between the semantically oriented, three-word-utterance level and later complex syntactic use. While, at the four-word level, there may be emerging forms of more complex language operations, it is the flexibility in early language that contributes to later flexibility in more complex processes, such as complementation, relativization, coordination, and passivization.

Development of Questioning

The development of questioning has been treated by Bloom and Lahey, 1978; Menyuk, 1969; and Trantham and Pedersen, 1976. Briefly, pragmatically oriented questions develop very early in the form of quizzical or questioning looks at the preverbal level, through the use of single words used as questions, through the development of question words (who? what? where?), to the use of question words with other structures. Two-word questions are often statements posed as questions (boy fall?). Later, question words are used with the semantic categories of action, modifier, location, time, and negative. Questions are developed as semantic relationships develop. Three-word questions are expansions of two-word questions and follow a progression similar to that from the two-word level, that is, from statements as questions to further refinement of Wh-type questions.

Summary

We should be able to summarize language data into a succinct description of a child's language system and the context in which that system is employed. This should lead directly to planning instruction and the facilitating of further language acquisition. The major questions asked in assessment are:

- Is the language used for communication and controlling the child's world?
- Does the child have some sense of discourse interaction?
- Is there flexibility in language use—across situations and the people with whom the language is used?
- Does the meaning come through?
- Is the language syntactically complete?
- Is the morphological system developing?
- Is the phonological system developing?

The problem-solving process should result in a summary of the language assessment information that illustrates the consistency in usage (although rapid changes may be occurring), the major restrictions in language usage, and the major communicative purposes for which the language is used. All communicative utterances have underlying intents, such as requesting, talking, asking, promising, allowing, and feeling (Searle, 1969). The purpose of the summary of the pragmatic assessment should be to judge the relative expertise of the language user in conveying these intents.

Discourse rules in communication convey social interaction behaviors that are necessary to communication process. Included among these are forms of turn-taking procedures for negotiating a conversation and for entering and leaving a conversation, forms for topics and changes, and various "polite forms."

The major question at the preverbal level with respect to assessment is, "Is there a communicative sense or desire to communicate, or is there evidence of communicative behavior?" The major question at the one-word level is, "Is there a sense of reference and are the referents used in a pragmatic or communicative way?" While the emphasis at the two-word level is on the development of those basic semantic relationships that form the foundation for all later language growth, the context for the use of those relationships must also be considered. At the three- and four-word levels and at the expanded levels of functioning, children gain more control of their world and then use that control to make their lives less complex and to serve their purposes.

In the following pages, scoring and summary forms for a language sample analysis using the BEAR approach are presented (see Exhibits 6–3, 6–4, 6–5, and 6–6).

Exhibit 6–3 BEAR Summary Form

SUMMARY SHEETS FOR LANGUAGE SAMPLE ANALYSIS
BARE ESSENTIALS IN ASSESSING REALLY LITTLE KIDS
(BEAR)

Name ______________________	Date of Birth _____
Examiner ______________________	Date Tested _____
Parents/Guardian ______________________	Phone __________
Address ______________________	Informant _______
Referred by ______________________	Age __________
Communication Mode ______________	Disability ________

Audiological Information:

Hearing Loss:

Date of Most Recent Evaluation:

Hearing Aid:

Etiology:

Comments:

Medical Information:

Present Health:

Medical History:

Comments:

Educational Information:

Present Placement:

Assessment Results:

Comments:

Language Information:

Present Status (General):

Other Language Evaluation Results:

Exhibit 6–4 Syntactic/Morphological Analysis: Scoring and Summary Form

SYNTACTIC/MORPHOLOGICAL ANALYSIS SUMMARY

I. One-Word Utterances

Record one-word utterances produced by the child.
Please transcribe in both international phonetic alphabet (IPA) and standard English notation.

Comments:

Exhibit 6–4 continued

II. Two-Word Utterances

Record the appropriate utterance example number from the sample transcription. Tally up to three (3) examples for each pattern represented

N + V	___	V + N	___
N + N	___	V + Adv pl	___
N + Adj	___		
N + Adv pl	___	Yes/no quest	___
		Wh-quest + X	___
Adj + N	___		
		Neg + X	___

Comments:

III. Expansion Level I

Record the appropriate utterance example number from the sample transcription. Tally up to three (3) examples for each rule represented.

Structural Elements			*Transformations*		
PN		___	T neg		___
CN		___	T do		___
Pron - subj	s	pl	T contr		___
	1 ___	___	T conj (and)		___
	2 ___	___	T poss Pron	s	pl
	3 ___	___		1 ___	___

		s.	pl.
obj	1	___	___
	2	___	___
	3	___	___
Def art			___
Indef art			___
D1			___
D2			___
Ddel (specify D1			___
or D2)			___
Tense reg past			___
Be + NP			___
Be + Adj			___
Be + Adv pl			___
V + ing			___
V + Adv pl			___
V + Adv t			___
V + Adv f			___
V + Adv m			___

	2	___	___
	3	___	___
T pos noun			___
T pos/del pron			
	1	___	___
	2	___	___
	3	___	___
T pos/del noun			
		___	___
T there			___
T imp			___
T got			___
T inv			___
T adj			___
T yes/no			
T wh-quest			
Who			___
What			___
What-do			___
Where			___
When			___
How			___
How +			___
How come			___

Comments:

Exhibit 6–4 continued

IV. Expansion Level II

Structural Elements		*Transformations*	
N pl irreg	___	T conj II	___
Indef pron	___	T conj/del	___
No. card	___	T tag quest	___
ord	___	T pronom	___
Tense irreg	___	TVT to + comp	___
M	___	TVT to comp/ del	___
QM	___	TVT ing + comp	___
Be + ing (aux)	___	TVT ing + com/del	___
Have + prt (aux)	___	TVT_3 + comp	___
V+ prt	___	Trel	
V + prt move	___	subj	___
VI + comp	___	obj	___
		pos	___
		NM/subj	___
		NM/obj	___
		T ind obj	___
		T ind obj/ del	___

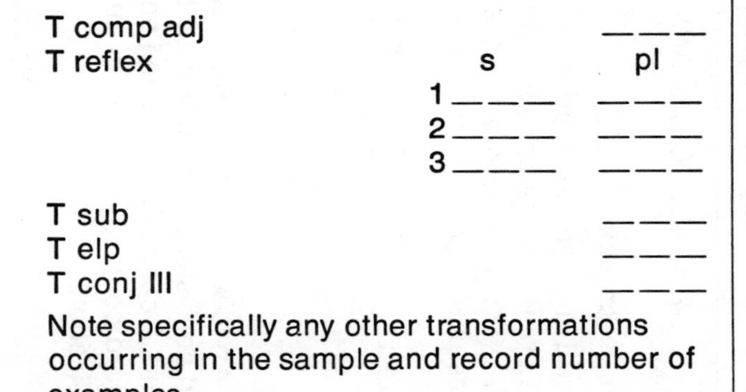

T adv clause
pl ___
t ___
m ___
other ___

Comments:

V. Expansion Level III

All structural elements are normally in use at this level.

Transformations

T comp adj ___

T reflex

	s	pl
1	___	___
2	___	___
3	___	___

T sub ___
T elp ___
T conj III ___

Note specifically any other transformations occurring in the sample and record number of examples.

Comments:

Exhibit 6–5 Phonological Analysis: Scoring and Summary Form

PHONOLOGICAL ANALYSIS SUMMARY

General Description

A. Record and attach a brief statement regarding the general development of the child's vocalizations.

B. *At or below one-word-utterance level:* Record vowels and syllables produced.

Vowels	CV	CVC

C. *At the two-word-utterance level and beyond:* Indicate phonemes used consistently and correctly in the sample. Note position of sound. A correctly articulated phoneme substituted for another in word context (/b/ for /p/ in puppy) is not considered correct application.

Vowels

Front	Mid	Back	Diphthongs
__ e/me	__ u/cup	__ oo/food	__ i/kite
__ i/bit	__ er/mother	__ oo/good	__ u/cute
__ a/cake	__ ir/first	__ o/coat	__ oi/boil
__ e/bed	__ ur/fur	__ a/father	__ ou/bout
__ a/cat	__ ar/car	__ o/hot	

Consonants

Voiceless	Voiced	Nasals/Glides
___ ___ ___ p	___ ___ ___ b	___ ___ ___ m
___ ___ ___ t	___ ___ ___ d	___ ___ ___ n
___ ___ ___ k	___ ___ ___ g	___ ___ ___ ng
___ ___ ___ f	___ ___ ___ v	
___ ___ ___ th (thin)	___ ___ ___ th (the)	
___ ___ ___ s	___ ___ ___ z	___ ___ ___ l
___ ___ ___ sh	___ ___ ___ zh (treasure)	___ ___ ___ r
___ ___ ___ wh		___ ___ ___ w
___ ___ ___ ch	___ ___ ___ j	___ ___ ___ y

Exhibit 6–5 continued

Distinctive Feature Analysis

I. Feature analysis worksheet for children *at or below two-word-utterance level*

1. Record phonemes uttered.
2. Determine + and – features of phonemes.

Phoneme	*Times*	*Voice*	*Vocalic*	*Low*	*High*	*Back*	*Front/Ant.*	*Round*	*Tense/Cont.*	*Nasal*	*Conson.*	*Strident*	*Coronal*

Exhibit 6–5 continued

IIA. Feature analysis worksheet for children *beyond two-word-utterance level*

1. Record target phoneme and the number of times it is produced (Column I).
2. Record substitutions and the number of times each occurs (Column II).
3. Record number of omissions and distortions (Column III).
4. Indicate + or − for each feature of target phoneme and substitutions.
5. Total across columns to determine number for correct feature use (Column IV).
6. Complete one copy of this sheet for each phoneme tested.

Feature	*I Target Phoneme no. of Times Correct*	*II Substitutions no. of Times Used*	*III no. of Omissions no. of Distortions*	*IV Total no. of Correct Feature Use*
Voice				
Vocalic				
Low				
High				
Back				
Anterior/Front				
Round				
Tense/Continuant				
Consonantal				
Nasal				
Strident				
Coronal				

Source: Based on forms developed by McReynolds and Engmann, 1975.

Exhibit 6–5 continued

IIB. Feature analysis worksheet for children *beyond two-word utterance level*

1. Record target feature.
2. Record phonemes that contain feature (+I for +feature; −I for − feature).
3. Record possible occurrences (PO) (+II for +feature; −II for − feature).
4. Record correct occurrences (CO) (+III for +feature; −III for − feature).
5. Total columns for + and − possible occurrences and correct occurrences.
6. Calculate percentages:
   % correct: CO/PO = % correct
   % incorrect: 100 = % correct = % incorrect
7. Complete one sheet for each feature present.

+I *Phonemes*	*+II* *Possible* *Occurrences*	*+III* *Correct* *Occurrences*		*−I* *Phonemes*	*−II* *Possible* *Occurrences*	*−III* *Correct* *Occurrences*
	Total____	Total____			Total____	Total____

% correct ____ % correct ____
% incorrect ____ % incorrect ____

Target Feature____________________

Source: Based on forms developed by McReynolds and Engmann, 1975.

Exhibit 6–5 continued

Summary of
Feature Production Information

Feature	+ % *Correct*	– % *Correct*
Voice	____	____
Vocalic	____	____
Low	____	____
High	____	____
Back	____	____
Anterior/Front	____	____
Round	____	____
Tense/Continuant	____	____
Consonantal	____	____
Nasal	____	____
Strident	____	____
Coronal	____	____

Comments:

Source: Based on form developed by McReynolds and Engmann, 1975.

III. Phonotactic Processes
   1. Note examples of the phonotactic processes.
   2. Record example phonetically (IPA) and in standard American English (SAE) notation.
   3. Indicate utterance number.

Variations	*Examples*		*Utterance No.*
	IPA	SAE	
Reduplication			
Simplification			

Exhibit 6–5 continued

Consonant cluster reduction
Voicing
Weak syllable deletion
Diminutive
Assimilation
Fronting
Glide/liquid substitution
Stop/fricative substitution
Comments:

Exhibit 6–6 Semantic/Pragmatic Analysis: Scoring and Summary Form

SEMANTIC/PRAGMATIC ANALYSIS SUMMARY

Part I

Indicate (√) number of examples of behaviors up to three at preverbal level. Indicate (√) number of examples of behavior up to three at one-word level, and record example as appropriate (example: Vocative - Hi).

Preverbal Level:

Communication behaviors:

Crying	___	Jargon	___
Gazing	___	Turn-taking	___
Facial expression	___	Touching	___
Posturing	___	Holding	___
Vocal play	___	Tugging	___
Pointing	___	Demonstrating	___
Gesturing	___	Asking	___
Babbling	___	Nodding (negation)	___

Cognitive/motor behaviors:

Body image	___	Embedding	___
Motor imitation	___	Categorization	___
Object permanence	___	Relational concept	___
Ordering	___		

Note: These behaviors may also be observed at higher language levels. Examples may be noted here with appropriate level indicated.

One-Word-Utterance Level:

Communication behaviors:

Imitation	———	Labeling	———
Vocative		Questioning	———
(attention/greeting)	———	Demanding	———
Protest	———	Description	———
Comment	———	Turn-maintaining	———

Note: These behaviors may also be noted at higher language levels. Examples may be noted here with appropriate level indicated.

Part II

Record the appropriate utterance example number from the sample transcription. Tally up to three (3) examples for each case represented.

Noun Cases:		*Verb Cases:*	
Agent	———	Action/causative	———
Object	———	Action/affect	———
Complement	———	Process/causative	———
Experiencer	———	Process/affect	———
Recipient	———	Stative	———
Possessor	———		
Entity	———	*Adverbial Cases:*	
Vocative	———	Location	———

Exhibit 6–6 continued

Modifier Cases:

Specification ____
Existence ____
Nonexistence ____
Recurrence ____
Disappearance ____
Condition/quality ____
Size ____
Shape ____
Color ____
Age ____
Position ____
Quantity ____

Time ____
Manner ____
Frequency ____

Other:

Rejection ____
Denial ____
Possession ____

Question Forms:

Yes/no ____
Who ____
What ____
What do/did ____
When ____
Where ____
How ____
Why (How come) ____

Part III

Record utterance number for each example noted in the language sample.

Two-Word-Utterance Level:

Comment + Topic ____
Topic + Comment ____

Possessive + X:

Noun ____
Pronoun ____

Agent/Experiencer/
  Entity + Action/ Process/ Stative ———
Action/Process/
  Stative + Object/Complement ———
Agent/Experiencer
  +Object/Complement/Entity ———
Agent/Object/
  Action/Entity + Location ———
X + Modifier:
  Existence/Specification ———
  Attribution
    (shape/color, etc.) ———
  Recurrence ———
  Disappearance ———
Entity + Entity/
  Modifier/Location ———

Three-Word-Utterance Level:

Agent + Action + Object ———
Agent + Location + X ———
Action + Location + X ———
Agent + Action + Location ———
Entity + Stative + Location ———
Agent + Be + Location ———
Entity + Modifier + Entity ———

X + Possessive:
  noun ———
  pronoun ———

Negative + X:
  Nonexistence ———
  Rejection ———
  Denial ———

X + Time ———

  Note Others ———
———
———

Agent + Modifier + X ———
Action + Modifier + X ———
Entity + Stative +
  Modifier/Entity ———
Agent + Negative + X ———
Action + Negative + X ———
Note Others ———
———
———

Exhibit 6–6 continued

Four-Word-Utterance Level:

Agent + Action + Object + X	____	Entity + Stative + Entity + X	____
Agent + Action + X + X	____	Agent + Action + Location + X	____
Entity + Stative + Modifier + X	____	Negation + X, etc. (at 4-word level)	____
Entity + Stative + Location + X	____	Note Others:	____
			____
			____

Record below additional examples not indicated on this form:

Successive Utterances:

List utterance number and specify level (two-, three-, four-, etc., word utterance) for each successive utterance.

Questions:

List utterance number and specify level (two-, three-, four-, etc., word utterance) for each question used.

Statements as questions:

Use of wh-questions:

(Example – wh + action/agent/location, etc.)

AN EXAMPLE OF A LANGUAGE SAMPLE ANALYSIS USING BEAR

The following language sample is an example of a narrative recording made by an observer in the nursery classroom over a 90-minute period. The sample is from Daphne, a hearing-impaired girl, aged 3 years, 2 months, with a bilateral sensorineural loss in the moderate-to-severe range. The exact cause of deafness is unknown, but Daphne's medical history presents a pattern of severe middle-ear and respiratory infections from the age of 4 weeks. She has worn binaural ear-level amplification since the diagnosis of hearing loss at 19 months of age. She has attended parent-infant or nursery school since that time. This sample illustrates the format presently in use at the University of Virginia for children enrolled in preschool programs and also those receiving evaluation services through the center.

The narrative recording, presented in Exhibit 6–7, must reflect exactly the context, stimulus, observed response, and related behavior in the observed situation. The language responses of the observed child should be recorded verbatim, or, if sign language is used, the exact signs should be noted. The use of cues and signs by the stimulus "speaker" should also be correctly noted. In this particular case, the child is using an aural/oral communication mode.

Following the narrative recording, the following elements in Daphne's language sample analysis are presented: the syntactic and semantic analysis of the language sample (Exhibit 6–8), the BEAR summary sheet (Exhibit 6–9), the snytactic/morphological analysis summary (Exhibit 6–10), the phonological analysis summary (Exhibit 6–11), and the semantic/pragmatic analysis summary (Exhibit 6–12).

Exhibit 6–7 Narrative Recording of a Language Sample from Daphne C. Kent

Setting	*Stimulus*	*Linguistic Response*	*Related Behavior*
Daphne walks into classroom. Teacher greets her and admires child's new coat.	Hi, Daphne. Is that a new coat?	1) Mommy buyed coat. MɔmI bad kot	Smiles and nods head to teacher.
	Very pretty. Let's hang up your new coat right here.	2) Me hang up mIɛ ng ʌp 3) Up, up here ʌp,ɛp h	Takes off coat and hangs it on hook marked with her name.
Teacher leaves to greet other children entering room.		4) My coat ma kot	Hugs and pats coat on hook.
Daphne admires her new coat.		5) Pretty coat pItI kot	
Daphne walks to child looking at a picture book of animals (child with normal hearing, age 3–6).	Daphne, look at the cow.	6) Where cow? whɛ kow	Sits next to child and looks at book.
Child points to picture of cow.	Right here.	7) No cow no kow 8) That horsey! dad hotI	Giggles at her "joke."

Exhibit 6–7 continued

Setting	*Stimulus*	*Linguistic Response*	*Related Behavior*
	It is not! It's a cow. Can't you tell?	9) No cow, horsey no kow, hotI	Gets up and walks away w/grin.
Teacher calls children to semicircle of chairs at one corner of the room.	OK, everybody come and sit down.	10) Me sit down now mI tI dow now	Walks to chair with her name and sits down.
Teacher holds up pictures of each child in class one at a time. Asks "Who is this?"			
Daphne ignores first picture and question.	Daphne, watch me, please.	11) Me watch mI w ɔ d	Nods head and returns attention to teacher.
	Paul, you watch too.	12) You watch ʊ w ɔ d	Looks at child next to her and points to teacher.
Teacher continues.	OK, everyone watch and listen. Who is this?	13) Billy BIwI	Waves hands in the air.
		14) Billy here? BIwIh	Looks around circle for Billy.
		15) No Billy no BIwI	Shakes head "no."
	Billy's not here today.	16) Him home Im om	

	Who is this?	17) Me, me, me mI, mI, mI 18) That's me daed mI	Waves hand.
	Put your picture up, D.	19) Me putted up mI pʊdʌd ʌp	Hangs picture on chart and returns to chair.
Outdoor play on the playground. Daphne runs for a swing, but other children reach them first.		20) Hey, no you swing he, no ʊ wIng	
		21) My turn ma t ʌ n	Voice becomes loud and angry.
		22) My swing ma wIng	
		23) Get off g ɔ f	Shakes fist at boy on swing.
Teacher comes over.	Daphne you can swing in a little while. Let them finish.	24) Me swing now! mI wIng now	

Exhibit 6–7 continued

Setting	*Stimulus*	*Linguistic Response*	*Related Behavior*
		25) You bad kid ʊ baed kId	Yells to boy on "her" swing.
Teacher stoops down to comfort Daphne.	You can swing later. Let's play in the sandbox for now.	26) No, no, no	
		27) Me swing mI wIng	
		28) No sandbox play no naenb ɔpe	
		29) Go 'way go we	Sits on ground with arms folded across chest and pouts.
Teacher walks away.	Ok, pout if you want to.	30) Bad baed	Pouts for a moment, then lies back on ground and "sings" to herself.
Snack time. Children are seated around a horseshoe table. Teacher has a basket with cookies and a	Look what I have.	31) ooooooooooo	Claps her hands.
		32) Cookie k ʊ kI	

container of juice on a tray.		33) Me want two cookie mI wɔ n t ʊ k ʊ kI	Holds up two fingers.
Child next to Daphne turns to her.	You gotta say "please" or no cookies for you.	34) Please cookie me pI k ʊ kI mI	
		35) Two cookie please k ʊ kI pI	
Teacher gives Daphne two cookies.	Good girl, Daphne. Here are two cookies for you.		
	Do you want juice?	36) Juice please ʊ pI	Nods head and holds out cup.
	Say "juice" pretty for me.	37) u	
	Very good.		
		38) Red juice w ɛ d u	
		39) What red juice? wha w ɛ d u	Looks in her cup, then at teacher.
	That's cranberry juice. It's red and it tastes very good. Drink some.	40) Red juice w ɛ d u	Looks skeptically at teacher and takes a small sip.

Exhibit 6–7 continued

	Is it good? Do you like that juice?	41) Good juice gʊ ʊ u	Nods head and finishes cup of juice.
		42) Me like red juice mI lak wɛ d u	
		43) More please mo pI	
		44) See all gone tI a g ɔ n	Holds up empty cup upside down.
		45) All gone juice a g ɔ n u	
		46) No more red no mo wɛ d	
Teacher aide is working with Daphne with a large puzzle board.	Ok, Daphne, let's take all the pieces out. We have four big pieces.	47) Out—ok ou—ode	Takes pieces out with both hands.
		48) All out a ou	
Aide points to apple piece.	What is this?	49) Apple aepo	

		50) Apple in? aepo In	Picks up puzzle piece and begins to put it in place.
	Right, you put the apple in.	51) Apple in now aepo In now	Pats puzzle piece in place.
		52) Me good girl mI g u g ɛ	Smiles at aide and leans back in chair.
Aide points to another piece.	Ok, what's this?	53) No	Shakes head.
		54) You what this. ʊ wha dI	Points to aide.
	No, you tell me.	55) No, you turn no ʊ t ʌ n	Leans elbows on table and grins.
Aide places puzzle piece.	It's my turn? Ok, it's an orange, and it goes here.	56) Good girl g ʊ g ɛ	Pats aide's hand.
		57) My turn ma t ʌ n	Picks puzzle piece shaped like a banana.
		58) Me know mI no	Places puzzle piece correctly.
		59) Banana nana	

Exhibit 6–7 continued

Aide points to last puzzle piece.	Very good. One more. What's this?	60) No	Shakes head.
		61) You turn ʊ t ʌ n	Points to aide.
	My turn again. This is a grape.	62) Grape? gep	
		63) No grape no gep	Takes puzzle piece from aide and places piece correctly in puzzle board. Voice displays impatience with aide.
		64) That pear. daed pe	

Exhibit 6–8 Syntactic and Semantic Analysis: Language Sample from Daphne C. Kent

SYNTACTIC AND SEMANTIC ANALYSIS OF THE LANGUAGE SAMPLE

Restrictions	*Syntactic and Semantic Rules*	*Transformations*
1. R.F. s/m: irreg past tense R.F. omission: art	P N + VT_1 + ccsn Mommy buyed coat Agent + action/causative + obj	
2. R.F. s/m: pron case (obj/subj) R.F. omission: modal or Q M noun or pron	pron 1st VT_2 + prt Me hang up Agent + action causative	
3.	adv pl UP, up, up here Location	
4.	pron poss 1st + ccsn My coat Possession + entity	T poss
5.	adj + ccsn Pretty coat Quality + entity	T adj
6. R.F. omission: form of "be" art (def)	wh-quest + ccsn Where cow? Wh-quest + entity	T wh/pl
7. R.F. misuse/pattern: That's not or That's no	neg + ccsn No cow Denial + entity	T neg
8. R.F. omission: form of "be" art (indef)	D_2/del + ccsn That horsey Specification + entity	
9. R.F. misuse/pattern: No. 7 or That's a__, not a__	No. 7 ccsn No cow, horse No. 7 entity Inferred specification	
10. R.F. s/m: pron case (obj/subj)	pron 1st + VI + prt + adv t Me sit down now Agent + action affect + time	

Exhibit 6–8 continued

	Restrictions	*Syntactic and Semantic Rules*	*Transformations*
11.	R.F. s/m: pron case (obj/subj) R.F. omission: modal or be+ ing	pron 1st + VI Me watch Experiencer + process affect	
12.		pron 2nd subj + VI You watch No. 11	T imp
13.		P N Billy Entity	
14.	R.F. omission: form of "be"	P N + adv pl Billy here? Entity + location (Inferred y/n quest)	Ty/n quest
15.		neg + P N No Billy Nonexistence (entity)	T neg
16.	R.F. s/m: Pron case (obj/ subj) R.F. omission: form of "be"	pron 1st + adv pl Him home Entity + location	
17.		pron 1st obj Me, me, me Entity	
18.	R.F. omission: form of be	D2 + 1st obj That me Spec + entity	
19.	R.F. s/m: Pron case-obj/ subj Past tense irreg verb	pron 1st subj + VI + adv pl Me putted up Agent + action affect + location	
20.	R.F. misuse/pattern: You can't . . . or, Don't you . . .	neg + pron 2nd subj + VI Hey, no you swing! Vocative + denial + agent + action affect	T neg

Exhibit 6–8 continued

Restrictions	*Syntactic and Semantic Rules*	*Transformations*
21. R.F. misuse/pattern: It's . . .	pos pron 1st + ccsn My turn Possession + entity	T poss
22.	No. 19 My swing No. 19	No. 19
23.	VI + prt Get off Action affect	T imp
24. R.F. s/m: pron case (obj/subj) R.F. omission: modal or QM	pron 1st + VI + adv t Me swing now agent + action affect + time	
25. R.F. omission: form of "be" art (indef.)	pron 2nd subj + adj + ccsn You bad kid Entity + quality + entity (equivalent)	T adj
26.	neg No, no, no rejection	T neg
27. R.F. s/m: pron case (obj/subj) R.F. omission: modal or QM	pron 1st + VI Me swing Agent + action affect	
28. R.F. misuse/pattern: syntactic order (I won't play in the sandbox)	neg + adv pl + VI No sandbox play Rejection + location + action affect	T neg
29.	VI + adv pl Go 'way Action affect	T imp
30.	adj Bad Quality	T adj
31.	Yaaa!	
32.	ccsn Cookie Entity	

Exhibit 6–8 continued

Restrictions	*Syntactic and Semantic Rules*	*Transformations*
33. R.F. s/m: pron case (obj/ subj) reg pl	pron 1st + VT + card # + ccsn Me want two cookie Experiencer + process causative + quantity + obj	
34. R.F. misuse/pattern: (You) give	ccsn + 3rd pron obj Please cookie me Obj + recipient	T imp
35. R.F. s/m: noun plural	# + ccsn Two cookie please. Quantity + obj. (cardinal #)	
36.	cncn Juice, please obj	
37.	Juice - cncn Entity	
38.	adj + cncn Red juice Quality entity (color)	T adj
39. R.F. omission: form of "be" demon (D_1)	Wh-quest + color (adj) + cncn What red juice? Wh-quest + color + entity	T wh/subj T adj
40.	Color (adj) + cncn Red juice Color + entity	T adj
41.	adj + cncn Good juice Quality + entity	T adj
42. R.F. s/m:	1st pron + VT + adj + cncn Me like red juice Experiencer + process causative + color + object	T adj
43.	adj More, please Recurrence	T adj

Exhibit 6–8 continued

Restrictions	Syntactic and Semantic Rules	Transformations
44. R.F. misuse/pattern: I am . . . . R.F. s/m: past tense reg form	(VI adj) See, finish Action affect, condition or quality	T imp
45.	All gone juice Disappearance (nonexistence)	
46.	No more red Disappearance (nonexistence)	
47.	adv pl Out, OK? Location	Ty/n (inferred)
48.	adj adv pl All out Quantity + adv pl	
49.	ccsn Apple Entity	
50. R.F. misuse/pattern: asking if apple should be placed in puzzle	ccsn + adv pl Apple in? Obj + location	Ty/n
51. R.F. omission: art R.F. omission: form of "be"	ccsn + adv-pl + advt Apple in now Entity + location + time	
52. R.F. s/m: Pron case (obj/subj) R.F. omission: form of "be"	pron 1st + adj + ccsn Me good girl Entity + quality + entity (equivalent)	T adj
53.	neg No Rejection	T neg
54. R.F. misuse/pattern: substitute quest form for command	pron 2nd subj + inference You what this Agent+ inferred: action causative + obj	T imp

Exhibit 6–8 continued

Restrictions	Syntactic and Semantic Rules	Transformations
55. R.F. s/m: Pron case (subj/ poss) R.F. misuse/pattern: neg It's not your turn	neg + pron. 2nd + ccsn No, you turn Denial + possession + entity	T poss T neg
56.	adj + ccsn Good girl Quality + entity	T adj
57.	pron 1st poss + ccsn My turn Poss + entity	T poss
58. R.F. s/m: Pron. case (obj/ subj)	pron 1st V_I Me know Experiencer + process affect	
59.	ccsn Banana Entity	
60.	neg No Denial	T neg
61. R.F. s/m: Pron case (subj/ poss)	pron 2nd poss + ccsn Your turn Poss + entity	T poss
62.	ccsn Grape? Question (entity)	Ty/n
63. R.F. misuse/pattern: neg That's not a pear	neg + ccsn No grape Denial + entity	T neg
64. R.F. omission: form of "be" art (indef)	D_2/del + ccsn That pear Specif + entity	

Exhibit 6–9 BEAR Summary Sheet: Language Sample from Daphne C. Kent

SUMMARY SHEETS FOR LANGUAGE SAMPLE ANALYSIS

BARE ESSENTIALS IN ASSESSING REALLY LITTLE KIDS
(BEAR)

Name Daphne C. Kent
Examiner Hasenstab/Laughton
Parents/Guardian M/M Chas. Kent
Address Box 6 Ruckersville, Va.
Referred by Routine Evaluation
Communication Mode Aural/Oral

Date of Birth 10/1/76
Date Tested 12/2/79
Phone (804) 555-3758
Informant __________
Age 3-2
Disability HI

Audiological Information:

Hearing Loss:
Bilateral sensory neural hearing loss in the moderate-to-severe range.

Date of Most Recent Evaluation:
11/15/79. See folder for full report.

Hearing Aid:
Binaural ear-level aids since 19 months of age—Audiotone 828S.

Etiology:
Unknown—Hearing loss suspected by parents at 15 months.

Comments:
Hearing loss diagnosed at 19 months followed by immediate fitting of aids. Monitored at 90-day intervals.

Medical Information:

Present Health:
Good

Medical History:
History of middle-ear infection since 6 months of age. See medical folder for details.

Exhibit 6–9 continued

Comments:

General history unremarkable except for above. Normal development in all areas to date except for language and speech.

Educational Information:

Present Placement:

University of Virginia Preschool for Hearing-Impaired and Language-Delayed Children—nursery level. Attends 5 days/ week for 3-hour sessions.

Assessment Results:

See McCarthy results 9/10/79 for details. All areas above mean except those related to language.

Comments:

Child was enrolled in Parent Infant Home Program from age 19 months to 23 months when she was transferred into the nursery level. Progress is continuous.

Language Information:

Present Status (General):

2/3-word-utterance level appropriate to context. Minimal gesturing. Generally intelligible speech. Consistent progress in development. Receptive language exceeds expressive (speech).

Other Language Evaluation Results:

See progress folder for all semester reports and individual therapy summaries. BEAR/CAPS indicates recognition of concepts through level I appropriate for chronological age.

Exhibit 6–10 Syntactic/Morphological Analysis Summary: Language Sample for Daphne C. Kent

SYNTACTIC/MORPHOLOGICAL ANALYSIS SUMMARY

I. One-Word Utterances

Record one-word utterances produced by the child. Please transcribe in both international phonetic alphabet (IPA) and standard English notation.

Child is beyond this level.

Comments:

II. Two-Word Utterances

Record the appropriate utterance example number from the sample transcription. Tally up to three (3) examples for each pattern represented.

N + V	11	12	27	V + N	__	__	29
N + N	__	__	__	V + Adv pl	__	__	__
N + Adj	__	__	__				
N + Adv pl	__	__	16	Yes/no quest	14	47	50+
				Wh-quest + X	__	6	36
Adj + N	5	38	40+	Neg + X	__	15	63

Exhibit 6–10 continued

III. Expansion Level I

Record the appropriate utterance example number from the sample transcription. Tally up to three (3) examples for each rule represented.

Structural Elements

		s	pl
PN			1 13 14+
CN			1 2 3+
Pron - subj		s	pl
	1	restricted	___ ___ ___
	2	12 ___ ___	___ ___ ___
	3	restricted	___ ___ ___
obj		s	pl
	1	___ ___ ___	___ ___ ___
	2	___ ___ ___	___ ___ ___
	3	___ ___ ___	___ ___ ___
Def art			restricted
Indef art			restricted
D1			
D2			8 64 ___
Ddel (specify D1 or D2)			___ ___ ___ 8 64 (D2)

Tense reg past	___ ___ ___
be + NP	___ ___ ___
be + adj	restricted
be + adv pl	___ ___ ___
V + ing	___ ___ ___
V + adv pl	29 ___ ___
V + adv t	10 24 51
V + adf	___ ___ ___
V + adv m	___ ___ ___

Comments: See following page.

Transformations

T neg	7 9 15+ some restr
T do	___ ___ ___
T contr	___ ___ ___
T conj (and)	___ ___ ___

		s	pl
T poss pron			
	1	4 21 22+	___ ___ ___
	2	restricted	___ ___ ___
	3	___ ___ ___	___ ___ ___
T pos noun			___ ___ ___
T pos/del pron			___ ___ ___
	1	___ ___ ___	___ ___ ___
	2	___ ___ ___	___ ___ ___
	3	___ ___ ___	___ ___ ___
T pos/del noun		___ ___ ___	___ ___ ___
		___ ___ ___	___ ___ ___
T there			___ ___ ___
T imp			11 23 29+
T got			___ ___ ___

T inv	___ ___ ___
T adj	5 25 38+
T yes/no	14 47 50
T wh-quest	___ ___ ___
Who	___ ___ ___
What	36 ___ ___
What-do	___ ___ ___
Where	6 ___ ___
When	___ ___ ___
How	___ ___ ___
How +	___ ___ ___
How come	___ ___ ___

IV. Expansion Level II

Structural Elements

N pl irreg	___ ___ ___	Tense irreg	___ ___ ___
Indef pron	___ ___ ___	M	___ ___ ___
No. card	35 33 ___	QM	___ ___ ___
ord	___ ___ ___	be + ing (aux)	___ ___ ___
		have + prt (aux)	___ ___ ___

Exhibit 6–10 continued

V + prt — — —
V + prt + move — — —
VI + comp — — —

Comments:

Restricted forms:
first person singular pronoun (obj/subj) No. 2 10 11+
third person singular pronoun (obj/subj) No. 16
irregular past tense verb No. 1
omission M/QM No. 2 10 11+
omission "be" No. 6 8 14+
omission article No. 6 8 23+
restricted neg No. 7 9 13+
noun plural regular + 31 33
word order No. 18 26 32+
second person singular possessive pronoun (subj/poss) No. 52 58

Transformations

T conj/del — — —
T conj II — — —
T tag quest — — —
T pronom — — —

TVT to + comp — — —
TVT to comp/del — — —
TVT ing + comp — — —
TVT ing + com/del — — —
TVT_3 + comp — — —

Trel
subj — — —
obj — — —
pos — — —
NM/subj — — —
NM/obj — — —

Trel/del — — —
Specify: — — —
T ind obj — — —
T ind obj/del — — —
T adv/clause
pl — — —
t — — —
m — — —

V. Expansion Level III

All structural elements are normally in use at this level.

Transformations			
T comp adj			___
T reflex		s	pl
	1	___	___
	2	___	___
	3	___	___
T tag			___
T sub			___
T elp			___
T conj III			___

Note specifically any other transformations occurring in the sample and record number of examples.

Comments:

Child exhibits no examples at this level.

Source: Based on form developed by Hannah, adapted by Suzanne Hasenstab.

Exhibit 6–11 Phonological Analysis Summary: Language Sample from Daphne C. Kent

PHONOLOGICAL ANALYSIS SUMMARY

General Description

A. Record and attach a brief statement regarding the general development of the child's vocalizations.

B. *At or below one-word-utterance level:* Record vowels and syllables produced.

Vowels	CV	CVC

C. *At two-word-utterance level and beyond:* Indicate phonemes used consistently and correctly in the sample. Note position of sound. A correctly articulated phoneme substituted for another in word context (/b/ for /p/ in puppy) is not considered correct application.

Vowels: Front	Vowels: Mid	Vowels: Back	Diphthongs
___ e/me	x u/cup	___ oo/food	x i/kite
x i/bit	___ er/mother	x oo/good	___ u/cute
x a/cake	___ ir/first	x o/coat	x oi/boil
x e/bed	___ ur/fur	x a/father	x ou/bout
x a/cat	___ ar/car	x o/hot	

Voiceless				Consonants Voiced				Nasals/Glides			
x	x	x	p	x	x	x	b	x	x	x	m
x			t*	x	x	x	d	x	x	x	n
x	x	x	k	x	x	x	g			x	ng
			f				v				
			th (thin				th (the)				
			s				z	1			l*
			sh				zh (treasure)				r
			wh					x			w
			ch				j				y
			h*								

*Omits in some contexts in positions not noted

Distinctive Feature Analysis

I. Feature analysis worksheet for children *at or below two-word-utterance level*

1. Record phonemes uttered.
2. Determine + and − features of phonemes.

Exhibit 6–11 continued

Phoneme	Times	Voice	Vocalic	Low	High	Back	Front/Ant.	Round	Tense/Cont.	Nasal	Conson.	Strident	Coronal

IIA. Feature analysis worksheet for children *beyond two-word-utterance level*

1. Record target phoneme and the number of times it is correctly produced (Column I).
2. Record substitutions and the number of times each occurs (Column II).
3. Record number of omissions and distortions (Column III).
4. Indicate + or − for each feature of target phoneme and substitutions.
5. Total across columns to determine number for correct feature use (Column IV).
6. Complete one sheet for each phoneme tested.

Feature	I Target Phoneme /r/ No. of Times Correct 0	II Substitutions /w/ No. of Times Used 5	III No. of Omissions 15 No. of Distortions	IV Total No. of Correct Feature Use
Voice	+	+		5
Vocalic	+	−		0
Low	−	−		5
High	−	+		0
Back	−	+		0
Anterior/front	−	−		5
Round	−	+		0
Tense/continuant	+	−		0
Consonantal	+	+		5
Nasal	−	−		5
Strident	−	−		5
Coronal	+	−		0

Exhibit 6–11 continued

IIA. Feature analysis worksheet for children *beyond two-word-utterance level*

1. Record target phoneme and the number of times it is correctly produced (Column I).
2. Record substitutions and the number of times each occurs (Column II).
3. Record number of omissions and distortions (Column III).
4. Indicate + or – for each feature of target phoneme and substitutions.
5. Total across columns to determine number for correct feature use (Column IV).
6. Complete one sheet for each phoneme tested.

Feature	I Target Phoneme /s/ No. of Times Correct 0	II Substitutions /t/ /n/ No. of Times Used 4 1	III No. of Omissions 14 No. of Distortions	IV Total No. of Correct Feature Use
Voice	–	– +		4
Vocalic	–	– –		5
Low	–	– –		5
High	–	– –		5
Back	–	– –		5
Anterior/Front	+	+ +		5
Round	–	– –		5
Tense/continuant	+	– +		1
Consonantal	+	+ +		5
Nasal	–	– +		4
Strident	+	– –		0
Coronal	+	+ +		5

IIA. Feature analysis worksheet for children *beyond two-word-utterance level*

1. Record target phoneme and the number of times it is correctly produced (Column I).
2. Record substitutions and the number of times each occurs (Column II).
3. Record number of omissions and distortions (Column III).
4. Indicate + or – for each feature of target phoneme and substitutions.
5. Total across columns to determine number for correct feature use (Column IV).
6. Complete one sheet for each phoneme tested.

Feature	I Target Phoneme /k/ No. of Times Correct 16	II Substitutions /d/ No. of Times Used 1	III No. of Omissions 1 No. of Distortions	IV Total No. of Correct Feature Use
Voice	–	+		16
Vocalic	–	–		17
Low	–	–		17
High	+	–		16
Back	+	–		16
Anterior/Front	–	+		16
Round	–	–		17
Tense/Continuant	–	–		17
Consonantal	+	+		17
Nasal	–	–		17
Strident	–	–		17
Coronal	–	+		16

Exhibit 6–11 continued

IIA. Feature analysis worksheet for children *beyond two-word-utterance level*

1. Record target phoneme and the number of times it is correctly produced (Column I).
2. Record substitutions and the number of times each occurs (Column II).
3. Record number of omissions and distortions (Column III).
4. Indicate + or – for each feature of target phoneme and substitutions.
5. Total across columns to determine number for correct feature use (Column IV).
6. Complete one sheet for each phoneme tested.

Feature	I Target Phoneme /t s/ No. of Times Correct 0	II Substitutions /d/ No. of Times Used 2	III No. of Omissions 0 No. of Distortions	IV Total No. of Correct Feature Use
Voice	–	+		0
Vocalic	–	–		2
Low	–	–		2
High	+	–		0
Back	–	–		2
Anterior/Front	–	+		0
Round	–	–		2
Tense/Continuant	–	–		2
Consonantal	+	+		2
Nasal	–	–		2
Strident	+	–		0
Coronal	+	+		2

IIA. Feature analysis worksheet for children *beyond two-word utterance level*

1. Record target phoneme and the number of times it is correctly produced (Column I).
2. Record substitutions and the number of times each occurs (Column II).
3. Record number of omissions and distortions (Column III).
4. Indicate + or – for each feature of target phoneme and substitutions.
5. Total across columns to determine number for correct feature use (Column IV).
6. Complete one sheet for each phoneme tested.

Feature	I Target Phoneme /ð/ No. of Times Correct 0	II Substitutions /d/ No. of Times Used 4	III No. of Omissions 0 No. of Distortions	IV Total No. of Correct Feature Use
Voice	+	+		4
Vocalic	–	–		4
Low	–	–		4
High	–	–		4
Back	–	–		4
Anterior/Front	+	+		4
Round	–	–		4
Tense/Continuant	+	–		0
Consonantal	+	+		4
Nasal	–	–		4
Strident	–	–		4
Coronal	+	+		4

Exhibit 6–11 continued

IIA. Feature analysis worksheet for children *beyond two-word-utterance level*

1. Record target phoneme and the number of times it is correctly produced (Column I).
2. Record substitutions and the number of times each occurs (Column II).
3. Record number of omissions and distortions (Column III).
4. Indicate + or − for each feature of target phoneme and substitutions.
5. Total across columns to determine number for correct feature use (Column IV).
6. Complete one sheet for each phoneme tested.

Feature	I Target Phoneme /t/ No. of Times Correct 8	II Substitutions /d/ No. of Times Used 4	III No. of Omissions 6 No. of Distortions	IV Total No. of Correct Feature Use
Voice	−	+		8
Vocalic	−	−		12
Low	−	−		12
High	−	−		12
Back	−	−		12
Anterior/Front	+	+		12
Round	−	−		12
Tense/Continuant	−	−		12
Consonantal	+	+		12
Nasal	−	−		12
Strident	−	−		12
Coronal	+	+		12

IIA. Feature analysis worksheet for children *beyond two-word-utterance level*

1. Record target phoneme and the number of times it is correctly produced (Column I).
2. Record substitutions and the number of times each occurs (Column II).
3. Record number of omissions and distortions (Column III).
4. Indicate + or – for each feature of target phoneme and substitutions.
5. Total across columns to determine number for correct feature use (Column IV).
6. Complete one sheet for each phoneme tested.

Feature	I Target Phoneme /l/ No. of Times Correct 1	II Substitutions /w/ /o/ No. of Times Used 3 3	III No. of Omissions 10 No. of Distortions	IV Total No. of Correct Feature Use
Voice	+	+ +		7
Vocalic	+	– +		4
Low	–	– – (mid)		7
High	–	+ –		4
Back	–	+ +		1
Anterior/Front	+	– –		1
Round	–	+ +		1
Tense/Continuant	+	– +		4
Consonantal	+	+ –		4
Nasal	–	– –		7
Strident	–	– –		7
Coronal	+	– –		1

Exhibit 6–11 continued

IIA. Feature analysis worksheet for children *beyond two-word-utterance level*

1. Record target phoneme and the number of times it is correctly produced (Column I).
2. Record substitutions and the number of times each occurs (Column II).
3. Record number of omissions and distortions (Column III).
4. Indicate + or − for each feature of target phoneme and substitutions.
5. Total across columns to determine number for correct feature use (Column IV).
6. Complete one sheet for each phoneme tested.

Feature	I Target Phoneme /i/ No. of Times Correct 0	II Substitutions /I/ No. of Times Used 30	III No. of Omissions 0 No. of Distortions	IV Total No. of Correct Feature Use
Voice	+	+		30
Vocalic	+	+		30
Low	−	−		30
High	+	+		30
Back	−	−		30
Anterior/Front	+	+		30
Round	−	−		30
Tense/Continuant	+	−		0
Consonantal	−	−		30
Nasal	−	−		30
Strident	−	−		30
Coronal	−	−		30

IIA. Feature analysis worksheet for children *beyond two-word-utterance level*

1. Record target phoneme and the number of times it is correctly produced (Column I).
2. Record substitutions and the number of times each occurs (Column II).
3. Record number of omissions and distortions (Column III).
4. Indicate + or – for each feature of target phoneme and substitutions.
5. Total across columns to determine number for correct feature use (Column IV).
6. Complete one sheet for each phoneme tested.

Feature	I Target Phoneme /u/ No. of Times Correct 5	II Substitutions /ʊ/ No. of Times Used 7	III No. of Omissions 0 No. of Distortions 2	IV Total No. of Correct Feature Use
Voice	+	+		14
Vocalic	+	+		14
Low	–	–		14
High	+	+		14
Back	+	+		14
Anterior/Front	–	–		14
Round	+	+		14
Tense/Continuant	+	–		5
Consonantal	–	–		14
Nasal	–	–		14
Strident	–	–		14
Coronal	–	–		14

Exhibit 6–11 continued

IIB. Feature analysis worksheet for children *beyond two-word-utterance level*

1. Record target feature.
2. Record phonemes in which feature is present: +I for + feature, −I for − feature.
3. Record possible occurrences from Worksheet IIA.: +II for + feature, −II for − feature.
4. Record correct occurrences from Worksheet IIA: +III for + feature, −III for − feature.
5. Total columns for possible occurrences (PO) and correct occurrences (CO) (+ and −).
6. Calculate percentages:

   % correct: CO divided by PO = % correct

   % incorrect: 100 − % correct = % incorrect

+I Phonemes	+ II Possible Occurrences	+III Correct Occurrences	−I Phonemes	−II Possible Occurences	−III Correct Occurrences
r	5	5	s	5	5
ð	4	4	k	17	17
l	7	7	tʃ	2	0
i	30	30	t	12	8
u	14	14			
	Total 64	Total 64		Total 36	Total 30

% Correct 100%
% Incorrect 0%

% Correct 83%
% Incorrect 17%

Feature: Voice

IIB. Feature analysis worksheet for children *beyond two-word-utterance level*

1. Record target feature.
2. Record phonemes in which feature is present: +I for + feature, −I for − feature.
3. Record possible occurrences from Worksheet IIA.: +II for + feature, −II for − feature.
4. Record correct occurrences from Worksheet IIA.: +III for + feature, −III for − feature.
5. Total columns for possible occurrences (PO) and correct occurrences (CO) (+ and −).
6. Calculate percentages:

   % correct: CO divided by PO = % correct

   % incorrect: 100 − % correct = % incorrect

+I Phonemes	+II Possible Occurrences	+III Correct Occurrences	−I Phonemes	−II Possible Occurrences	−III Correct Occurrences
r	5	0	s	5	5
l	7	4	k	17	17
i	30	30	tʃ	2	2
u	14	14	ð	4	4
			t	12	12
	Total 56	Total 48		Total 40	Total 40

% Correct 86%
% Incorrect 14%

% Correct 100%
% Incorrect 0%

Feature: Vocalic

Exhibit 6–11 continued

IIB. Feature analysis worksheet for children *beyond two-word-utterance level*

1. Record target feature.
2. Record phonemes in which feature is present: +I for + feature, −I for − feature.
3. Record possible occurrences from Worksheet IIA.: +II for + feature, −II for − feature.
4. Record correct occurrences from Worksheet IIA.: +III for + feature, −III for − feature.
5. Total columns for possible occurrences (PO) and correct occurrences (CO) (+ and −).
6. Calculate percentages:

   % correct: CO divided by PO = % correct

   % incorrect: 100 − % correct = % incorrect

+I Phonemes	*+II Possible Occurrences*	*+III Correct Occurrences*	*−I Phonemes*	*−II Possible Occurrences*	*−III Correct Occurrences*
			r	5	5
			s	5	5
			k	17	17
			tʃ	2	2
			ð	4	4
			t	12	12
			l	7	7
			i	30	30
			u	14	14
	Total ____	Total ____		Total 96	Total 96

% Correct ______ | % Correct 100%

% Incorrect ______ | % Incorrect 0%

Feature: Low

IIB. Feature analysis worksheet for children *beyond two-word-utterance level*

1. Record target feature.
2. Record phonemes in which feature is present: +I for + feature, −I for − feature.
3. Record possible occurrences from Worksheet IIA.: +II for + feature, −II for − feature.
4. Record correct occurrences from Worksheet IIA.: +III for + feature, −III for − feature.
5. Total columns for possible occurrences (PO) and correct occurrences (CO) (+ and −).
6. Calculate percentages:

   % correct: CO divided by PO = % correct

   % incorrect: 100 − % correct = % incorrect

+I Phonemes	+II Possible Occurrences	+III Correct Occurrences	−I Phonemes	−II Possible Occurrences	−III Correct Occurrences
k	17	16	r	5	0
tʃ	2	0	s	5	5
i	30	30	ð	4	4
u	14	14	t	12	12
			l	7	4
	Total 63	Total 60		Total 33	Total 25

% Correct 95%*   % Correct 76%

% Incorrect 5%   % Incorrect 24%

*This percentage of correct occurrences is somewhat misleading since the substitutions for /i/ and /u/ are /I/ and /ʊ/, respectively, which depart from the target phoneme in *degree* of highness.

Feature: High

Exhibit 6–11 continued

IIB. Feature analysis worksheet for children *beyond two-word-utterance level*

1. Record target feature.
2. Record phonemes in which feature is present: +I for + feature, −I for − feature.
3. Record possible occurrences from Worksheet IIA.: +II for + feature, −II for − feature.
4. Record correct occurrences from Worksheet IIA.. +III for + feature, −III for − feature.
5. Total columns for possible occurrences (PO) and correct occurrences (CO) (+ and −).
6. Calculate percentages:

   % correct: CO divided by PO = % correct

   % incorrect: 100 − % correct = % incorrect

+I Phonemes	+II Possible Occurrences	+III Correct Occurrences	−I Phonemes	−II Possible Occurrences	−III Correct Occurrences
k	17	16	r	5	0
u	14	14	s	5	5
			tʃ	2	2
			ð	4	4
			t	12	12
			l	7	1
			i	30	30
	Total 31	Total 30		Total 65	Total 54

% Correct 99%
% Incorrect 1%

% Correct 83%
% Incorrect 17%

Feature: Back

IIB. Feature analysis worksheet for children *beyond two-word-utterance level*

1. Record target feature.
2. Record phonemes in which feature is present: +I for + feature, −I for − feature.
3. Record possible occurrences from Worksheet IIA.: +II for + feature, −II for − feature.
4. Record correct occurrences from Worksheet IIA.: +III for + feature, −III for − feature.
5. Total columns for possible occurrences (PO) and correct occurrences (CO) (+ and −).
6. Calculate percentages:
   % correct: CO divided by PO = % correct
   % incorrect: 100 − % correct = % incorrect

+I Phonemes	+II Possible Occurrences	+III Correct Occurences	−I Phonemes	−II Possible Occurrences	−III Correct Occurrences
s	5	5	r	5	5
ð	4	4	k	17	16
t	12	12	tʃ	2	0
l	7	1	u	14	14
i	30	30			
	Total 58	Total 52		Total 38	Total 35

% Correct 90%
% Incorrect 10%

% Correct 92%
% Incorrect 8%

Feature: Anterior/Front

Exhibit 6–11 continued

IIB. Feature analysis worksheet for children *beyond two-word-utterance level*

1. Record target feature.
2. Record phonemes in which feature is present: +I for + feature, −I for − feature.
3. Record possible occurrences from Worksheet IIA.: +II for + feature, −II for − feature.
4. Record correct occurrences from Worksheet IIA.: +III for + feature, −III for − feature.
5. Total columns for possible occurrences (PO) and correct occurrences (CO) (+ and −).
6. Calculate percentages:

   % correct: CO divided by PO = % correct

   % incorrect: 100 − % correct = % incorrect

+I Phonemes	+II Possible Occurrences	+III Correct Occurrences	−I Phonemes	−II Possible Occurrences	−III Correct Occurrences
u	14	14	r	5	0
			s	5	5
			k	17	17
			tʃ	2	2
			ð	4	4
			t	12	12
			l	7	1
			i	30	30
	Total 14	Total 14		Total 82	Total 71

% Correct 100 %
% Incorrect 0 %

% Correct 87%
% Incorrect 13%

Feature: Round

IIB. Feature analysis worksheet for children *beyond two-word-utterance level*

1. Record target feature.
2. Record phonemes in which feature is present: +I for + feature, −I for − feature.
3. Record possible occurrences from Worksheet IIA.: +II for + feature, −II for − feature.
4. Record correct occurrences from Worksheet IIA.: +III for + feature, −III for − feature.
5. Total columns for possible occurrences (PO) and correct occurrences (CO) (+ and −).
6. Calculate percentages:

    % correct: CO divided by PO = % correct

    % incorrect: 100 − % correct = % incorrect

+ Phonemes	+II Possible Occurrences	+III Correct Occurrences	−I Phonemes	−II Possible Occurrences	−III Correct Occurrences
r	5	0	k	17	17
s	5	1	tʃ	2	2
ð	4	0	t	12	12
l	7	4			
i	30	0			
u	14	5			
	Total 65	Total 10		Total 31	Total 31

% Correct 15% % Correct 0%

% Incorrect 85% % Incorrect 100%

Feature: Tense/Continuant

Exhibit 6–11 continued

IIB. Feature analysis worksheet for children *beyond two-word-utterance level*

1. Record target feature.
2. Record phonemes in which feature is present: +I for + feature, −I for − feature.
3. Record possible occurrences from Worksheet IIA.: +II for + feature, −II for − feature.
4. Record correct occurrences from Worksheet IIA.: +III for + feature, −III for − feature.
5. Total columns for possible occurrences (PO) and correct occurrences (CO (+ and −).
6. Calculate percentages:

   % correct: CO divided by PO = % correct

   % incorrect: 100 − % correct = % incorrect

+I Phonemes	+II Possible Occurrences	+III Correct Occurrences	−I Phonemes	−II Possible Occurrences	−III Correct Occurrences
r	5	5	i	30	30
s	5	5	u	14	14
k	17	17			
tʃ	2	2			
ð	4	4			
t	12	12			
l	7	4			
	Total 52	Total 49		Total 44	Total 44

% Correct 94% % Correct 100%

% Incorrect 6% % Incorrect 0%

Feature: Consonantal

IIB. Feature analysis worksheet for children *beyond two-word-utterance level*

1. Record target feature.
2. Record phonemes in which feature is present: +I for + feature, −I for − feature.
3. Record possible occurrences from Worksheet IIA.: +II for + feature, −II for − feature.
4. Record correct occurrences from Worksheet IIA.: +III for + feature, −III for − feature.
5. Total columns for possible occurrences (PO) and correct occurrences (CO) (+ and −).
6. Calculate percentages:

   % correct: CO divided by PO = % correct

   % incorrect: 100 − % correct = % incorrect

+I Phonemes	+II Possible Occurrences	+III Correct Occurrences	−I Phonemes	−II Possible Occurrences	−III Correct Occurrences
			r	5	5
			s	5	4
			k	17	17
			tʃ	2	2
			ð	4	4
			t	12	12
			l	7	7
			i	30	30
			u	14	14
	Total ______	Total ______		Total 126	Total 125

% Correct ______ % Correct 99%

% Incorrect ______ % Incorrect 1%

Feature: Nasal

Exhibit 6–11 continued

IIB. Feature analysis worksheet for children *beyond two-word-utterance level*

1. Record target feature.
2. Record phonemes in which feature is present: +I for + feature, –I for – feature.
3. Record possible occurrences from Worksheet IIA.: +II for + feature, –II for – feature.
4. Record correct occurrences from Worksheet IIA.: +III for + feature, –III for – feature.
5. Total columns for possible occurrences (PO) and correct occurrences (CO) (+ and –).
6. Calculate percentages:
   % correct: CO divided by PO = % correct
   % incorrect: 100 – % correct = % incorrect

+I Phonemes	+II Possible Occurrences	+III Correct Occurrences	–I Phonemes	–II Possible Occurrences	–III Correct Occurrences
s	5	0	r	5	5
tʃ	2	0	k	17	17
			ð	4	4
			t	12	12
			l	7	7
			i	30	30
			u	14	14
	Total 7	Total 0		Total 89	Total 89

% Correct 0%
% Incorrect 100%

% Correct 100%
% Incorrect 0%

Feature: Strident

IIB. Feature analysis worksheet for children *beyond two-word-utterance level*

1. Record target feature.
2. Record phonemes in which feature is present: +I for + feature, −I for − feature.
3. Record possible occurrences from Worksheet IIA.: +II for + feature, −II for − feature.
4. Record correct occurrences from Worksheet IIA.: +III for + feature, −III for − feature.
5. Total columns for possible occurrences (PO) and correct occurrences (CO) (+ and −).
6. Calculate percentages:
   % correct: CO divided by PO = % correct
   % incorrect: 100 − % correct = % incorrect

+I Phonemes	+II Possible Occurrences	+III Correct Occurrences	−I Phonemes	−II Possible Occurrences	−III Correct Occurrences
r	5	0	k	17	16
s	5	5	i	30	30
tʃ	2	2	u	14	14
ð	4	4			
t	12	12			
l	7	1			
	Total 35	Total 24		Total 61	Total 60

% Correct 69%
% Incorrect 31%

% Correct 98%
% Incorrect 2%

Feature: Coronal

Exhibit 6–11 continued

Summary of Feature Production Information

Feature	+ % Correct	– % Correct
Voice	100	83
Vocalic	86	100
Low	—	100
High	95* (32%)	76
Back	99	83
Anterior/front	90	92
Round	100	87
Tense/continuant	15	100
Consonantal	94	100
Nasal	—	99
Strident	0	100
Coronal	69	98

Comments:

Analysis indicates that the target features to emphasize with Daphne would be –high, +coronal, +continuant/tense, +strident. The feature + high is misleading in percentage of correct utterances due to the fact that she substitutes /I/ for /i/ and /ʊ/ for /u/, whereas these vary only in degree of height of tongue. A more realistic percentage would be 32%. Order of emphasis would be the contrast of high feature + and –, the + coronal, and + tense/continuant. The strident feature comes later in phonological development and therefore should not be emphasized at this time.

III. Phonotactic Processes
1. Note examples of the phonotactic processes.
2. Record example phonetically (IPA) and in standard American English (SAE) notation.
3. Indicate utterance number.

Variations	Examples IPA	Examples SAE	Utterance No.
Reduplication	nana	banana	59
	no no no	no no no	26
	mI mI mI	me me me	17
	ʌ p ʌ p ʌ p	up up up	3
Simplification	sI	sit	10
	dou	down	10
	naenbɔ	sandbox	28
	mo	more	43, 46
	gʊ	good	52, 56
	gɛ	girl	52, 56
	dI	this	54
	pɛ	pear	64
	wa	what	39, 54
	μ	juice	36, 37, 42, 45
	pI	please	34, 35, 36, 43
	wɛ	where	6
	hɛ	here	3, 14

Exhibit 6–11 continued

Consonant cluster reduction	pItI	pretty	5
	w ɔ d	watch	11, 12
	wIng	swing	20, 21, 24, 27
	p ɛ	play	28
	w ɔ n	want	33
	pI	please	34, 36, 43
	aepo	apple	49, 50, 51
Voicing	gep	grape	62, 63
No voicing demonstrated in this sample.			
Weak syllable deletion			
	naenb ɔ	sandbox	28
	nana	banana	59
Diminutive	m ɔ mI	mommy	1
	hotI	horsey	8, 9
Assimilation:			
Forward	p ʊ d ʌ d	putted	19
	naenb ɔ	sandbox	28
Backward	daed	that	8, 18, 65
Fronting	ode	okay	47

Glide/liquid substitution			
	BIwI	Billy	13, 14, 15
	w ε d	red	38, 39, 40, 42,46
Stop/fricative substitution			
	dI	this	54
	daed	that	8, 18, 65
	tI	see	4
	hotI	horsey	8
	tI	sit	10

Comments:

The phonotactic analysis indicates that the articulation errors displayed in this child's speech are developmental rather than deviant. Processes in greatest evidence are simplification and consonant cluster reduction.

Exhibit 6–12 Semantic/Pragmatic Analysis Summary: Language Sample from Daphne C. Kent

SEMANTIC/PRAGMATIC ANALYSIS SUMMARY

Part I

Indicate (√) number of examples of behaviors up to three at preverbal level. Indicate (√) number of examples of behavior up to three at one-word level, and record example as appropriate (example: Vocative - Hi).

Preverbal Level:

Communication behaviors:

Behavior				Behavior			
Crying	√			Jargon			
Gazing	√	√	√	Turn-taking	√	√	√
Facial expression	√	√	√	Touching	√	√	√
Posturing	√	√	√	Holding	√	√	
Vocal play	√	√	√	Tugging	√		
Pointing	√	√	√	Demonstrating	√	√	√
Gesturing	√	√	√	Asking	√	√	√
Babbling				Nodding (negation)	√	√	√

Cognitive/motor behaviors:

Behavior				Behavior			
Body image				Embedding			
Motor imitation				Categorization			
Object permanence				Relational concept			
Ordering							

[Child is beyond preverbal level. The behaviors indicated are used correctly at other language levels with verbalization, which is acceptable.]

One-Word-Utterance Level:

Communication behaviors:

Behavior				Behavior			
Imitation				Questioning	62		
Vocative (attention/greeting)				Demanding			
Protest	53			Description	30		
Labeling	32	49	59	Turn-maintaining			

(These behaviors are also evident at higher language levels for this child.)

Part II

Record the appropriate utterance example number from the sample transcription. Tally up to three (3) examples for each case represented.

Noun Cases:				*Modifier Cases:*			
Agent	1	2	10 +	Specification	8	18	64
Object	1	33	34 +	Existence	15		
Complement				Nonexistence			
Experiencer	11	12	33 +	Recurrence	43		
Recipient	34			Disappearance	44	45	46
Possessor				Condition/quality	5	25	41 +
Entity	4	5	6 +	Size			
Vocative	20			Shape			
				Color	39	40	42
				Age			

Exhibit 6–12 continued

Position				*Other:*			
Quantity	33	35		Rejection	28	26	53
Verb Cases:				Denial	7	9	20 +
Action/causative	1	2		Possession	4	21	22 +
Action/affect	10	19	24 +	*Question Forms:*			
Process/causative	33	42		Yes/No	14	47	62 +
Process/affect	11	12	58	Who			
Stative	inference only			What	39		
Adverbial Cases:				What do/did			
Location	3	14	16	When			
Time	10	24	51	Where	6		
Manner				How			
Frequency				Why (How come)			

Part III

Record utterance number for each example noted in the language sample.

Two-Word-Utterance Level:

Comment + Topic				Action/Process/Stative + Object/Complement			
Topic + Comment	36			Agent/Experiencer + Object/Complement/ Entity	34		
Agent/Experiencer/Entity + Action/Process/Stative	2	12	11 +				

Agent/Object/Action/Entity + Location	16	51	23
X + Modifier, Modifier + X:			
Existence/Specification	8	18	64
Attribution (shape/color, etc.)	25	5	38 +
Recurrence	43		
Disappearance	44	45	46
Entity + Entity/Modifier/ Location			
Possessive + X:			
noun			
pronoun	4	21	22 +
X + Possessive			
noun			
pronoun			
Negative + X:			
Nonexistence	15		
Rejection	26	28	53
Denial	7	20	55 +
X + Time:			
Note Others			
Three-Word-Utterance Level:			
Agent + Action/Process + Object	1	33	42 +
Agent + Location + X	51	10	
Action + Location + X			
Agent + Action + Location	19		
Entity + Stative + Location			
Entity + Modifier + Entity	inferred	only	
Agent + Modifier + X	52	25	
Action + Modifier + X	44		
Entity + Stative + Modifier/ Entity	25 (omits *be*)		
Agent + Negative + X			
Action + Negative + X			
Note Others:			
No. 24 Agent + Action + Time			
No. 39 Wh-quest + Modifier + Object			
Four-Word Utterance Level:			
Agent + Action + Object + X	33	42	
Agent + Action + X			
Entity + Stative + Modifier + X			
Entity + Stative + Location + X			
Entity + Stative + Entity + X			

Exhibit 6–12 continued

Agent + Action + Location + X	10	___	___
Negation + X, etc. (at 4-word level)	___	___	___

Note others:

No. 20 Vocative + neg + agent + action	___	___	___

Sentence Summary—Daphne

One-Word Utterances

9. Horse (successive utterance)
13. Billy
23. Getoff
30. Bad
32. Cookie
36. Juice (please)
37. Juice
43. More
44. See } successive
44. Finish } utterance
47. Out
49. Apple
53. No
55. No (successive utterance)
59. Banana
60. No
62. Grape?

Two-Word Utterances

2. Me hang up
4. My coat
5. Pretty coat
6. Where cow?
7. No cow .
8. That horsey
9. No cow (successive utterance)
11. Me watch
12. You watch
14. Billy here?
15. No Billy
16. Him home
18. That me
21. My turn
22. My swing
27. Me swing
29. Go 'way
35. Two cookie (please)
38. Red juice
40. Red juice
41. Good juice

45. Allgone juice
46. Nomore red
48. All out
50. Apple in
55. You turn (successive utterance)
56. Good girl
57. My turn
58. Me know
61. You turn
63. No grape
64. That pear

Three-Word Utterances

1. Mommy buyed coat
19. Me putted up

24. Me swing now
25. You bad kid
28. No sandbox play (successive utterance)
34. Please cookie me (successive utterance)
39. What red juice?
51. Apple in now
52. Me Good girl
54. You what this (successive utterance)

Four-Word Utterances

10. Me sit down now
20. Hey, no you swing
33. Me want two cookie
42. Me like red juice

Successive Utterances:

List utterance no. and specify level (two-, three-, four-, etc. word utterance) for each successive utterance.

Examples: boy girl
Mommy home cry
#9 No cow, horse (2 word + 1 word)
#28 No sandbox play
#34 Please cookie me
#44 See, finish (1 word + 1 word)
#54 You what this
#55 No, you turn (1 word + 2 word)

Exhibit 6–12 continued

Questions:

List utterance # and specify level (two-, three-, four-, etc. , word utterance) for each question used.

Statements as questions:

#14 Billy here?

#47 Out-ok? (request for affirmation of correct behavior)

#50 Apple in?

#62 Grape?

Use of wh-questions:

#6 Where cow? (wh/location + cow)

#39 What red juice? (wh/object + modifier + entity)

REFERENCES

Ault, R. *Children's cognitive development.* New York: Oxford University Press, 1977.

Axline, V. M. *Play therapy.* New York: Ballantine Books, 1947.

Bangs, T. E. *Vocabulary Comprehension Scale.* Boston, Mass.: Teaching Services Corporation, 1975.

Bates, E. *Language and context: The acquisition of pragmatics.* New York: Academic Press, 1976.

Bates, E., & Johnston, J. *Pragmatics in normal and deficient child language.* Paper presented at American Speech and Hearing Association annual convention, Chicago, 1977.

Bloom, L. *One word at a time: The use of single word utterances before syntax.* The Hague: Mouton, 1973.

Bloom, L., & Lahey, M. *Language development and language disorders.* New York: John Wiley & Sons, 1978.

Boehm, A. *Boehm Test of Basic Concepts.* New York: Psychological Corporation, 1971.

Brown, R. *A first language.* Cambridge, Mass.: Harvard University Press, 1973.

Cazden, C. The situation: A neglected source of social class differences in language use. *Journal of Social Issues,* 1970, *26,* 35–60.

Chafe, W. *Meaning and the structure of language.* Chicago: University of Chicago Press, 1970.

Chomsky, N., & Halle, M. *The sound pattern of English.* New York: Harper & Row, 1968.

deVilliers, J. G., & deVilliers, P. A. *Language acquisition.* Cambridge, Mass.: Harvard University Press, 1978.

Dore, J. A pragmatic description of early language development. *Journal of Psycholinguistic Research,* 1974, *3,* 343–350.

Englemann, S. *Basic Concept Inventory* (Field research ed.). Chicago, Ill.: Follett Educational Corporation, 1967.

Feagans, L. *Babbling in discourse: A way to skip the two-word utterance stage in language development.* Paper presented at the fourth annual Boston University Conference on Language Development, 1979.

Fillmore, C. The case for case. In E. Bach & J. Harms (Eds.), *Universals in linguistic theory.* New York: Holt, Rinehart, and Winston, 1976.

Greenfield, P., & Smith, H. *The structure of communication in early language development.* New York: Academic Press, 1976.

Hannah, E. *Applied linguistic analysis II.* Pacific Palisades, Calif.: Sencom, 1979.

Hannah, E., & Gardner, M. *Preschool Language Screening Test.* Northridge, Calif.: Joyce Publications, 1974.

Hargis, C. *English syntax.* Springfield, Ill.: Charles C Thomas, 1977.

Huttenlocher, J. The origins of language. In R. Solso (Ed.), *Theories in cognitive psychology.* New York: John Wiley & Sons, 1974.

Ingram, D. *Phonological disability in children.* New York: Elsevier, 1976.

Jakobson, R., Fant, C. G., & Halle, M. *Preliminaries to speech analysis.* Cambridge, Mass.: MIT Press, 1952.

Kagan, I., Rosman, B., Day, D., Albert, J., & Phillips, W. Information processing in the child. *Psychological Monographs,* 1964, *78* (1, Whole No. 578).

Kretschmer, R., & Kretschmer, L. *Language development and intervention with the hearing impaired*. Baltimore, Md.: University Park Press, 1978.

Lee, L. Developmental sentence types: A method for comparing normal and deviant syntactic development. *Journal of Speech and Hearing Disorders*, 1966, *31*, 311–330.

Lee, L. *Developmental sentence analyses*. Evanston, Ill.: Northwestern University Press, 1974.

Leonard, L. *Meaning in child language*. New York: Grune and Stratton, 1976.

McCarthy, D. Language development in children. In L. Carmichael (Ed.), *Manual of child psychology* (2nd ed.). New York: Wiley Publishers, 1954.

McReynolds, L., & Engmann, D. *Distinctive feature analysis of misarticulations*. Baltimore, Md.: University Park Press, 1975.

Menn, L. Phonotactic rules in beginning speech: A study in the development of English discourse. *Lingua*, 1971, *26*, 225–251.

Menyuk, P. *Sentences children use*. Cambridge, Mass.: MIT Press, 1969.

Muma, J. R. *Language handbook, concepts, assessment, intervention*. Englewood Cliffs, N.J.: Prentice-Hall, 1978.

Poole, I. Genetic development of articulation of consonant sounds in speech. *Elementary English Review*, 1934, *71*, 159–161.

Searle, J. *Speech acts*. London: Cambridge University Press, 1969.

Skarakis, E., & Prutting, C. Early communication: Semantic functions and communicative intentions in the communication of preschool children with impaired hearing. *American Annals of the Deaf*, 1977, *122*, 382–391.

Templin, M., and Darley, F. L. *The Templin-Darley Tests of Articulation* (2nd ed). Iowa City, Iowa: University of Iowa Bureau of Educational Research and Service, 1957.

Trantham, C., & Pedersen, J. *Normal language development*. Baltimore, Md.: Williams and Wilkins, 1976.

Tyack, D., & Gottsleben, R. *Language sampling, analysis and training: A handbook for teachers and clinicians*. Palo Alto, Calif.: Consulting Psychologists Press, 1974.

Winitz, H. *Articulation, acquisition and behavior*. New York: Appleton-Century-Crofts, 1969.

Part II

Intervention

Assessment in itself is incomplete. It must necessarily be seen as an initial step in an intervention program and as an integral part of ongoing educational programming. As indicated in the previous chapters, the purpose of assessment is to provide an informational foundation on which intervention can be based and a reference point for beginning programming. The purpose then expands to include provision for determining the progress of the child and the appropriateness of the program designed for that child.

The results of the assessment strategies already discussed, combined with intensive observation, provide guideline information for the development of an individualized program for each child, including long-range or general goals and more specific immediate objectives. Placement and scheduling needs must also be based on assessment information.

The remainder of this book will focus on educational intervention programming, or on what happens after initial assessment is completed. A central tenet to the purpose of educational programming is that, if educators, clinicians, or other related professionals are to provide the optimal learning environment for infants and preschool children with hearing impairment and/or language delay, assessment and educational practice must be intimately bound together.

As summarized by Northcott (1973), educational practice and management include the following provisions:

- parents, including guidance counseling and education
- listening, language, and speech procedures
- experiential inductive approaches to learning
- early amplification and management
- exposure to hearing children in an integrative setting

The focus of preschool intervention thus includes aspects of early intervention, early diagnosis of hearing loss or language delay, subsequent provision of amplification if necessary, parent training, and emphasis on the positive aspects of what a child can do and hear, in order that larger numbers of hearing-impaired and language-delayed children may be successfully placed in regular classrooms in the elementary school setting.

The results of effective infant and preschool intervention will be evidenced in kindergarten and the primary levels of the elementary school. Many children may be able to function in the regular academic setting with supplementary services, such as a modified curriculum, speech and language therapy, regular classroom teacher orientation, and educational support and instruction from a resource or itinerant teacher of the hearing impaired. The structure and format represented by the Comprehensive Services Program will, we hope, be beneficial to teachers and clinicians in any setting that provides services to infants and preschool children with hearing or language difficulties.

Chapter 7

Infancy

M. Suzanne Hasenstab

PRESCHOOL PROGRAMS

In the United States, education has traditionally begun at age 6 with entry into that memorable experience known as first grade, where the secrets of knowledge are revealed through the mastery of reading, 'riting and 'rithmetic. Gradually, in general education a concern for children before the first grade emerged. In an effort to provide a school-experience orientation and establish a "readiness" for academic subjects, kindergartens have become commonplace and, in some instances, are compulsory before formal entry into first grade.

Growth of Preschool Programs

Gradually over the past 40 years, concern for providing a school-oriented environment for children under age 6 has been nurtured, developed, and expanded by psychologists and educators. Efforts to alleviate the school problems related to poverty and early environmental deprivation were directed toward programs for preschool children that would provide early stimulation (Bereiter & Engelmann, 1974; Haring, 1976; Karnes, 1973; Parker, 1972). The premise on which these programs were based was that if a child could be exposed to stimulating learning experience through the early years, the necessity of requiring long-term special education services could be reduced. Early education was to be both remedial and preventive. This elaborated notion of education has now reached downward to include the period of infancy or, for the purposes of this text, the time between birth and about 30 months of age.

Preschool Services for Handicapped Children

Throughout the past 20 years, federal and state legislation, coupled with increased accountability in special education, has fostered an emphasis on locating and educating handicapped infants and preschool children under the age of 5. In November 1975, Public Law 94–142, the Education of All Handicapped Children's Act, was signed, This law stated that, as national policy, all handicapped children were entitled to a free and appropriate education. Further, by 1980, all handicapped children between the ages of 3 and 21 years were assured of the right to free public education, including special services appropriate to their needs.

Child Find programs have been initiated in many areas to locate children with disabilities who are not receiving services. Still, large numbers of preschool children and infants, estimated at roughly one million (Garwood, 1979), remain unidentified and/or unserved. Because federal legislation includes children beginning at age 3, a large proportion of these unserved children are included in the under-age-3 group. In some states, the age of eligibility for educational services from public schools extends to age 2. However, this still excludes infants with handicapping conditions from local educational services or free public education.

Preschool Programs for the Hearing Impaired

Specifically in the area of hearing impairment, there has been for some time an awareness of the crucial need for the earliest possible intervention. Programs such as the John Tracy Clinic have provided support and education for infants and preschool children and their parents, both at clinics and through correspondence programs.

Both center-based and home-based intervention programs, with services aimed at the population of hearing-impaired children under the age of 2½ years, emphasize parent participation through guidance and education (Hasenstab & McElroy, 1980; Horton, 1975; McConnell & Horton, 1970; Miller, 1970; Pollack, 1970). The role of the parent in programming, as well as goals related to parent "education," will be discussed later in this chapter.

Despite the awareness of the need for early intervention programming and existence of several well-designed and well-implemented facilities, far too many hearing-impaired children are still not being reached. At present, there is no nationwide, coordinated early-intervention system to determine high-risk neonates or the hearing status of babies at birth and shortly thereafter or to ensure that children at risk or those with evident hearing loss are referred to appropriate clinics and centers (Oyer & Hardick, 1976). The task of locating hearing-impaired infants still rests primarily with alert parents and knowledgeable pediatricians who are aware of the importance of early amplification and education. The field of pediatric intervention requires increased numbers of trained and qualified teachers, audiologists, support personnel, and programs designed for infants who demonstrate hearing and language difficulties.

THE PERIOD OF INFANCY

The first 24 to 30 months of an individual's life is known as the period of infancy. During this time, the child undergoes rapid changes in all areas of development. Except for adolescence, infancy is unrivaled as the period of most rapid growth in human life. From a virtually totally dependent being at birth, the normal child develops through infancy and emerges by age 2½ years as a mobile, social, communicating, thinking individual with a firm foundation for further growth and perfection of abilities.

We hold to the tenet in education and psychology that early experiences in life are capable of producing an effect on later development, although there is debate over the degree to which such influence is carried. As Kagan, Kearsley, and Zelazo (1979) point out, this premise is not new; it has in fact been assumed throughout our country's history, even 200 years ago. Thus, there is general agreement as to the importance of early experiences in infancy. As Caldwell (1974) notes, the early years of life are crucial in developing the child's cognitive, emotional, and social behaviors. Further, it is at this time that the environment exerts a maximum effect on the child's developmental potential. Hunt (1961) also stresses the importance of these very early months, especially if, with respect to the environment, the child is deprived in some way. With the hearing-impaired infant, such deprivation is evident in the lack of auditory stimulation from environmental experiences. Increased research on development in infancy and the results of various intervention strategies will provide much needed information regarding this period that is still to a great extent shrouded in mystery.

Theories of Development

In examining theories of developmental psychology, three general approaches or categories emerge: psychoanalytical, behavioristic, and cognitive. The absence of a single unifying theory is probably best explained by the fact that human development displays many facets. And, although these various facets interact, they exist independently enough to warrant separate study. Each theory, whether contemporary or now considered passé, tends to focus on one or two facets of development and does not attempt to explain the entire continuum of human behavior. For example, psychoanalytic theory attempts to explain how various states of emotion affect behavior and personality development. Behavioristic theory stems from a concern with learning and socialization. Finally, the cognitivists are largely concerned with the issue of thought as related to behavior.

In general, two theoretical positions have dominated the study of infant behavior. The first centers about the maturation of the child as a physiological being. This theory provided the foundation for the work of such pioneers in child development as Gesell and Thompson (1938) and Cattell (1940). Simply stated, this theoretical position states that the child's environment is relatively unimportant except for being generally attending and supporting. Maturation is considered to be inevitable, and heredity determines the outcome. On the other side of what has been termed the "nature-nurture controversy" are Watson and Watson (1928), perhaps the most radical in their pronouncements, and Skinner (1938, 1953). The foundation of this second orientation is the environment; this theory emphasizes the importance of experience in infancy. In fact, these two extreme emphases on heredity and environment have now been merged somewhat and are seen as cooperative elements in infant and child development. However, the exact degree and specific role of each factor is still the subject of interesting debate.

Various theories of development have been advanced throughout history. Some have exerted a profound effect on psychological and educational thought and practice; others have merely passed as fads. In the present text, it is neither possible nor desirable to present an exhaustive explanation of developmental theory. However, the teacher/clinician must be aware of the fact that theoretical tenets affect what is carried out in practice.

Freudian Theory

Freud's work (Brill, 1938) was primarily concerned with the development of personality from infancy to adulthood as related to psychosexual growth. Freud's infant personality was primitive, undeveloped, and simple. This early personality, labeled the *id,* encompasses basic or instinctive urges. From early infancy the id clashes with reality, and, according to Freud, the second level of personality emerges. This second level is called the *ego,* which appears at about 8 months of age. The baby begins to learn what is possible and what is not regarding the gratification of needs. The id and ego remain dominant through early childhood, until the *superego* emerges at about 6 years of age. This third level of development involves the ethical and moral aspects of personality and is concerned with social reality. In addition to the three levels of personality, Freud describes five stages in the psychosexual development of personality. Of the five, the first two, the oral phase and the anal stage , relate to infancy.

Although Freudian theory provides interesting reading and indeed may be helpful in understanding some aspects of personality, especially pathological or abnormal personality, the contemporary view of infancy is that there is more to this period than primitive, somewhat seething behavior.

Social Learning Theory

Bandura and Walters (1963) have attempted to explain what is termed *social learning* in children. Their theory is founded on the assumption that a great amount of social learning occurs through imitation. Further, the effects of imitation can be explained, based on the principles of operant conditioning. The three basics that underlie social learning theory are: (1) children imitate, (2) imitative behavior is considered operant, and (3) reinforcement often follows imitation.

Anyone who has spent time in the company of a very young child can attest to the fact that they do indeed imitate. The effects of imitation have been described by Bandura and Walters (1963) and Bandura (1969). The modeling effect, or the acquisition of new responses, has been applied to several aspects of child behavior, including the development of language. Although simplistic in this respect, this effect may account for some aspects of language learning. Further effects of imitation are evidenced in the inhibitory effect, the suppression of deviant behavior, and the disinhibitory effect, the appearance of previously suppressed deviant behavior. These particular effects center on the reward or punishment received by the model for certain behavior. Quite simply, with the inhibitory effect children may stop a certain behavior not because punishment is directed to them but because they observe a type of punishment being given to somebody else. On the other hand, reinforcement of another's behavior, which children may consider inappropriate for themselves, may still induce imitation of such behavior. This theory, which emphasizes observational learning, is helpful because children do imitate. But caution in its application is necessary until issues concerning the degree, amount, and types of learning are resolved.

Piagetian Theory

Though, as we have noted, numerous theories of development have been advanced to explain the process of change and growth from child to man, Piaget's theory of cognitive development has perhaps exerted the greatest influence on psychologists and educators who are concerned with infancy and development during preschool years. Although it has not been able to answer all the complex questions concerned with cognitive development in infancy, Piagetian theory has made us aware that infancy is a much more active period than previously believed.

Sensorimotor development. The period of infancy coincides with Piaget's sensorimotor stage, which is from birth to about age 2 or 3. However, at each of the Piagetian stages, the ages are approximations, and, as Lefrancois (1974) emphasizes, it is the order of appearance of behavior rather than the age that is important. The reflexes, or schemata, that a child is born with limit the child's world to the present. At first, objects exist only immediately; they cease to exist when they are out of the realm of the child's senses. In the beginning, the schemata are separate and discrete, but as the infant interacts with the environment in the period of infancy, they become coordinated and related. Soon, as the child develops a notion of object permanence, several activities can be coordinated and performed on a single object. Object permanence is the realization that objects continue to exist even when they are not a part of one's sensory awareness. In other words, objects have an identity of their own and are separate from the child and the behavior and activity of the child.

Substages of sensorimotor development. Piaget divides the period of sensorimotor development into six substages (Flavell, 1963). Each of these stages indicates how the infant reacts to and understands the world. Briefly, the six substages may be described as follows:

1. The period from birth to 1 month: The child exercises reflexes and behaviors with which the child was born. During this substage, the baby can execute only one activity at a time. For example, the child may visually attend to an attractive object within the sensory realm but cannot reach for it.
2. The period from 1 to 4 months: The notable behavior during this period is called primary circular reactions. These are behaviors that begin as accidental responses. However, these responses have the capacity to cause their own repetition; the response stimulates its repetition. Primary circular reactions center about the child's own body.
3. The period from 3 to 8 months: At this third substage, secondary circular reactions occur. Although similar in principle to primary circular reactions, they involve acting upon objects within the child's immediate environment rather than the child's own body.
4. The period from 8 to 12 months: Flavell (1963) notes two important developments during this fourth stage of the sensorimotor period. First, the infant masters the coordination of behaviors that were

initially unrelated, then uses these newly coordinated actions toward a particular goal. The child can successfully coordinate looking, grasping, and mouthing to get a toy into the mouth. This event signals the realization that objects can exist separate from an action. The second important development is the infant's recognition of an activity as a sign for an upcoming event. This is basic to an understanding of causality. For example, a baby at this stage anticipates being fed when placed by the parent in the high chair.

5. The period of 12 to 18 months: At this substage, more sophisticated circular reactions, called tertiary circular reactions, develop. The difference from earlier circular reactions lies in the modification the child employs to determine an effect. The behavior still causes its own repetition, but modifications are made for exploratory reasons. At this stage the child initiates truly active investigation of the environment.
6. The period from 18 to 24 months: The final substage of sensorimotor development serves as a transition period when the child begins truly to conceptualize the surrounding environment. This signals the move from the motoric and perceptual intelligence of the preceding stages to the more cognitive intelligence that characterizes the preoperational period in Piaget's theory.

Moral Development

Other theories have attempted to define various aspects in the development and manifestation of human behavior. Kohlberg (1964) has constructed six stages of value or moral development, extending from a punishment and obedience orientation, in which goodness or badness is based on physical consequences of behavior, to the universal ethical-principle orientation, in which what is right is defined on the basis of abstract and ethical ideas such as justice and respect for human dignity. The infant and really young child start at the first stage and will hopefully attain the sixth stage as an adult.

Societal Behavior

Erickson (1963) explains development in terms of societal expectations balanced with individual maturation. The individual passes through eight stages, beginning in infancy and reaching completeness in what is called maturity. Behavior is learned or adapted based on society's demands on the individual at various stages. If one does not conform to the demands of each succeeding stage, difficulties and unhappiness ensue. Although this is an interesting approach, it is much too simplistic to account for the complex interrelationships of individual and society.

Learning Theory

Operant conditioning. One basic form of learning has been described as operant conditioning. In this process, an action by the infant (or any other individual) is followed by some environmental alteration, which, if positive, is called a reinforcer. The effect of the reinforcer is to increase the response occurrence. Recent research demonstrates that even neonates can master an operant conditioning sequence. The nature and effectiveness of reinforcers constitute a large area of examination. What is reinforcing for an infant is not always reinforcing for a 3-year-old. Although some aspects of learning can be explained as operant conditioning, many more cannot. Thus, this paradigm must be regarded as only one facet contributing to learning.

Self-generated learning. Another facet of learning may be explained as problem-solving behavior manifested in infants. Investigations like those of Papousek (1967) indicate that motivation for learning, even in young infants, can stem from the activity of solving a problem in mastering a task. This view attributes considerable ingenuity to the infant and infers much concentration on active thinking.

Summary

Although the various theories relating to the multifactor questions of development, behavior, and learning fail to supply all the answers, they do provide some insight into the mysterious period of infancy. The evolution of theory and research investigations based on theory will continue to provide new information to assist the infant interventionist in the task of providing the environment and experiences that will be most conducive to the growth and development of the hearing- or language-handicapped child and increasing our knowledge regarding "normal" infants. Although the foregoing discussion of theory related to infancy is merely an overview, it should serve to illustrate that theory does indeed affect practice and, perhaps more important, the philosophic base from which one interacts with children.

DEVELOPMENT IN INFANCY

The newborn infant, although physically dependent on others for food, care, and protection, enters the world armed with particular responsive behaviors that assist in the adaptation to the new world. Within a few hours after birth, the baby is capable of visually tracking a moving object within its field of vision (Wertheimer, 1961). The child is auditorily sensitive (Eisenberg, 1969; Eisenberg, Griffin, Coursin, & Hunter, 1964). A sudden loud noise quickly produces a Moro reflex or startle response. Even an infant as young as 12 hours old can discriminate sound variation in consonants. Odors and tastes are salient to the newborn infant; the neonate responds instantly to touch. When the palm of a neonate's hand is touched, the Darwinian reflex or grasp occurs. A stroke across the sole of the foot will result in a Babinski reflex with upturned toes. A light touch on a baby's mouth or cheek produces a search for nourishment or rooting reflex.

Other reflexes or behaviors are crucial to the newborn's survival. For example, coughing, sneezing, and yawning are respiratory functions that assist in keeping air passages clear. The child turns its face to one side or the other to avoid smothering when placed on the stomach. Sucking of course is crucial to the intake of food, but it also tends to soothe the infant and to induce sleep. Reflexive crying is the infant's first vocalization and quickly expands in use to signal discomfort and a need state.

Development of the Auditory System

By the 20th week of prenatal development, the inner-ear mechanism has completed maturation. By the 37th week, the middle-ear conductive structures are complete and functioning. Although the auricle and auditory canal will continue to grow until the child is 8 or 9 years old, the adult configurative ear is complete by midterm of pregnancy (Northern & Downs, 1978). The hearing child enters the world with a completely developed and functioning auditory system.

Studies by Eisenberg (1970) and Eimas, Sigueland, Juscyzk, and Vigorit (1972) indicate that neonates can discriminate sound on the basis of intensity, frequency, and stimulus dimensionality. Perhaps Eisenberg's most important indication is that infants respond most effectively to speech-like auditory stimuli (Eisenberg, 1976). Spring and Dale (1977) have demonstrated that linguistic stress is discriminated by infants between 1 and 4 months of age. Northern and Downs (1978) concluded that infants are able to produce discriminatory responses for the suprasegmental features of speech, including intonation, rhythm, stress, intensity, and duration. The importance of such knowledge for the clinician/teacher is emphasized by Ling (1976), who notes that these features can be audible through amplification for the majority of hearing-impaired children, even for those who display only low-frequency residual hearing. The logical conclusion from these observations is that infants employ cognitive abilities in their selective listening activity. This represents a much greater degree of intellectual activity than is credited to the infancy period by the Piagetian sensory motor stage.

Studies of babies between 9 and 18 months of age by Friedlander (1970) indicate that listening is indeed a salient activity for infants, that they display a large range of discriminative listening to auditory stimuli, including natural and synthetic speech. Studies by Kagan et al. (1979) and Irwin (1952) illustrate that from an early age babies are quite active in the use of incoming auditory events. However, all sounds are not easily or equally discriminated by infants. Eilers' (1977) investigation of discriminatory abilities of babies aged 1 to 3 months, 6 to 8 months, and 12 to 14 months with regard to specific consonant-vowel (CV) and vowel-consonant (VC) syllables indicates that, for some contrasts, discriminatory evidence is obvious from birth and across older babies, for example, /sɑ/ versus /ʃɑ/ and /sɑ/ versus /vɑ/. She further noted that other contrasts, /fi/ versus /θi/ and /sɑ/ versus /zɑ/, became easier as babies neared 14 months of age. One additional contrast pair, /fɑ/ versus /θɑ/, was found to be difficult at all ages. This study and others indicating similar results suggest a developmental factor or listening-experience factor for various features of speech sounds. For example, when the syllable pairs used by Eilers are examined, relative ease of discrimination was noted for contrasts of vowel duration and consonant voicing. When vowel duration was equalized and the VC syllable ended with a contrasting voice/nonvoice fricative, ease of discrimination was still evident. However, if the final voice/nonvoice consonants were stops, difficulty in discrimination was noted, even for many older babies. This finding is even more interesting if one examines the occurrence of various speech sounds in the child's developing repertoire and of misarticulations noted in the early speech of children. It is difficult to examine auditory development without considering the question of how it is related to language and speech acquisition through infancy.

Infancy as the Basis for Linguistic Development

The beginnings of language commence with the first sound uttered as a reflex cry by the infant at birth. From this initial vocalization, one of the most intriguing accomplishments of the human species develops: the use of spoken (and written) language in communication. The importance of the auditory system in the development of this ability becomes obvious when one is concerned with hearing-impaired children, who do not talk because they do not hear.

For a period, the hearing-impaired infant shows some parallels with the normal child in the use and development of various vocalizations. Still, it must be noted that many infant interventionists, including ourselves, have observed much variation in the quantity and quality of the vocalizations of some congenitally hearing-impaired babies, compared with the vocalizations of their hearing peers.

The teacher/clinician who requires a foundation in language and speech acquisition should examine carefully the available literature and research on this subject. In this section, we can present only an overview. Yet, it is important to grasp the developmental aspects of language and speech if we expect to intervene in such developmental areas.

As noted in the discussion of auditory processing, the initial perceptual or listening distinction a baby must make is that between the sounds of environment and the sounds of speech. This distinction the infant appears to master quite early, as demonstrated by the saliency of human voices. A further distinction that is imperative in language and speech development is that between true speech information and the sounds people make that are not particularly relevant. In a revealing study, Condon and Sander (1974) examined films of neonates frame by frame as they were exposed to a tape of adult voices. The film analysis showed that these very young babies synchronized movement with the articulated patterns of adult speech. At this point, there is general agreement that the human infant comes equipped with an auditory system that is particularly sensitive to human voices and speech. This conclusion might also indicate an innate capacity for the acquisition of a spoken language. If one is involved with infant programs for hearing-impaired or language-deficient children, this issue becomes a philosophical as well as practical focal point of concern.

Infant Prespeech Vocalizations

The stages of development in phonetic control presented by Oller (1980) are most helpful in aiding professionals in the understanding of sequence in infant vocalization. The reflex cry at birth soon expands by 4 weeks of age to crying variations. Oller (1980) defines this phase of phonetic development as the phonation stage, which is characterized by quasi-resonant nucleus (QRN) vocalization. In these nonreflexive utterances, the infant is not utilizing the full capacity or resonance of the vocal tract and the mouth is closed or nearly closed.

Between 2 and 3 months of age, the gooing stage emerges. Now the baby combines the QRN with velar, uvular, and epiglottal vocalization. At this stage, the child alternates the opening and closing of the vocal tract in back positions.

The next stage, at 4 to 6 months of age, is the expansion stage. This includes six substages that may occur in various order, except for the final one, marginal babbling, which marks the transition into future stages. The six expansion-stage components are:

1. The fully resonant nuclei (FRN) substage, in which the infant opens the mouth more completely in vocalization. This allows for the possibility of resonant type contrasts.
2. The raspberry (RSP) substage, in which the baby uses front closure as opposed to the back closure noted in the gooing stage.
3. The squeals (SQ) substage, characterized by a high pitch and low growls (GRL), marking the use of pitch contrast.
4. The yelling (YEL) substage, introducing contrasts of amplitude.
5. The ingressive-egressive sequence (IES) as a possible further control of the breath stream within the vocal tract. This is characterized by in-out breathing accompanied by vocalization.
6. The marginal babbling (MB) substage, which combines all of the foregoing substages. Here the infant produces a series of articulatory contrasts. This differs from the true babbling in that the timing framework is absent and the quality of syllables noted in true babbling is not present.

Between the ages of 7 to 10 months, true babbling, or the canonical stage, is reached. This stage is characterized by reduplicated babbling sets in which time constraints are imposed on the contrasts, variations, openings, and closures that have appeared earlier in the child's vocal repertoire.

Oller's final stage before one-word utterances is the variegated babbling stage, occurring between 11 and 12 months. This stage includes consonantal and vocalic feature contrasts in sequences of various syllables, as well as gibberish (GIB), which includes variations of stress in intonation contour.

Oller's stages of development in phonetic control should not be viewed as contradicting the stages outlined by Menyuk (1972) or those described by distinctive feature analysis (Jakobson, 1968) in Chapter 6. Rather they serve as an additional descriptive classification for the professional who must observe, assess, and then program, based on the utterances made by a young baby.

The teacher/clinician must also be aware of the pragmatic behaviors demonstrated by infants, as listed and defined in Chapter 6. Early pragmatic behaviors are a major part of the communication process employed in infancy. Almost from birth, babies attend to a speaker's face and approximate facial gestures (Reddy & Rao, 1977). This natural attending behavior and other behaviors exhibited by infants can be used to advantage by parents and interventionists in stimulating communication foundations.

As can be seen from this overview of auditory language development during the prespeech stage, from birth to about 12 months of age, the baby proceeds rapidly in both the reception and early mastery of abilities that will allow verbal expression. Amplification and stimulation of these early behaviors during the first 12 months of development can provide a growth period for the hearing-impaired child that parallels that of normally hearing peers.

First Words

In the latter part of the babbling stage, roughly between 12 to 14 months of age, the infant begins consistently to apply vocalization patterns to actions or objects. This period is commonly referred to as the one-word utterance level or the period of holophrastic speech. These early word approximations are usually CV utterances, as in /no/, or CVCV reduplicated combinations, such as /dʌ dʌ/. In the early semantic and pragmatic stages, one-word utterances serve the child in a wide range of communication functions, as indicated in Chapter 6.

DeVilliers and deVilliers (1978) have characterized the single-word utterance as distinctive in two ways. There is a recognizable approximation to some adult word; and the child consistently applies a word to a particular object, action, or event. Children's use of single-word utterances is an interesting subject for study in regard to the form and function of early language. In Nelson's (1973) study of the first 50 utterances of 18 children between the ages of 12 and 24 months, the children's words were categorized in six form classes. These categories were based not on adult form but on classes of words as they were used functionally by the subjects. These form classes are as follows:

1. Specific nominals:	(Specific nominals include names of particular people or objects within the child's environment, such as Mama, Rex, etc.)
People	
Animals	
Objects	
2. General nominals:	
Objects	ball
Substances	milk
Animals	doggie people - boy
Letters	numbers - one
Abstractions	birthday
Pronouns	he
3. Action words:	
Demand/descriptive	up
Notice	look
4. Modifiers:	
Attributes	pretty

States	all gone
Locatives	outside
Possession	mine
5. Personal-social words:	
Assertion	no
Social/expressive	please
6. Function words:	
Questions	where
Miscellaneous	not be applicable to above classes

It should be noted that, in Nelson's study, of the above word categories, the first three comprised 80 percent of the subjects' utterances.

One-word utterances can also be viewed according to semantic function classes, as in Bloom's (1973) analysis. Bloom's concern is primarily with the referential function of early words or the aspects of the child's surroundings to which words refer. A customary note of caution must be made regarding the meaning of words for a child; they may not have the same meaning for a child as for an adult. The interventionist must be conscious of this fact and, through careful and continuous observation, determine exactly what the child means.

Bloom suggests eight word functions or relationships in one-word utterances, similar to those outlined by Brown (1973). Bloom's functions are:

1. Existence	there	the function being to point out an object
2. Recurrence	more	the function being to request or comment on the recurrence of an action or object
3 Disappearance	all gone	the function being to comment on the disappearance of an object previously present
4. Nonexistence	no	the function being to comment on nonexistence where presence was expected
5. Rejection	no	the function being to protest
6. Cessation	stop	the function being to comment on an activity to be closed

7. Action	up	the function being to request or comment regarding movement
8. Location	up	the function being to comment on spatial positioning

Bloom (1970) also suggests two broad categories of first utterances that can serve as a helpful focal point. She divides words into those that are substantive and serve as labels for actions and objects in the child's environment and those that are relational and describe a relationship between objects or actions. Substantive *words* such as "mama," "ball," "run," and "bye-bye" would coincide with Nelson's nominal classes, specific and general, and action-word class. Relational words, such as "more," "all gone," and "there" are similar to Nelson's modifier, personal-social, and function-word classes.

The period of one-word utterances may continue from 6 to 12 months. Although there are similarities among children as to classes and functions of words used during this period, the child's surroundings should determine the target words for the teacher/clinician to select in programming. For example, "Mama" and "Dada" are generally accepted early references for parents, but for one child, "Duffy," a dog's name, may be important, while for another child, "Bunny," referring to a favorite toy may be a priority. McLean and Snyder-McLean (1978) emphasize that one important aspect of this stage is that the child's expressive language expands not only in quantity, or the number of words produced, but also in variation of meaning for words within the child's repertoire. In other words, semantic function increases. Therefore, it is important not only to develop a useful vocabulary but also to apply words to various context.

Successive Utterances

As vocabulary and meaning develop throughout the stage of one-word utterances, the child gradually begins to sequence two words that do not quite conform consistently to rules of grammar, for example, "cookie eat" instead of "eat cookie." Examination of these utterances based on intonation and timing (Bloom, 1973) indicates that they are more appropriately defined as two one-word utterances uttered in succession. Recently, attention has been focused on this transition period between one- and two-word utterances (Braine, 1976; Greenfield & Smith, 1976). The major characteristic appears to be that the multiple word combinations are inconsistent grammatically but that, unlike a series of one-word utterances a child might produce, successive utterances are related in a specific way.

In this phase of successive utterances, the child combines related words in what Bloom refers to as a chained utterance or a topic-comment pattern.

Braine (1976) suggests that a "groping pattern" may also occur in successive utterances. During this time, the child is searching to express a meaning but has not yet grasped how to carry out the expression. The chaining form predominates initially but is gradually overtaken by Bloom's second form, the holistic utterance. McLean and Snyder-McLean (1978) compare this second form with Braine's (1976) positional-productive, in that, in both cases, the child combines words in consistent sequence and pronounces them as a common entity. This period of successive utterances should be of interest to those involved in the education of the hearing impaired, since it contains many utterances produced not only by young children with hearing loss but also by many school-age students with limited spoken language.

Two-Word Utterances

At approximately 18 to 24 months of age, the child with normal hearing and language acquisition begins to combine words that form the first representation of grammar. In contrast to successive utterances, these multiple word combinations display consistent word order combined with phrasing and intonation contour suggestive of a sentence. This stage of two-word utterances, also referred to as telegraphic speech, has received much attention from those interested in child language (Braine, 1963; Brown & Bellugi, 1964; McNeill, 1970; Miller & Ervin, 1964).

As deVilliers and deVilliers (1978) point out, the term *telegraphic* is quite appropriate in defining this stage. The words that the child uses are content words, or those which are most pertinent in the situation. These words are primarily nouns, verbs, and some modifiers, while articles, prepositions, elements of the auxiliary, and so on, are omitted. The selection of content words results in an economical representation of adult grammar.

In actuality however, the two-word sentence represents more than an efficient or economical production of a longer adult sentence. In two-word utterance combinations, the child expresses particular semantic relationships between the words that are partially evident by the word order. By the selection of word order, such as agent-patient or agent-action, the child expresses the same semantic relation that adults produce in more sophisticated sentences. (The semantic relationships and syntactic patterns evidenced most often at the two-word-utterance stage were presented in Chapter 6.)

Several characteristics emerge in this stage of linguistic development. These are well summarized by McLean and Snyder-McLean (1978). First, the types of utterances at this stage are quite often extensions or elaborations of single-word utterances. Relationships regarding existence, nonexistence, recurrence, and so forth, are also evident at this stage. Second, the child's language serves to relate the specificity of objects, actions, and events, or their relationships, that are within the context of the child's immediate or recent experience. Third, the major portion of words used are nouns and verbs, with functional words omitted. However, these nouns and verbs are used in various semantic roles. As limiting as it may initially appear, the capacity of a young child for communication at this level is very large.

Although the emergence of two-word utterances normally occurs between 18 and 24 months of age, in the infant with hearing impairment or language delay, this stage may not be noted until later. The possibility of occurrence close to normal development naturally depends on a multitude of factors, such as degree of loss, amplification, time of intervention, additional handicaps, parental support, and so on. However, this stage can represent for the infant interventionist a goal toward which to work. A firm understanding of these early linguistic and auditory stages will assist the teacher/clinician in setting forth appropriate and sequential objectives in language development.

Vocalization Selection

Having examined the sequence pattern of infant vocalization, a logical question arises as to why such a sequence exists. Menyuk (1972) suggests that the sequence may be due to the factor of ease of production, that is, that some sounds are simply easier for the child to produce. The physical structure of the infant's vocal apparatus—for example, the relatively high positioning of the larynx (Lieberman, Harris, Wolff, & Russell, 1971; Murai, 1960), the small pharynx, and large tongue that nearly fills the baby's mouth—suggests a possible partial explanation in ease of production. However, auditory sensitivity and discrimination ability, as illustrated by the Eilers study (1977) mentioned earlier, suggest that the auditory system and the vocal system actually interplay in the determination of vocalization sequence.

If this is true, then there is a critical need for early amplification and aural habilitation to coincide with early language development programming for the hearing-impaired infant. Northern and Downs (1978) and Ling (1976) emphasize that sensory deprivation of the auditory system will, over time, result eventually in the inability of the system to perceive contrasts of speech sounds. Moreover, this devastation is felt to be irreversible. This view relates closely to the theory of critical periods, which states that, at certain times during development, the child is best suited to receive and use certain stimuli. Beyond the critical period, the stimuli will have a gradually reduced effect on the particular area in question. In the present case, we are concerned with auditory stimuli and linguistic information received auditorily. Based on the critical period hypothesis, if auditory-linguistic intervention is not done during infancy and early preschool years, the chances for optimal language, speech, and listening behaviors are greatly reduced. Northern and Downs (1978) sum it up precisely: "The best potential language development can be secured only by applying the proper training procedures at an age which will take advantage of critical periods for prelinguistic and linguistic skills" (p. 93).

Other Developmental Areas

Although the prime emphasis in this section is on auditory and linguistic development, the infant interventionist is naturally concerned with all other areas of child development. Children who demonstrate hearing loss or language delay may have normal development in other areas, such as cognition (although related to language, it is not synonymous) and motor abilities. The interventionist's role with such infants is to help maintain this normal growth by providing experiences for the child to use the newly developing abilities. Babies, too, may demonstrate multiple handicaps that will affect other developmental areas. In these cases, unless the teacher/clinician is familiar with multiple handicaps, it is best to secure the help of other professionals and to exercise the intervention program from a team approach.

It is helpful to record data pertaining to developmental areas other than language and audition. This information will be of value to the teacher at the preschool level and will also aid in documenting overall progress for parents as well as for the teacher/clinician. We have found three approaches that are helpful in this regard, depending on the age and needs of the baby and the parents.

The first, Northcott's (1977) *Curriculum Guide for Hearing Impaired Children (0–3 Years) and Their Parents,* contains sequenced forms for recording general developmental progression in the areas of personal-social, perceptuo-cognitive, self-help, gross-motor, fine-motor, speech- and language-expressive, speech- and language-receptive, and auditory communication. Three to four skills are listed from ages 3 to 60 months in sequential order with space for recording date of observation and comments.

The second aid, *Developmental Programming for Infants and Young Children, Early Intervention Developmental Profile* by Schafer and Moersch (1978), was noted in Chapter 4. It contains many items from the Bayley Scales of Infant Development (Bayley, 1969) but categorizes the behaviors into areas of development from birth through 36 months of age.

The developmental areas that are addressed are perceptual/fine motor, cognition, language, social-emotional, self-care, and gross motor. Record forms are contained in a convenient booklet with space for recording dates of behavior observed and comments.

The third system, *Behavioral Characteristics Progression (BCP)*, developed by the VORT Corporation (1973) for Santa Cruz County, California, is most helpful with infants who demonstrate handicaps in addition to hearing loss or who are having a particularly slow start in development. BCP offers 59 developmental areas or "strands" that relate to various handicapping conditions. Specific areas that apply to objectives for a specific baby can be selected. Each area contains behaviors in developmental sequence up to 50 steps. Ages are not presented, and the record sheets are criterion-referenced. Record sheets and explanations are contained in individual notebooks.

There are of course other systems of recordkeeping that might serve programs as well or better. This will obviously depend on the infants serviced, the program structure, and so on. However, the three presented here have been found to accommodate the needs of the Comprehensive Services Parent Infant Program quite well.

PARENTS

Any discussion of infant intervention programming naturally concerns the involvement of parents, especially the mother who is the traditional caretaker during the period of infancy. There still is strong support for the belief that the home is the optimal setting for infant education and that the parent, through guidance and instruction, is the optimal teacher. The goal of parental involvement is to ensure greater success in early programming by addressing the child's education through the parents.

Parents as Teachers

Educating infants through their parents raises an interesting point. Turnure (1969) found that by the age of 3 months babies could recognize their own mothers' voices and preferred them to unfamiliar voices. This was true even when the mothers' voices were altered by filters. Her study employed as subjects babies aged 3, 6, and 9 months of age. Although responses to the voices varied with age, the mothers' voices were always preferred.

From a practical point of view, the mother is in most cases the primary source of stimulation during infancy. By assisting and guiding her, we can facilitate the natural mother-child interaction and produce a rich experiential and educational environment. However, caution must be observed. Individual differences must always be a consideration; these include personality, motivation, and confidence, as well as such factors as the quality and quantity of the time a mother may have. Realistically, over the years, the roles of parents have changed in many instances. Fathers may be primary caretakers, and both parents or single mothers may charge the care of even very young infants to day-care centers or baby sitters. This does not negate the possibility of successful infant intervention, but it may require some adjustments. We have found that fathers who are primary caretakers, or perhaps equal caretakers as in the case of staggered work schedules, are as competent as mothers in working with young babies. The majority of day-care centers and baby sitters are also willing to cooperate with intervention strategies and goals.

Factors in Parental Involvement

Attitudes

An important aspect in parent involvement is the parents' attitudes and goals. Pollack (1970) categorizes parents into two main groups: those who "show readiness" to partake in parent-infant programming and those who for various reasons do not. She suggests several factors that in part determine success in parent involvement in an intervention program. The first relates to the parental attitude or image of the infant. Amidst all of the confusion and frustration of discovery and awareness that a handicap exists, parents form feelings toward the disability and their child. The results may be positive, or they may be quite negative. Despite the common fact of parenthood, little education has been provided to assist individuals to adapt to this role, let alone to prepare to meet the difficulties that a handicapped child presents. Safford and Arbitman (1975) caution that professionals must be careful not to oversimplify or overgeneralize the feelings of parents of special children. The child's handicap raises various personal as well as family concerns. The presence of a handicapped child and the adjustments that may be necessitated because of it are often not as obvious or as simple as professionals might assume.

Parental attitudes in infancy and early childhood will eventually affect children's views of themselves. All children need to feel successful, competent, and of value. This positive concept of self develops largely through children's perceptions of how others view them. These perceptions are based on the behavioral and attitudinal messages of parents and others intimately involved with the child (Ferholt and Solnit, 1978; Safford, 1978). Reactions of pity, overprotection, rejection, or scorn are neither helpful nor constructive. What is needed is respect, love, and acceptance of children in their own right. Yet many parents may need guidance and support in achieving these positive attitudes.

Expectations

Pollack's (1970) second factor centers around parental expectations. This affects not only immediate goals for the child but the long-range ideas that parents hold. It is not unusual for parents to set unrealistic expectations for their hearing-impaired or language-delayed child, either by expecting too much too soon or, more commonly, by not expecting enough. If too little achievement is expected because of a handicap, then little will be accomplished.

Realistic ideas about what can be expected for an individual infant will evolve when appropriate and honest information, coupled with support, is provided by the teacher/clinician. Positive attributes of the child should be emphasized and the child's potential stressed. Problem areas resulting from the hearing or language disorder must be addressed honestly, but without pessimism.

Parent expectations are not limited to the area affected by the handicap, in this case hearing and language skills. It is vital for parents to realize early that, although some areas may be delayed in relation to normal developmental schedules, others will not. The fact that a child is hearing impaired does not mean that the child's motor development will also be delayed, unless of course a multihandicapping condition exists. Parents should be reminded of the accomplishments that their baby will achieve despite the disability.

Expectations should also be addressed specifically for the handicapping areas. As we have already noted, the goals and objectives must be honest and realistic. Emphasis on small steps and accomplishments makes the baby's progress more evident to the parents. By pointing out progress and explaining the importance of each emerging behavior in development, the parents will be assured that their baby is advancing. Explanation of short-term objectives, or where the baby goes next, will present a goal toward which the parents and the interventionist can direct effort and attention.

Expectations that are centered on discipline, toilet training, and other self-help skills and acceptable social behavior are also of importance. In most cases, what is expected of children with normal hearing should also be expected of a child with a hearing impairment. Lessened expectations in these areas will result in overprotectiveness of a young child, which is not healthy either for the parent or for the baby. Such a situation becomes tremendously taxing to the parents and other family members, and the child may become unbearable to live with. Young children have the need and right to be taught acceptable social behavior and independence in self-care. It is an injustice to neglect this because of oversolicitousness. Professionals must realize that for various reasons—pity, guilt, concern, sorrow—they can easily slip into overindulgence and overprotectiveness of a small baby who is known to have an area of deficit. Whatever prompts the reaction, the fact remains that at some point the baby will have to come in contact with other people in situations outside the child's home; and no one appreciates an undisciplined, spoiled, domineering child!

It behooves the infant interventionist to discuss expectations and goals, both immediate and future, with the parents, with attention directed to their perceptions of what the baby might be expected to accomplish. Self-fulfillment of either the parent's or the teacher/clinician's ego must be avoided; the baby and the baby's future must remain the central focus at all times.

The Parent-Interventionist Relationship

The third factor suggested by Pollack (1970) to be a determiner of a parent's success as an educator of the infant is the relationship that is established between the teacher/clinician and the parent. The quality of this relationship is an integral part of a successful infant intervention program and is a major responsibility of the teacher/clinician. Parents need to feel that they are respected as parents, that they truly have a vital contribution to make in their baby's progress, and that they can trust the professionals involved in the infant's program. As Ferholt and Solnit (1978) emphasize, parent involvement is most beneficial when the focus is on the child's resources rather than the handicap. In order to achieve this focus, a firm bond of trust must exist between the parents and the interventionist.

Professional teacher/clinicians must examine their own motivations in their vocation. A frustrated "mothering complex" or do-good attitude has no place in parent-infant programs. The teacher/clinician involved in an ego trip is a detriment to both self and clients. Pride in one's work is essential, but seeing oneself as the saviour of little handicapped children is overdoing it.

Professionals must find within their own personalities those qualities that best promote trust and rapport with parents. Some professionals are animated and outgoing, while others present a more controlled or aloof image. But either of these types of personalities can interact well with parents if honesty, directness, and tact are maintained and combined with understanding, support, and genuine interest.

Some Easy Ways to Alienate Parents

Talk down to parents. Fallen (1978) cautions that lectures are out of place in addressing parents. Parents deserve respect as parents who have helpful knowledge about their baby. Also parents will not be impressed by the use of technical or professional terms that are unfamiliar and have no meaning for them. Converse with and educate parents at a level which they can grasp and utilize. Take time to make explanations, and allow them to pose questions to clear up uncertainties.

Try to be forcibly convincing. This tactic, known as "bulldozing," will win very little cooperation from parents. The teacher/clinician may be correct on an issue with parents but in such cases must allow the parents themselves to reach an acceptance or understanding of the teacher/clinician's viewpoint. This can be aided by providing the parents with documented literature to supplement the information provided by the interventionist. Conferences with other professionals may also be of value. In many instances, parents may hold onto certain beliefs, which, although possibly inappropriate, is their privilege. The old adage that "one can catch more flies with sugar than with vinegar" might well apply in such cases.

Push your personal philosophy. This is closely related to the foregoing tactic but is more concerned with parental attitudes, feelings, and fears about the child and with the parents' decisions based on such attitudes and emotions. The teacher/clinician must be very cautious about making decisions that involve primarily parental responsibilities. Overdependent parents are as undesirable as overdependent children. Listen to the parents' needs and assist them in decision making and problem solving without personal bias clouding the issues.

Compete with parents. Fallen (1978) and Bromwich (1977) emphasize that professionals must avoid competition with parents and interference with the parent-infant attachment. It is imperative that professionals remember at all times that, regardless of any particular home situation, the baby belongs to its parents and that the parents are of ultimate importance throughout the child's infancy and development to adulthood. The fact is that the baby's parents are more important to the child than the interventionist and will exert a powerful influence on the child throughout the growing years. Competition with a parent can result in alienation of the parent, parent feelings of inadequacy, or the parent's dependence on the interventionist (Fallen, 1978; Garwood, 1979; Safford, 1978). Parents, both mothers and fathers, have a need to feel important and necessary in their child's life. It is the professional's responsibility to support those feelings, not to usurp them.

Summary

Parents are indeed important in the implementation of a parent-infant program. It is the responsibility of the infant interventionist to promote a relationship of cooperation and a sense of teamness with the parents in the operation of that program. Mutual trust, respect, and support will best meet the needs and goals of all involved, especially of the infant, who is after all the central focus.

ASPECTS OF PROGRAMMING

In the planning and designing stage of a parent-infant program, several aspects must be considered to shape the overall structure and the ultimate delivery of services that the program will provide. It is a pleasurable luxury to indulge oneself in the conceptualization of the ideal parent-infant program. However, as many program developers will attest, the program's actual existence must rest on the cold (and sometimes cruel) reality of situational limitations.

Finances, Funding, and Budgets

Perhaps the most important reality that a parent-infant program faces in the planning stages is in the area of finances. Without money for personnel, materials, travel, and so on, the program cannot exist. The amount of funds a program has at its disposal will determine the number of teachers, and therefore the number of clients that may be served. Programs may receive financial support from various federal and state funding agencies or private funding sources, or they may operate with tuition income or financial support from various other sources. However the funds are obtained and financial support maintained, this is surely a bottom-line concern for administrators and other personnel.

Personnel

Teachers

At least two concerns arise regarding personnel: the qualifications and the number of teacher/clinicians needed to maintain a program effectively. For some time, teacher competency has been an issue in general and special education. Many states continue to upgrade certification requirements. However, in most cases, these requirements are focused on the levels that affect teachers in classrooms only down to the kindergarten level. There are minimal or no requirements for preschool practitioners who service children under kindergarten age, as specified by state certification standards.

In many universities, undergraduate and graduate training programs offer preschool specialist courses of study for both normal and handicapped children, but in most cases the emphasis in these courses is on the time period following infancy, that is, ages 3 through 5. In some instances, short-term programs and even degree programs are focused on infant specialists in a cross-categorical approach. However, although beneficial from the viewpoint of general infant stimulation, these programs fail to present and promote those aspects that are specific to intervention in cases of hearing loss. Training programs for infant specialists in hearing impairment and language delay are few and far between. Universities that do offer such training programs often couple them with a parent-infant program that serves as an experiential setting for prospective teachers and also as an educational program for infants and their families. This is the type of arrangement in effect in the Comprehensive Services Program.

The number of teacher/clinicians that are required in a parent-infant program will depend on the number of families requiring such service. Ideally, in a home-based program, a teacher is assigned to four or five families. This allows the equivalent of one full day per family, though additional home visits might also be scheduled. In a center-based infant program, larger numbers of children can be serviced, either in small groups or individually. One reason, for this, of course, is that travel time is reduced or eliminated for the interventionist. However the program is structured, teachers must be allotted ample time to devote themselves to the families to which they are assigned. This includes not only actual contact time but also time for planning, recordkeeping, professional development, and so on. The teacher-client ratio is indeed an important consideration. Overburdened teacher/clinicians cannot implement a program efficiently and productively.

Support Personnel

In addition to the teacher/clinicians who actually carry out program directives, a system of support personnel positioned within the program or serving in a consultancy or cooperative capacity is vital to effective programming. Audiologists, members of the medical profession, and family counselors are important contributors to parent-infant programs. Teacher aides can assist in center-based programs. A secretarial and clerical staff are also necessary. The coordination of all this effort is the task of a competent administration.

Scheduling, staff meetings, staff development, individual personnel responsibilities, space, and materials—all of these considerations will also affect parent-infant programming. However, each of these is best addressed with respect to the specific organization and needs of individual programs rather than in terms of a general approach.

Curriculum

The purpose of this text is not to serve as a curriculum guide or to suggest that a single format or set of operational procedures will apply to all parent-infant programs. Our intent at this point is rather to provide the reader with information concerning the curriculum developed in the Comprehensive Services Parent-Infant Program based on the needs of the children it serves. Hopefully, this information will serve as a catalyst in the development of other home-based program curricula.

The curriculum of the Comprehensive Services Parent-Infant Program is altered to accommodate the specific capabilities and needs of each child. Family objectives are based on each parent-child unit being served, resulting in a highly individualized curriculum. However, the same general areas are addressed for each child. The curriculum areas and the specific objectives, activities, and materials developed in each area of course involve both the parents and the child.

Cognition and Concept Development

The central focus in the curriculum area of cognition and concept development is on the promotion and provision of experiences for the infant that will stimulate early cognitive development and comprehension in concept formation. There is general agreement among linguists and psychologists that, although language and cognition are not synonymous terms, a close developmental relationship exists between them during the period of infancy (Muma, 1978). It is not known if language activates cognition or vice versa, if there is mutual activation, or if other variables also may be involved. But a relationship does exist. Vygotsky's (1962) premise is that language and cognition initially develop in parallel and merge early in childhood. Bloom's (1972) concept of "crossover" in language and cognition supports this idea. The concept is illustrated in Bloom's (1973) semantic categories of existence, nonexistence, and recurrence that occur at the one-word-utterance stage, as compared with Piaget's notion of object permanence. If these categories did not exist cognitively in the young child, it would not be possible for the relationship between language and cognition to be expressed verbally. Initially, thought is essential to language, but later language becomes paramount over thought (Garwood, 1979).

As noted earlier, the concept of sensory motor development does not provide all of the answers to cognitive and language development in infancy, but it can serve as a useful guideline in targeting objectives in infant programming. Initially, cognitive development is based on information available to the infant through the sensory channels. Thus, even a baby with one deficient input channel, in this case hearing, is able to receive other types of sensory information. Lenneberg (1972) posited that very early cognitive development is relatively unimpaired if only one sensory channel is deficient. Therefore, hearing-impaired infants should proceed through the first five stages of sensory motor development in much the same way as their hearing peers. The progression through these stages can be monitored to determine development. However, language enters in very early and should receive simultaneous stimulation from the beginning of intervention.

The development of concept understanding of course proceeds throughout early childhood, but it begins in infancy in conjunction with language and cognitive development. The acquisition of concepts allows the child to gain perspective on the environment and forms a basis for early expressive language. Concepts are defined by Nelson (1974) in terms of logical relationships. Concept awareness or comprehension implies an understanding of functional or relational rules. The principles of cognitive organization that apply to sensorimotor stages can also be applied to concept development. In other words, concepts are formed in a manner similar to that for sensory schemes. Children explore and investigate functions of objects and then classify, based on functional use rules (McLean & Snyder-McLean, 1978). This notion of semantic concepts relates well to single-word utterances and their meanings.

In very early cognitive and concept development, the baby relates, manipulates, and interprets environment via experiences that allow such interaction. These experiences are important because what a child knows influences how the child receives and uses information. In turn, new experiences alter what the child knows and create new knowledge. By encouraging parental interaction and promoting a variety of environmental experiences in which the infant is free to observe and explore, opportunities will be created for the development of cognition and concepts that are the foundations for later linguistic and cognitive development.

Audition and the Development of the Listening Function

The primary focus in the curriculum area of audition and the listening function is to ensure early adjustment to amplification and the consequent use of residual hearing. We have seen that hearing is of prime importance in the development of early language learning. It is only natural, therefore, that this area is emphasized. The sense of hearing allows the infant to gain auditory information of a nonlinguistic nature. Sounds in the child's environment from toys, pets, household surroundings, and so forth, although nonlinguistic, are meaningful and contribute to the child's growing knowledge and understanding of the world.

Goals for parents are centered on the care and maintenance of aids, on understanding what the child's hearing loss and residual hearing permit or inhibit, and on principles of auditory stimulation. Objectives for infants include wearing the aids successfully and developing listening skills as far as the child is able to progress, based on the steps presented in Chapter 3.

Expressive Language and Prespeech Ability

The curriculum areas of cognition and audition are coordinated and form the basis for expressive language development. The goal of developing the foundations of communication between the infant and people within the child's environment is central to a parent-infant program. Communication involves expression as well as reception. The curriculum area of expressive language thus relates to preverbal motor behaviors, to early pragmatic, semantic, and phonological expressive modes of communication that can be fostered in the infant. The debate between seemingly diametrically opposed factions in the area of hearing impairment has no place in the programming of the infant. Whether an aural/oral approach, total communication, or cued speech is used with the baby, the principles of early amplification and language and an emphasis on prespeech should be the foundation for expressive language development. Most parents want their child to learn to talk, but without amplification and direct attention to speech development, apart from the use of signs or cues, the baby will have little success in that domain.

If provided with opportunities for experiential cognitive encounters and consistent auditory stimulation, the hearing-impaired or otherwise language-delayed child has the potential to develop rich expressive language, including speech. Input by parents and the encouragement of infant vocalization and imitation during the prespeech stages can and should be fostered. The hearing-impaired or language-delayed child may not proceed to one- and two-word utterances as rapidly as the child with normal hearing and language ability, but consistent and continual progress toward these expressive language levels can be observed.

Fine- and Gross-Motor Abilities

If the infant is not demonstrating any evident lag, the areas of motor development are monitored to ensure continuous progression. It is important for parents to see their child develop and change through infancy; and, aside from language behavior, motor behaviors provide the most obvious evidence of maturation. If multihandicapping conditions exist that involve motor development, as for example in many postmeningeal children, specific objectives are developed to assist in accommodating needs in this area.

Self-Help Skills and Socialization

As the child increases in motor ability and in language understanding and use through infancy, independence and responsibility for self-care should be encouraged. This includes such areas as self-feeding, toileting, discipline, and acceptable social behavior, both at home and in other environmental settings. Allowing small children to experiment in feeding or undressing themselves, for example, promotes not only practice in coordination but also a feeling of accomplishment in mastering a task alone or with minimal assistance.

Visual Abilities

A final area of curriculum concerns the monitoring of a child's vision. Visual handicaps are often found in conjunction with hearing impairment. Therefore, close attention must be given to this important sense modality. Because vision is vital to the hearing-impaired child, any indications of visual difficulty should be immediately referred for diagnosis and possible treatment or remediation.

A particular aspect of visual abilities that should be emphasized is visual attention, especially as it involves communication. Although far from a complete visual message, speech reading provides the visual information necessary for the reception of language. If signs or cued speech are used, they represent another area that is dependent on visual attention and other visual abilities.

Summary

The above areas form the core of the program curriculum employed in the Comprehensive Services Parent-Infant Program. Specific areas are prioritized depending on the age of the infant, the degree of handicap, child and parent needs, and other factors that would affect progress in development. A firm grasp of the aspects of infant development in these areas is a prerequisite for the infant interventionist. Although there is much knowledge yet to be gained and many questions still to be answered, existing information can assist the teacher/clinician in developing realistic and appropriate objectives and experiences that will ensure progress and maturation in developmental areas.

CONCLUSION

The period of infancy, while still posing numerous unanswered questions, has revealed much valuable information to investigators regarding its role in the developmental process. During this period, babies are active learners, exploring their surroundings and utilizing the information they acquire in the formation of new knowledge. The period of infancy is crucial for the child with a hearing or language difficulty because the critical foundations are laid during this time. However, babies are far from ideal students. They are limited in communicating to their teachers exactly what and how much they actually know. In addition, they present behaviors, such as falling asleep or fits of crying, that totally devastate our most ingeniously planned activities. Nevertheless, by employing parents as educational allies, intervention is possible. With the aid of parents, great strides can be made in the development of the crucial areas of audition and language.

REFERENCES

Bandura, A. *Principles of behavior modification*. New York: Holt, Rinehart, and Winston, 1969.

Bandura, A., & Walters, R. *Social learning and personality development*. New York: Holt, Rinehart, and Winston, 1963.

Bayley, N. *Bayley Scales of Infant Development (BSID)*. New York: Psychological Corp., 1969.

Bereiter, C., & Engelmann, S. An academically oriented preschool for disadvantaged children: Results from the initial experimental group. In G.R. Lefrancois (Ed.), *Little George*. Belmont, Calif.: Wadsworth Publishing Co., 1974.

Bloom, L. *Language development: Form and function in emerging grammars*. Cambridge, Mass.: MIT Press, 1970.

Bloom, L. *Cognitive and linguistic aspects of early language development, short course*. Paper presented at American Speech and Hearing Association convention, 1972.

Bloom, L. *One word at a time: The use of single word utterances before syntax*. The Hague: Mouton, 1973.

Braine, M.D.S. The ontogeny of English phrase structure: The first phrase. *Language*, 1963, *39*, 1–13.

Braine, M.D.S. Children's first word combinations. *Monographs of the Society for Research in Child Development*, 1976, *164*.

Brill, S.S. (Ed.). *The basic writings of Sigmund Freud*. New York: Random House, 1938.

Bromwich, R. Stimulation in the first year of life: A perspective on infant development. *Young Children*, 1977, *32*, 71–82.

Brown, R. *A first language: The early stages*. Cambridge, Mass.: Harvard University Press, 1973.

Brown, R., & Bellugi, U. Three processes in the child's acquisition of syntax. *Harvard Educational Review*, 1964, *34*, 133–151.

Caldwell, B. M. The fourth dimension in early childhood education. In G. R. Lefrancois (Ed.), *Little George*. Belmont, Calif.: Wadsworth Publishing Co., 1974.

Cattell, P. *The measurement of intelligence in infants*. New York: Psychological Corporation, 1940.

Condon, W. S., & Sander, L. W. Neonate movement is synchronized with adult speech: Instructional participation and language structure. *Science*, 1974, *183*, 99–101.

deVilliers, J. G., & deVilliers, P. A. *Language acquisition*. Cambridge, Mass.: Harvard University Press, 1978.

Eilers, R. Developmental changes in speech discrimination in infants. *Journal of Speech and Hearing Research*, 1977, *20*, 766–780.

Eimas, P. D., Sigueland, E. R., Juscyzk, P., & Vigorit, J. Speech perception in infants. *Science*, 1972, *171*, 303.

Eisenberg, R., Griffin, E., Coursin, D., & Hunter, A. Auditory behavior in the human neonate: A preliminary report. *Journal of Speech and Hearing Research*, 1964, *7*, 245–269.

Eisenberg, R. B. Auditory behavior in the human neonate: Functional properties of sound and their ontogenetic implications. *International Audiology*, 1969, *8*, 34–45.

Eisenberg, R. B. The development of hearing in man: An assessment of current status. *Journal of the American Speech and Hearing Association*, 1970, *12*, 119–123.

Eisenberg, R. B. In R. E. Stark (Ed.), *Sensory capabilities of hearing impaired children*. Baltimore, Md.: University Park Press, 1976.

Erickson, E. H. *Childhood and society* (2nd ed.). New York: Norton, 1963.

Fallen, N. H. *Young children with special needs*. Columbus, Ohio: Charles E. Merrill, 1978.

Ferholt, J. B., & Solnit, A. J. Counseling parents of mentally retarded and learning disabled children. In L. E. Arnold (Ed.), *Helping parents help their children*. New York: Brunnar/ Mazel Publishers, 1978.

Flavell, J. H. *The developmental psychology of Jean Piaget*. Princeton, N.J.: D. Van Nostrand, 1963.

Friedlander, B. Z. Receptive language development in infancy. *Merrill Palmer Quarterly of Behavior and Development*, 1970, *16*, 7–51.

Garwood, S. G. *Educating young handicapped children, a developmental approach*. Germantown, Md.: Aspen Systems Corporation, 1979.

Gesell, A., & Thompson, H. *The psychology of early growth*. New York: Macmillan, 1938.

Greenfield, P., & Smith, J. *The structure of communication in early language development*. New York: Academic Press, 1976.

Haring, N. G. Assessment and diagnosis of severely handicapping conditions. In M. A. Thomas (Ed.), *Hey, don't forget about me*. Reston, Va.: Council for Exceptional Children, 1976.

Hasenstab, M. S., & McElroy, M. D. Assessment of hearing impaired children under age three—A process. *Hearing Aid Journal*, 1980, *33*(9): 38–39.

Horton, K. B. Early intervention through parent training. *Otolaryngological Clinic of North America*, 1975, *8*, 143–157.

Hunt, J. McV. *Intelligence and experience*. New York: Ronald Press, 1961.

Irwin, O. C. Infant speech, the effect of occupational status and of age on use of sound frequency. *Journal of Speech and Hearing Disorders*, 1952, *13*, 320–323.

Jakobson, R. *Child language, aphasia and phonological universals*. The Hague: Mouton, 1968.

Kagan, J. B., Kearsley, R. B., & Zelazo, P. R. *Infancy: Its place in human development*. Cambridge, Mass.: Harvard University Press, 1979.

Karnes, M. Implications of research with disadvantaged children for early intervention with the handicapped. In J. B. Jordan & R. F. Dailey (Eds.), *Not all little wagons are red: The exceptional child's early years*. Reston, Va.: Council for Exceptional Children, 1973.

Kohlberg, L. The development of moral character and ideology. In M. Hoffman (Ed.), *Review of child psychology*. New York: Russell Sage Foundation, 1964.

Lefrancois, G. R. *Little George, a survey of child development*. Belmont, Calif.: Wadsworth Publishing Co., 1974.

Lenneberg, E. H. Prerequisites for language acquisition by the deaf. In T. J. O'Rourke (Ed.), *Psycholinguistics and total communication: The state of the art*. Washington, D.C.: American Annals of the Deaf, 1972.

Lieberman, P., Harris, K. S., Wolff, P., & Russell, L. H. Newborn infant cry and non-human primate vocalization. *Journal of Speech and Hearing Research*, 1971, *14*, 718–727.

Ling, D. *Speech and the hearing impaired*. Washington, D.C.: A.G. Bell Association for the Deaf, 1976.

McConnell, F., & Horton, K. B. *A home teaching program for parents of very young deaf children: Final report*. Nashville, Tenn.: Vanderbilt University, School of Medicine, 1970.

McLean, J. E., & Snyder-McLean, L. K. *A transactional approach to early language training*. Columbus, Ohio: Charles E. Merrill, 1978.

McNeill, D. *The acquisition of language*. New York: Harper & Row, 1970.

Menyuk, P. *The development of speech*. New York: Bobbs-Merrill Co., 1972.

Miller, J. B. *A demonstration home training program for parents of preschool deaf children: Final report*. Kansas City: Kansas University, Medical Center, 1970.

Miller, W., & Ervin, S. The development of grammar in child language. *Monographs of the Society for Research in Child Development*, 1964, *29*(92): 9–34.

Muma, J. *Language handbook, concepts, assessment, intervention*. Englewood Cliffs, N.J.: Prentice Hall, 1978.

Murai, J. I. Speech development in infants. *Psychologica*, 1960, *3*, 27–35.

Nelson, K. Structure and strategy in learning to talk. *Monographs of the Society for Research in Child Development*, 1973, *38*, 149.

Nelson, K. Concept, word and sentence: Interrelations in acquisition and development. *Psychological Review*, 1974, *81*, 267–285.

Northcott, W. N. *The hearing impaired child in a regular classroom: Preschool, elementary and secondary years*. Washington, D.C.: A.G. Bell Association for the Deaf, 1973.

Northcott, W. N. *Curriculum guide for hearing impaired children (0-3 years) and their parents*. Washington, D.C.: A.G. Bell Association for the Deaf, 1977.

Northern, J. L., & Downs, M. P. *Hearing in children*. Baltimore, Md.: Williams and Wilkins, 1978.

Oller, D. K. *Interpretation of infant vocalizations: Short course*. Paper presented at A.G. Bell Association for the Deaf convention, 1980.

Oyer, H. J., & Hardick, E. J. Communication for hearing handicapped people in the United States. In H. J. Oyer (Ed.), *Communication for the hearing handicapped: An international perspective*. Baltimore, Md.: University Park Press, 1976.

Papousek, H. Conditioning during early post-natal development. In Y. Brackbill & S. G. Thompson (Eds.), *Behavior in infancy and early childhood*. New York: Free Press, 1967.

Parker, R. K. (Ed.). *The preschool in action*. Boston: Allyn & Bacon, 1972.

Pollack, D. *Educational audiology for the limited hearing infant*. Springfield, Ill.: Charles C Thomas, 1970.

Reddy, J. K., & Rao, M. S. Imitation of facial and manual gestures by human neonates. *Science*, 1977, *198*, 75–79.

Safford, P. L. *Teaching young children with special needs*. St. Louis, Mo.: C.V. Mosby, Co., 1978.

Safford, P. L., & Arbitman, D. C. *Developmental intervention with young physically handicapped children*. Springfield, Ill.: Charles C Thomas, 1975.

Schafer, D. S., & Moersch, M. S. (Eds.). *Developmental programming for infants and young children, early intervention developmental profile*. Ann Arbor: University of Michigan Press, 1978.

Skinner, B. F. *The behavior of organisms*. New York: Macmillan, 1938.

Skinner, B. F. *Science and human behavior*. New York: Appleton-Century-Crofts, 1953.

Spring, D. R., & Dale, P. A. Discrimination of linguistic stress in early infancy. *Journal of Speech and Hearing Research*, 1977, *20*, 224–232.

Turnure, C. *Response to voice of mother and stranger by babies in the first year*. Paper presented at Society for Research in Child Development meeting, Santa Monica, Calif., March, 1969.

VORT Corporation. *Behavioral characteristics progression (BCP)*. Palo Alto, Calif.: Author, 1973.

Vygotsky, L. *Thought and language*. Cambridge, Mass.: MIT Press, 1962.

Watson, J. B.. & Watson, R. R. *Psychological care of infant and child*. New York: Norton, 1928.

Wertheimer, M. Psychomotor co-ordination of auditory and visual space at birth. *Science*, 1961, *134*, 1692.

Chapter 8

Nursery-Level Programming

M. Suzanne Hasenstab

A comprehensive preschool experience for hearing-impaired and language-delayed children demands a continuous and coordinated learning environment that will promote a smooth transition for a young child from a parent-infant orientation to a center-based, class orientation. For the purpose of this text, nursery level is defined as that level of preschool education that is designed to meet the developmental needs of children with hearing impairment and/or language delay between the ages of 30 and 48 months. Actual ages may, however, vary from child to child, depending on individual maturation levels.

The nursery-level program is a planned educational experience for young preschool children that emphasizes the continuation of parental cooperation and involvement. The emphasis is therefore twofold. A central emphasis is of course on intervention strategies and objectives to enhance and develop the individual child in all areas of growth. Of equal importance, however, is attention to nurturing the parent role in the effort to further the child's progress through preschool years in order that a firm foundation may be established in the child's educational career.

The fact that the nursery level program in this context pertains particularly to the educational needs of children, hearing and nonhearing, who display language delay makes it imperative that language be the central issue throughout all aspects of programming. This precludes viewing language as encompassing all aspects of the child's life experiences. It must be viewed in relation to cognitive prerequisites and parallel development. Moreover, language must be approached as related to social and emotional areas of development. McLean and Snyder-McLean (1978) present a three-dimensional matrix as a basis for a language-oriented program that includes the functions, content, and structure of communicative acts. They emphasize that, if language is not viewed in broad perspective, optimal linguistic-related programming cannot be attained.

THE INTEGRATED NURSERY SCHOOL

The question of appropriate educational placement that includes the interaction of hearing- and language-handicapped children with their normal peers is indeed one of great concern for preschool interventionists. Although at preschool the majority of these children require the intensive linguistic and auditory attention afforded by a self-contained unit, they also require exposure to hearing children of like age. The reason for integration is at least twofold: the presence of normal peers in a nursery setting provides age-appropriate language models, and it also provides play and social behavior in line with developmental age. In regard to the development of language, Northcott (1973) advocates the interaction of hearing-impaired children with hearing peers to facilitate the development of listening ability as well as the exposure to normal speech and language. Simmons (1968) and Pollack (1967) support this position and also emphasize the value of interaction with hearing children as related to the exposure to a truly auditory environment, which in turn encourages the use of aided residual hearing. As this occurs and listening ability develops, the acquisition of language and speech is enhanced.

The issue of interaction with hearing children has been addressed in the Comprehensive Services Program by enrolling hearing children from the surrounding community as full-time members of the preschool classes at both nursery and prekindergarten levels. Since the usual enrollment does not exceed 10 children for any one class session (some nursery children may attend part-time), a maximum of 3 children with normal language and speech and social development is enrolled at each level. This situation has been beneficial to all concerned. The handicapped children are receiving necessary interaction experiences with hearing peers; the hearing children receive a richly educational preschool experience; parents feel that the small groups, comprehensive curriculum, and extensive individual attention are beneficial to all the children; and teachers and teachers in training are constantly made aware of appropriate developmental behaviors at all ages. This option should be seriously considered in planning and implementing preschool services for hearing-impaired and language-delayed children, since it clearly provides extensive advantages for all children involved.

DEVELOPMENT AT NURSERY LEVEL

Physical Growth and Motor Development

Physical Changes

At the nursery level, the rate of physical growth begins to slow, as compared with infancy, although continuous height and weight gains will occur. Physical appearance begins to change as limbs lengthen and the baby look begins to diminish. Motor abilities will increase in complexity; and large muscle control, general body coordination, and fine-motor ability are achieved. The repertoire of walking, running, and climbing expands to include more skillful performance of such activities and also new motor accomplishments, such as riding a tricycle.

Although the young preschool child is actually making astounding gains in the area of motor growth, professionals must remember that increased control and use of the muscular system, as in other developmental areas, is systematic and dependent on other areas of maturation. Hurlock (1972) cautions that attempts to develop motor abilities beyond a child's maturation level will meet with failure until the musculature and the neurological systems are ready to accomplish such tasks. It is therefore important that the nursery-level teacher be acquainted with developmental stages and accomplishments appropriate for the child between 30 and 48 months of age.

Motor Development of Hearing-Impaired and Language-Delayed Children

The motor development of hearing-impaired and language-delayed children generally parallels the rate and sequence of normal peers unless an additional debilitating condition exists, as in the case of cerebral palsy or mental retardation. It should also be noted that children with hearing impairment as a result of spinal meningitis may display difficulty in balance and orientation in space, due to the involvement of the vestibular mechanism during illness. Teachers must be aware of the individual abilities of each child in their charge, including motor abilities or deficits and rates of growth.

Environmental Factors Affecting Motor Growth

A further consideration in motor development involves the variables related to a child's environment (Fallen, 1978). Although a child may have the potential for certain physical abilities, the environment may impose limitations on the actualization of that potential. Opportunities must be provided at home and in preschool that allow young children to exercise and practice coordination, strength, and endurance by use of their growing bodies. Environmental limitations may be imposed through lack of opportunity, parent or teacher attitudes, overprotection, cultural or sexist attitudes toward behavior, exposure to other male or female child models, or unrealistic expectations by adults. The responsibility of the nursery staff is to provide experiences for young hearing- and language-impaired children that will stimulate a natural and free use of the body within the surroundings. A variety of materials, equipment, and activities that foster experimentation and motivation throughout the nursery day will promote normal and natural motor development. The nursery level is far different from a teacher lecture at which students sit passively.

Development of the Auditory System

Physical Development

In our discussion of the development of the auditory mechanism in Chapter 7, it was noted that the formation and maturation of the auditory structures were functionally accomplished by prenatal midterm. Although the newborn enters the world with the auditory system in full operation (unless of course the child is congenitally hearing impaired), some structures will continue to develop throughout childhood.

The auricle achieves adult form by the 20th week of pregnancy but will continue to grow in size until the child is 9 or 10 years old. The external auditory canal in the young child differs from the longer, curved form of the adult ear. Also, the short and straight external auditory canal of the young child is without the bony portion along the floor of the canal. The development of this bony portion is completed by about the 7th year. There is also a slight variation in the positioning of the tympanic membrane in early childhood. This membrane takes an oblique horizontal position that makes it somewhat difficult to view in examination (Northern & Downs, 1978).

The middle-ear structures have also been completed before birth, but the stapes will continue to refine into adulthood. Northern and Downs (1978) show that the stapes in the middle ear of a young child is actually less delicate and finely formed than the normal stapes in an adult middle ear. Similarly, the Eustachian tube changes in size and position as the child matures and will lengthen and narrow as it moves in a more vertical position between the middle ear and throat.

Otitis Media

An increasingly recognized cause of language and speech delay—and therefore of great concern medically, educationally, linguistically, and audiologically—is the high incidence of middle-ear infection during the preschool years. Middle-ear infection or otitis media may be classified into three conditions, all of which involve the presence of fluid in the middle-ear cavity.

The purpose of the Eustachian tube is to allow for equalization of air pressure in the middle ear. If it becomes blocked or closed, the middle-ear cavity becomes a sealed space. Air that usually fills the cavity becomes absorbed and is not replaced. Negative middle-ear pressure is then created, and fluid exudes from the surrounding tissue. The negative pressure also causes the tympanic membrane to retract. This condition is defined as *serous otitis media*. Hearing loss can result and, since little or no pain may be experienced, the condition could continue undetected and become more extensive. Impedance audiometry is utilized to detect this condition, and medical intervention should be secured, although serous otitis media may often present difficulty in clearing.

Acute otitis media, as opposed to serous otitis media, is usually accompanied by pain and discomfort for the child. Pain may subside if the tympanic membrane ruptures due to the condition. The fluid that has accumulated within the middle-ear cavity becomes suppurative and may drain through the perforated ear drum, producing a "runny" ear.

When this condition continues to recur, it is called *chronic otitis media*. Northern and Downs (1978) note that, in addition to possibly presenting an interruption in hearing, if chronic middle-ear infection continues, the middle-ear tissues will constantly undergo a cycle of damage, healing, and scarring. In addition, other secondary middle-ear disorders may result from damage caused by recurrent otitis media, such as cholesteatoma or polyps. Severe otitis media for long periods of time has the potential to damage ossicles and may actually contribute to an eventual sensory neural hearing impairment.

Our great concern with otitis media among young children is twofold. First, hearing-impaired children with sensory neural hearing loss actually have their critically needed residual hearing reduced when middle-ear functioning is interrupted due to otitis media. The hearing loss becomes a combined conductive and sensory neural condition in which the resulting loss is additive. Second, the presence of chronic middle-ear infection during preschool years, in addition to creating a potential for damage to the middle ear and possibly an acquired sensory neural hearing loss, makes a child with normal hearing virtually hearing impaired for periods of time. During the vital years of language acquisition, the presence of mild to moderate, although temporary, hearing loss can inhibit the normal development of language and speech. This population of children deserves increased attention regarding intervention and treatment of their condition as well as continual monitoring to ensure a healthy ear and appropriate linguistic growth. Indeed, a large number of children now enrolled in the Comprehensive Services Program for language delay have been diagnosed as displaying chronic otitis media.

Development of Listening Ability

In Chapter 3, in connection with auditory processing, we noted that children with auditory deficits must be assisted in learning to use amplified or otherwise residual hearing. For the child with normal hearing and a normal processing function, listening ability develops through daily living experiences and becomes more sophisticated throughout preschool years. However, this does not occur with hearing-impaired and many language-delayed children. The provision of an "auditory environment" with constant attention to stimulation of listening ability is crucial in the nursery level program and is intimately interwoven with growth in the area of language.

Language Development

Beyond Two-Word Utterances

In the preceding chapter, language acquisition was seen to include the two-word-utterance level. In this chapter, examination of the linguistic process will continue, to include expansions of three-, four- and five-word utterances and descriptions of the language components as they are displayed at nursery level. It should be borne in mind that the child with hearing and/or language impairment will not be likely to perform linguistically at levels indicated and described as age appropriate in the present context. However, the normal language development for nursery age is critical knowledge for preschool professionals in order that objectives, goals, and sequential steps in fostering continued linguistic growth may be optimal. Indeed, studies of young hearing-impaired children indicate that spoken language development can parallel that of normal children, even though it evolves at a slower rate (Smith, 1972; West & Weber, 1974).

Three-Word Utterances

Syntax. As the child gradually extends utterances from the two-word to the expanded three-word stage, certain similarities may be observed. Utterances continue to consist primarily of content words, mainly nouns and verbs, with the omission of grammatical function words such as prepositions, articles, and the verb auxiliaries. In other words, speech is still telegraphic. Function words that do appear possess semantic content (deVilliers & deVilliers, 1978) and are important to the child. Certain descriptors, pronouns in the possessive case, and the demonstrative this/that are function words commonly found at early language levels. Although syntax is emerging, semantic complexity is still predominant.

Although consistencies may appear across various stages, each stage of language development we have examined is marked with particular characteristics that specify growing mastery of the linguistic system. The three-word-utterance level presents two noted progressions. Brown (1973), in his extensive study of child language, indicates that the young child at this stage employs an embedding process. Specifically, a functional relationship is embedded into a grammatical relationship. Kretschmer and Kretschmer (1978) present the following example: The grammatical relation "hit ball" is embedded with the functional relation "no ball" to produce the three-word utterance "hit no ball." Thus, two ideas are merged into one longer utterance.

The second process employed at this language level is the conjoining of two grammatical relations that share a common word or idea. Thus "mommy go" and "go bye-bye" are conjoined to produce "mommy go bye-bye." The conjoining of the utterances "Patty eat" and "eat cookie" would produce "Patty eat cookie." This is an initial step toward language economy and efficiency, and it is an important one in the development of syntax.

Semantics. Concurrent with increased length of utterance is the expansion of the child's expressive lexicon. Semantically, the child adds new words to an existing repertoire and in addition, adds new meanings for words previously mastered. Words also begin to be used in varying semantic roles. Sentences of three words expand previous utterances semantically and include expressions of such underlying semantic relations as agent-action-object, agent-action-locative, and so on (see Chapter 6). The nursery-age child also employs three-word utterances in request, question, denial, and other functions. As pointed out in Chapter 6, this represents the pragmatic aspect of early sentences.

Semantic development is indeed overwhelming. Children do not merely acquire new words, but words that vary greatly in their complexity. DeVilliers and deVilliers (1978) suggest four levels of word complexity, the simplest being *proper names*. In this case, there is only one referent for each word. In the examination of first words it was noted that Mommy and Daddy, proper names, were among the first used. Common nouns may occur by adult definition but in child use have only one referent. "Dog" in this case means only one specific dog. This use is termed overspecification.

At a slightly more difficult level is the true use of *common nouns,* in that they represent a category of similar objects. Thus, "dog" includes not only the child's dog but all other dogs as well. These classifications are based on the child's awareness of functional or perceptual similarity. Simple verbs and descriptors are also included in this level.

Relational words, which Bloom (1978) states depend on object reference and context, present still greater complexity. This level too is highly dependent on conceptual knowledge and coincides with the linguistic refinement and expansion stage discussed in the next section.

The fourth level represents complex relational words called *deictic expressions*. These include the demonstratives this/these and that/those, the location adverbs here and there, as well as time expressions that vary in regard to the location in time or place of the speaker. The shifting reference criteria make for the complexity of such words.

Semantic development through the three-word-utterance stage involves the process of adopting or acquiring labels for objects, ideas, or categories on the basis of perceptual or functional similarities (Clark, 1973; Nelson, 1974). A common element serves to link together experiences, actions, objects, and so forth, into a certain category. However, these categories may differ from adult classes, and a child may overgeneralize or overspecialize in use of a word. In either case, closer and closer modification toward the adult standard signifies mastery.

Phonology. The development of phonology is concurrent with the expansion of syntax and semantics in the normal acquisition of language. Phonological development is actually a two-part consideration. Speech perception involves the auditory processing of the connected spoken language of others (see Chapter 3). Speech production allows for the actual expression, via articulatory programming, of words and sentences (see Chapters 5 and 6). Both phases are dynamic in nature and constitute a long-term process of acquisition.

Three important distinctions must be focused upon when discussing the linguistic component of phonology (deVilliers & deVilliers, 1978; Kretschmer & Kretschmer, 1978; Muma, 1978). Phonetic or segmental distinctions concern phonemes or phoneme clusters, the "raw speech sounds," as Kretschmer terms them, and how they are produced. This includes, for example, the manner and place of articulation. Phonological distinctions, on the other hand, relate to rules for the combination of segmental features or speech sounds in meaningful context and as part of the language system. The third distinction is in respect to suprasegmental or prosodic features, which are defined by intonation, pitch, rhythm, stress, and timing constructs. All three of these distinctions play their respective roles in the mastery of phonology.

This area of language development has long been a central issue in programming for children with hearing impairment and other representations of language delay. It involves the most obvious display of nontypical language growth: the child does not speak at all or the speech is highly unintelligible. Success in the development of clear and understandable spoken language obviously depends on a multitude of factors particular to each child, and individual programs must be specifically designed. However, study of normal phonological acquisition aids in the understanding of the sequential process as well as the dynamics of phonology.

Muma (1978) outlines four general stages in the development of speech:

1. Birth to 12 months	Foundation stage Control of vocational mechanism Selective imitation Speech perception
2. 12 to 18 months	Development of first words Single-syllable utterances Continued speech perception
3. 18 months to 4 years	Mastery stage for most of phonological system Words primarily single syllables, occasional two- or three-syllable words
4. 4 years +	Mastery stage for more difficult speech sounds Acquisition of complex words

It thus may be seen that the acquisition of speech is not a process in which there is a sudden development of speech sounds. The process occurs gradually over time and is affected by several interactional factors.

Acquisition of phonology depends upon the perception of speech that is based in auditory processing and auditory acuity. We have already discussed the critical nature of auditory considerations. Speech development is also founded on the child's increased control and maturation of the vocal apparatus, which includes respiration, musculature, and neurological systems. For example, children with motor involvements display speech difficulty even if hearing and other language aspects are normal. Phonology is further affected by the interrelationship of the other linguistic components with the factor of cognition. Menyuk (1971) has shown that children with difficulty related to syntax also display errors in speech articulation. There is also strong evidence of speech problems among children with limited or delayed cognitive abilities. (Cruickshank, 1971; Hewitt & Forness, 1974; Kirk, 1972). Phonological development must therefore be viewed in the overall context of the child's linguistic and cognitive growth.

Traditionally, mastery of speech and phonemes that are produced in spoken language has been viewed in normative terms. Based on such an approach, nursery-age children should have initiated production of the following sounds in order:

Phoneme	*Average Age (Months)*
all vowels and /p/, /m/, /h/, /n/, /w/, /b/	18
/k/, /g/, /d/, /t/, /ŋ/	24
/f/, /y/	30
/r/, /l/, /s/, /ʃ/	36

However, mastery of these sounds in all positions or in all phonetic contexts is not expected until later (Ingram, 1976).

Phoneme	*Age of Mastery (Years)*
all vowels and /p/, /m/, /h/, /n/, /w/	3
/b/, /k/, /g/, /d/, /f/, /y/	4
/t/, /ŋ/, /r/, /l/	6
/ʃ/, /s/	7–8

Other normative references (McCarthy, 1954; Poole, 1934; Templin, 1957) may serve as helpful guidelines in a general sense but fail to supply necessary information that describes a child's use of phonological aspects.

We can also view phonological development at the nursery level by the acquisition of distinctive features. Menyuk's (1972) rank order in production sequence is nasality, voice, stridency, continuant, and place. Menyuk indicates that fine development of these features (beyond /p/, /b/, /m/, /t/, /d/, /n/, /f/, /v/, /k/, /g/, and /ŋ/) is dependent on skill in manipulation of the tongue in conjunction with other articulatory apparatus.

Here again, there is only a partial view of a child's phonological production, for although feature analysis provides more helpful information, gaps are still obvious in attempting to describe child phonology. DeVilliers and de Villiers (1978) suggest word form as a basis for selective production by children. As mentioned in Muma's summary stages (1978), children at nursery level tend to produce single-syllable words or simple two- or three-syllable words. These word forms are usually CV, CVC, or CVCV productions. Children will reduce adult words to these more simplified forms.

Another dimension for the observer of child phonology is through phonological processes that typify child rules in speech production. The advantage of this approach is that it allows the explanation of child phonology based on consistent substitution and systematic strategies that children employ in the simplification of adult pronunciation (deVilliers & deVilliers, 1978). Children consistently use particular forms at various stages of phonological development (see Chapter 6).

As noted in Chapter 6, Ingram (1974, 1976) has defined the several phonological or phonotactic processes that are present in utterances of nursery-aged children:

- diminutive—the addition of /i/ to the end of a word (mommy, puppy)
- voicing—the voicing of initial consonants and the unvoicing of final consonants (cat = /gaet/, bed = bet, cookie = /d ʊ tI/)
- consonant cluster reduction—deletion of cluster features (stop = /top/, first = /f ʌ s/)
- weak syllable deletion—simplification of multisyllable words (banana = /naen ʌ /, potatoe = /teto/)
- assimilation—substitution of one phonetic activity for another (forward: coat = /tot/, doggy = /g ɔ ggI/; backward: kitty = kikky, top = /t ɔ t/)
- reduplication—syllable repetition (mama, bye-bye)

DeVilliers and deVilliers (1978) list additional phonotactic processes:

- fronting—substitution of front consonants for back consonants (go = /do/, soap = /top/)
- simplification—reduction of CVD to CV syllable (dog = /do/, boat = /bo/)
- glide for liquids—substitution of glides for consonants for liquid forms (love = /w ʌ v/, run = /w ʌ n/)
- fricative/stop exchanges—substitution of stop consonants for fricatives in initial positions (sunny = /p ʌ nI/); substitution of fricatives for stop consonants in final positions (neck = /nes/)

Based on phonological or phonotactic processes that are consistent and systematic, the "errors" of child production are a normal aspect of phonological development. Although exhibited in varying degrees by different children, they are evident in the speech of nursery-age children.

Expansion and Refinement Stage

Syntax and morphology. As the young child develops linguistically beyond three-word utterances, there is increased expansion and refinement in syntax. At earlier levels, semantic complexity played a vital central role in acquisition, but, as utterances lengthen and ideas and words are combined, syntactic complexity becomes the focal point. The most notable aspect of this expansion and refinement is the addition of the inflectional morphemes acquired and manifested by children in linguistic development.

This addition of morphological markers affords the child mastery of more subtle shades of meaning in expression.

Brown's (1973) in-depth studies on the morphological acquisition of children indicate uniformity in the mastery of such grammatical units and the acquisition of morphemes in a predictable order. In the longitudinal studies by Brown and his colleagues, 14 morphemes were identified and ranked in terms of acquisition (see Table 8–1). The order of acquisition was based on the increased complexity underlying each morpheme. This complexity was analyzed and identified in two ways: by the number of transformations inherent, and by the meanings contained in each morpheme produced. The first consideration, related to syntax, indicated that morphemes involving one transformation were acquired earlier than those demanding an additional transformation. The second aspect, based on cumulative semantic complexity, involves the degree of necessary information that the child must take into account. DeVilliers and deVilliers (1978) cite the example of the morpheme *-ed* for the regular past form of verbs, wherein the form need not change based on the subject (I walk*ed,* you walk*ed,* they walk*ed*). However, to use the copula *be* correctly, the child must first consider the subject (am/is/are), the number (is/are), and the tense (is/was). In actuality, it is the combination of these complexities that determines the order of acquisition.

Another form of expansion beyond the three-word-utterance level is the addition of function words previously omitted in the expressive language

Table 8–1 Brown's Fourteen Grammatical Morphemes

Morpheme	*Form*	*Example*
Present progressive	-ing	Bobby runn*ing*.
In-on (prepositions)	in, on	Book *on* table. Book *in* box.
Plural (regular)	-s, -es, etc.	See boys.
Past irregular	ran, went, etc.	Bobby *ran*.
Possessive	-'s	Bobby's shoe.
Uncontractible copula	is, am, are	Mommy *is* pretty.
Articles	a/an, the	Pet *the* kitty.
Past regular	-ed, -d, -/t/	Bobby walk*ed*.
Third person regular	-s	Bobby walk*s*.
Third person irregular	has, does, etc.	Bobby goes.
Uncontractible auxiliary	be + ing	Bobby *is* runn*ing*.
Contractible copula	's, 're, 'm	Bobby's big.
Contractible auxiliary	be + ('s, 're, 'm) + ing	Bobby's runn*ing*.

Source: Based on data from Brown (1973).

of the young child. This, of course, is closely related to morphological aspects but also includes an increased number of descriptors and the initiation of specific interrogative forms. Single verbs expand by inflection and also by the addition of elements in the auxiliary, such as the modal (can go) and have + participle (have gone). With refinements and expansions, the child's linguistic system becomes more efficient in allowing the communication of extensive ideas, more economical in requiring fewer utterances to present ideas, and more interpretable by allowing greater information available to the listener.

Semantics. From the three-word-utterance stage through the stage of refinement and expansion, the preschool child rapidly acquires the productive use of vocabulary. Children appear to use many words, even though minimal exposure may have occurred. They also employ words long before the words have acquired complete adult meaning. We still lack the necessary knowledge to explain exactly what strategies and how such strategies are employed in the development of semantic complexity and in the child's comprehension and expression of words.

There is some understanding in this area, however. Semantic relations are related to concepts that children form, and we assume that cognitive awareness of the environment accounts in part for the child's interpretation of words and the meaning attached to words when the child expresses them. Although it has been observed that children do not imitate new syntactic constructions, imitation may assist in the expansion of new vocabulary (Kretschmer & Kretschmer, 1978).

As the child masters increasingly sophisticated sentences and varies the use of words in differing semantic roles and relationships, the child is allowed more complete expressive talent. This is the linguistic goal of the nursery-age child. The greater command the child has over language, the greater the ability for learning new information, using previously acquired information, expressing ideas, needs, and desires, and interacting with others in the environment.

Pragmatics. The summation and application of the nursery-age child's language ability evolves in an increasing ability to communicate functionally with those nearby. Acquisition of conversational skills is another aspect of growing linguistic sophistication. The understanding of conversational cues and correctly responding to them signal pragmatic development. Kretschmer and Kretschmer (1978) state that pragmatic sophistication occurs over time. As children mature in the other linguistic components, they will also acquire facility in conversational interaction. This is the comprehension of how language is used in a social function.

As may be observed even in this brief overview of linguistic development between the ages of 30 to 48 months, the nursery-age child makes extensive strides in the acquisition of language. The child with normal hearing and language functioning proceeds in a relatively short period of time from the telegraphic expressions of two- and three-word utterances to the use of sentences comprised of descriptors, qualifiers, actions, processes, and other relational uses of words. The child graduates from a naming and topic/comment format to utilize questions and requests for information, directives, and explanation.

The child with hearing and/or language impairment will vary in language functioning based on the extent of the handicap. Nevertheless, the emerging language behaviors of normal children at this level should remain the goal, either immediate or in the near future, for nursery-level professionals.

Emotional and Social Maturation

The entry into the age referred to as nursery level in this text expands the young child's social interaction to include other children of the same age. Even though other children may be present in the family or extended family with whom the child is familiar, the nursery school will usually represent the first exposure to a group of children of one's own age. On the other hand, nursery teachers may have in their charge young children who have been primarily or totally surrounded by adults and who have no experience involving children of any age. In any case, social development is an important aspect of the nursery-level experience of a handicapped child (Cruickshank, 1948). Formal and informal interactions through planned activities and play must foster opportunity for growth in socialization.

The nursery level should not mean merely a teacher interacting with a child or vice versa; it should also encourage child-to-child socialization exchanges. Planned activities such as snacks or beginning-of-the-day procedures provide excellent opportunities to encourage the development and appreciation of acceptable social behavior between children. As mentioned in regard to infants, handicapped children as well as their normal peers must operate day to day in a world that demands certain social responsibilities toward themselves and others. Unless children are provided with settings conducive to such learning, they may become socially handicapped as well.

Socialization and Hearing or Language Impairment

The area of social development is a critical area for children with hearing and/or language disorders. Much social learning takes place in situations where communication is intimately interwoven. Indeed, although socially appropriate behavior comes about through modeling and experimenting, a large degree of verbal guidance and feedback is associated with social learning and emotional expression.

Due to the lack of age-appropriate linguistic and communicative behavior, many hearing-impaired and language-delayed nursery children also display immature or inappropriate social and emotional behaviors. Absence of a system for communication inhibits interaction, both responsive and initiated. Words supply an acceptable expression of needs. If there are no words (or signs), a more direct route is taken, usually through physical avenues. Words express emotions, and the frustration of such vital displays can result in rather physically direct information.

Supplying a communication system to foster interaction and expression of natural emotion is a prime objective of nursery programs for children with limited language performance. Equally important for children is learning to understand and deal with childhood emotions in themselves and their peers. Joy, fear, anger, and sadness are all aspects of daily life for everyone, but many hearing- and language-impaired children cannot realize that fact unless they are provided with sufficient experience and explanation to secure the relevant knowledge.

Play as a Facilitator of Social and Emotional Development

The universal activity of young children, indeed the business of childhood, is play (Hasenstab, 1975). Preschool professionals have long recognized the fact that play provides the opportunity for a variety of learning experiences—linguistically, intellectually, and socially. Fallen (1978) describes play as the avenue by which a child discovers facets of self, emotion, personality, language, and other persons. Lindberg (1971) explains that as young children play they develop foundations crucial to survival in later school years. The notion of "mere play" is contested by Murphy (1971), who states that such activity involves the integration of many awarenesses and the continuous development of new insight into one's surroundings.

Depending on the nursery child's previous experiences, environment, and of course the extent of handicap, the developmental progression of social play from solitary, to parallel, and then to cooperative play may be delayed or distorted (Safford, 1978). Indeed, it is our experience that some children's play experiences have been so deprived that they are rendered incapable of objective investigation. For this reason, guidance in teaching young preschoolers how to play, especially with other children, is a necessary and integral function that permeates all aspects of the nursery program. A healthy balance of time for experimentation on one's own and for interaction at whatever level of social play a child may be involved in is a paramount consideration. The nursery staff should be aware of the value of "free play" as well as organized planned activities. Overstructure is as debilitating to learning as understructure. Teachers must be sensitive as to when their intervention is needed and when children should be allowed to solve a play dilemma, either with an object or in social context, by themselves.

The Problem of Separation from Parent

All preschool professionals can attest to the display of tears, clinging, and total rejection of the teacher when a young child fears separation from the parent. Parents naturally are paramount in the child's life at this early age; in some cases, separation of any form may never have occurred. However, other children may have experienced a departure from the family under not so pleasant circumstances, as in the case of hospital confinement. In such instances, removal of the mother or father may be all the more frightening to the child. Even for a child not particularly prone to fear of separation, the first few days in nursery school, with new people, adults, and children and a new environment, may be awesome.

Allowing gradual separation is often helpful in effecting a smooth entry to the nursery level. "Mom time" for a few minutes each session at the beginning of the school day has been shown to be beneficial. This time can then be gradually decreased until the child feels confident that mother will return. Since many parents observe during the session, allowing a child to escort a parent to the observation room and then retrieve the parent when school is over has also proved to be of assistance.

Not all children will exhibit difficulty in separating from the parent, and degrees of anxiety will vary; but the preschool staff should be sensitive to the child's perception of the new situation and resulting apprehension. Preschool teachers should also bear in mind that the separation anxiety may also exist with the parent and that guidance and support may be necessary to prevent the mother or father from fostering a fear of detachment. Assurance that the child will function satisfactorily without the presence of the parent and encouragement of parental observation of the preschooler involved in daily routine will help allay qualms that parents may have about leaving their little ones.

Emotional Development and the Self Concept

Young preschool children become increasingly aware of themselves as individuals in the development of a self concept. This is in part due to reactions and interactions of the family, other significant adults, and peers. Therefore, a secure and accepting environment in the preschool is critical.

Teachers and other preschool staff members must remember that children with hearing and language problems are children first and that the factor of their handicap does not lessen their value as human beings. Professionals must also assist parents in maintaining such an attitude. Expectations should be positive, realistic, and appropriate.

The self concept or a self-image, Hurlock (1972) explains, includes both a physical and a psychological domain. The physical self-image for young preschool children involves an awareness of their sex, their bodies, and various body parts and of the use of their bodies within the environment. The psychological self-image is concerned with thoughts and feelings about qualities or limitations of one's self. This "thought" activity occurs somewhat later, but even the young child begins to react according to attitudes displayed toward the child since infancy.

The self concept directly affects a child's social and emotional growth, which in turn fosters either a positive or negative self concept. Young children at age 2 or 3 are still primarily egocentric in nature, and therefore ideas of self emerge before ideas, attitudes, or concepts of others. Self-opinion influences socialization and emotional reaction to other persons, since the self is used as the judgment standard for all behavior.

The development of the self concept is naturally affected first by the home and family; but, for children with whom early intervention occurs, the input information quickly expands to include children and adults outside the home setting. All aspects of the child—personality, physical appearance, abilities, and limitations—cause reactions from surrounding persons and therefore influence the self concept. For the hearing- or language-handicapped child, the additional factor of the disability also plays a role in the development of a self-image. Self-acceptance, expectations, self-motivation and self-confidence all have roots in development during early childhood.

CURRICULUM

The curriculum for the nursery level in the Comprehensive Services Program is constructed on a basis of five major areas: language-cognition-comprehension, audition, language communication, motor abilities, and social-emotional behavior. As in the parent-infant program, the curriculum is adapted to the individual needs of each child. In this section, we provide a description of each curriculum area; as noted earlier, our purpose is not to provide a curriculum guide, but rather to present objectives and activities that may be helpful as starting points in creating ideas and activities in other intervention settings.

Language-Cognition-Comprehension

The purpose of the language-cognition-comprehension component in the nursery curriculum is to provide linguistic and cognitive experiences that will foster the child's mastery of comprehension and understanding of the surrounding world. The component includes the reception of sensory information through all of the input channels, with extensive emphasis on audition and vision. It also pertains to the development of conceptual understanding and comprehension of relationships between objects as they exist in the environment.

This primary component of curriculum is further delineated to include specific attention to particular areas and the language and concepts related to them. Self-awareness is one subcategory. This aspect, highly coordinated with both the development of the self concept and motor abilities, involves children's cognitive discovery of their bodies, how they may use their bodies in goal attainment, and the language and vocabulary that represent parts and functions of themselves. Since the child at nursery age is naturally ego-centered, the child's own body provides motivation for discovery and learning. An understanding of words, cues, or signs for facial and body parts is a continuing objective. Another objective is comprehension of associated sensory activity (taste, smell, hear, etc., as actions and words depicting action) and of the actions the child's body is able to perform (run, walk, jump, etc.).

Stimulation for conceptual understanding is initiated in parent-infant programming but continues to be vital at the nursery level. The relationship of the child to the environment and of objects to objects in the surroundings includes various relationships that must be understood cognitively and linguistically. Concepts of, and words, cues, or signs representing, relationships of position, location, size, quality, and so forth are richly represented in daily activities of an experience-oriented nursery school. The provision of opportunities for children to discover such relationships and to receive information about representational symbols is an important aspect of this area of curriculum, based on the language development appropriate to this age level.

The principal objectives of this curriculum area thus are:

- development of the child's cognitive and linguistic understanding of the environment
- development of concepts and language related to self
- development of concepts and language related to object relationships
- development of strategies for the reception of language information

The central emphasis is on input comprehension. During the parent-infant program, much stimulation was provided so that the young baby would be exposed to a variety of sensory and cognitive experiences. At the nursery level, the purpose is to build upon and expand that cognitive foundation with increased emphasis on aspects of receptive language development and the understanding of words, cues, or signs in communication.

This language-cognition-comprehension component has important implications for nursery-level personnel regarding their language sophistication in communicating with hearing- and language-disordered children. Adjustment of the sophistication of one's spoken language to allow comprehension by the particular audience being addressed is an important strategy to be mastered by the preschool teacher. Olson (1970) indicates that listeners must have a comparable language base to that which is being directed to them or comprehension cannot take place. The purpose of verbal information is to communicate the speaker's intent or idea to the listener. The responsibility of the speaker is to at least anticipate the listener's knowledge of the referent. In other words, the preschool teacher must direct spoken or signed information to a child at a linguistic level that the child can understand. Appendix B presents suggested language objectives and activities suitable for young children.

Audition

Audition is closely related to—actually an integral part of—the comprehension of language. The major goal for children at the nursery level is to develop an awareness of sounds within the surrounding environment and to develop an awareness of spoken language through the use of amplified residual hearing. Miller and Lehman (1970) state that, since sound of one sort or another is always present in a child's surroundings, learning to interpret such auditory information can be beneficial to the child, even though the auditory message is altered due to hearing loss. However, as mentioned in the previous chapter, unless the auditory function is actively stimulated from early in life, the auditory system will fail to respond effectively.

The primary emphasis, therefore, is on establishing an auditory environment to serve the needs of the handicapped children who fall into three basic categories, all of which require auditory stimulation. The first category includes those with diagnosed sensory neural hearing impairment. The need for auditory stimulation in this case is obvious. Subcomponents include adjustment to amplification if fitting has just occurred, simple care of the aid, consistent and constant use of amplification, development of listening, localization of sounds, and other processing-related abilities.

The second group of children, those with language delay as a result of chronic middle-ear problems, also, as noted, requires an auditory environment. Although in most cases middle-ear problems that are closely monitored will not cause lasting damage to the auditory system, for periods of time these children are functionally hearing impaired. The development of listening ability and attention to speech are critical in the child's mastery of receptive and expressive language during the linguistically critical preschool years.

The third group of children manifests language delay concurrent with auditory problems related to the processing of auditory information. These children must be guided through the interdependent levels of auditory processing in order to enhance both listening and linguistic ability.

An environment that capitalizes on all aspects of sound is critical for each of these groups of children if significant gains are to be made in the growth of auditory and linguistic development. Pollack and Ernst (1973) offer 10 suggestions to aid in the establishment of an auditory environment in the nursery setting:

1. Develop an attitude of readiness to listen.
2. Use auditory stimuli (speech, environmental sounds).
3. Use speech in communicating with the child (aural/oral, total communication, or cued speech).
4. Allow time for processing of auditory information.
5. Maintain face-to-face proximity when speaking to a child.
6. Use normal conversational intensity and rate.
7. Use appropriate speech and language models.
8. Utilize linguistic redundancy.
9. Orient the child to the activity context.
10. Involve parents.

A final suggestion pertains to the physical structure of the nursery-level classroom: Provide an optimal sound setting, including acoustic tile, carpeting, draperies, and so forth. Although general in nature, these suggestions provide a framework in which to develop more program- and child-specific goals.

Language Communication

The third curriculum area concerns the expressive aspect of language. The language experiences that are provided at the nursery level must enable the child to internalize linguistic rules that will allow the production of language in communication. Additional emphasis is placed on fostering an awareness of the role of language and speech in the communication process. Kretschmer and Kretschmer (1978) indicate that communication competence appears to be poorly developed in young children with hearing loss. One purpose of this curriculum area is to aid in the reduction of that deficit.

Obviously, this curriculum component is initiated at the level at which a particular child is functioning. Much variation from child to child can occur, due to differences in degree of hearing loss, hearing age, onset of hearing loss, quality of experiences previous to the nursery level, and so on. Continual progress is the goal for all children, but the amount of progress and the rate will depend on the individual characteristics of each child.

Many children may require intervention at the prespeech stage. Until prosody, control of breath flow and musculature of the oral apparatus, especially the tongue, is gained, intelligible speech is not possible. Spontaneous vocalizations are stimulated and rewarded when used in appropriate situations in combination with gestures. For example, at the prespeech stage, a child may extend an open palm and utter /m/ /m/ to request a cookie at snack time. Basically, prespeech attention is similar to that in parent-infant programming, except that the activities and experiences are more appropriate to nursery-age children.

When children consistently use one-word utterances, they are considered to be at the speech stage, though prespeech strategies will still be used. Here, the emphasis is on the semantic content and pragmatic function of words for the child. Articulation expectations are based on the child's age and hearing level. Syntactic patterns enter in at the two- and three-word-utterance level. At all levels, the interrelationship of the linguistic components remains central.

As noted in Chapter 6, continuous language samples are maintained on all children enrolled in the preschool programs. Each week, approximately 15 to 25 utterances are recorded in various situations for each child. These "mini-samples" are analyzed and collected in each semester. This provides an ongoing record of the children's linguistic progress over time and allows the staff to evaluate progress and make curriculum adjustments as needed.

Expression through oral communication and an aural/oral approach are fostered by the Comprehensive Services Program, although we do employ cued speech and sign language in a total-communication approach. We believe that there is no one communication system that can apply generally to all children with hearing loss. Because this is a hearing-speaking world, we also believe that all children deserve the right to use their capacity to speak and hear, no matter how limited. The goal is competence in communication; arguments over methodology do little to achieve that end.

In summary, the curriculum area of language communication is concerned with fostering the child's oral and/or manual facility in communication with others in the environment. It is aimed at the integration of all linguistic components to produce competent communicative performance. It thus permeates all phases and experiences in the nursery-level program.

Motor Development

A curriculum for nursery-age children would not be complete without consideration of motor development. In the period before the fourth birthday, the young child gains increased control over the body, in both large- and fine-muscle abilities. These two areas are integrated into all aspects of the child's nursery-level program. Motor activities are coordinated with activities designed for cognitive and linguistic discovery, movement in space helps to demonstrate active words, and increased mastery of musculature and movement allows success in self-help areas.

The motor area of curriculum emphasizes the child's developing skills in the use of arms and legs in strength, endurance, and coordination. It also focuses on the child's ability to maneuver in space and to walk, run, change position, and so on, smoothly and rapidly. Fine-muscle ability is also stressed so that children develop eye-hand coordination and finger dexterity as well as control of face musculature and the tongue in speech production.

In addition to its general curriculum, the Comprehensive Services Program has the advantage of participation in a motor development clinic on the University of Virginia campus. Each class participates in this experience for 60 minutes each week, with activities designed specifically for each age group. Teachers, parents, and children have found this to be a valuable additional service.

It may be said in summary that goals in the motor development area of the curriculum are generally age appropriate unless an additional debilitating circumstance is evident that limits the hearing-impaired or language-delayed child's motor growth.

Social and Emotional Maturation

As indicated earlier, various aspects of a language delay resulting from a hearing impairment or other disability may cause retardation in the area of social and emotional maturity. This fifth area of curriculum is thus geared to promote social competence and healthy emotional displays of nursery-age, hearing-impaired and language-delayed children. It is designed to foster relationships both with other children and with adults, including those in school and at home.

Socially, the child is encouraged to develop self-confidence, independence, a foundation of responsibility, and successful social interaction with others. The emotional domain is concerned with the realization of feelings and their healthy and appropriate expression. These goals are often "taught" as incidental learning in the context of the nursery school's daily routine, as conducive situations arise.

Fallen (1978) supports the tenet that preschool programs for handicapped children can facilitate emotional and social development and suggests four factors that are implicit in this support:

1. Preschool experience: The preschool can provide social experiences and interactions to aid in overcoming or preventing social immaturity.
2. Significant adults: adults, as models, can foster emotional and social development.
3. Peer relationships: Peer interaction can foster social and emotional development. Nonhandicapped children make favorable social models.
4. Curriculum and materials: a curriculum should be designed to assist children in social and emotional development, emphasizing acceptable social behavior, emotional expression via acceptable means, independence, and responsibility. A general, affective approach is beneficial.

The end goal is a healthy well-adjusted, socially competent adult. This area thus must be addressed early in order that experiences can be provided or acted upon that will stimulate growth toward this outcome.

Self-Help Skills

Independence and self-confidence grow from an ever-increasing awareness that one can care for one's self with decreasing dependence on others. The self-help curriculum area capitalizes on this assumption. Self-help skills range from toileting to mastery of an activity or game without assistance from others, but it also includes the awareness that help may sometime be necessary and beneficial.

Children who enter the nursery level vary greatly in this area, depending on age, maturation in other areas, and home environment. Often self-help includes educating parents regarding the expectations of their children and allowing the child freedom to accomplish such tasks as dressing and undressing or putting away toys. This is an area that integrates well into the total preschool scheme.

Summary

The curriculum designed for use at the nursery level of the Comprehensive Services Program is based on those aspects that relate specifically to the needs of the hearing-impaired and language-delayed children and also those aspects that pertain to child growth in general. Although goals are developed in each area, as part of the child individual educational plan (IEP), actual experiences cross over and foster development across areas. It is vitally important that attention in the preschool curriculum go beyond the handicap and span all areas of child development.

In implementing the curriculum, teaching is done primarily with a unit approach, wherein a topic is selected that is of interest to the children, such as seasonal occurrences or holidays, and objectives in various areas are implemented through appropriately related activities. For example, a unit developed around Halloween over a two-week period can successfully integrate objectives of the five major component areas as well as each subcategory to provide individual and group experiences for each child at his level of performance.

PARENTS AND THE NURSERY SCHOOL

In the preschool years, although the instructional environment has shifted from the home to the classroom setting, parents are far from excluded in the process of their children's education and development. If the parents have graduated from a parent-infant home program they will most likely be well along in working cooperatively with the staff in providing experiences for the child. They must be encouraged to continue to carry out goals and objectives outside the preschool setting to foster continued progress in all areas of development

The preschool staff must bear in mind that, traditionally, parenting has been a private and personal endeavor. The goal is thus to work with parents, not to usurp their position. Educational programs do intrude on families, but such intrusion need not be negative. Professionals have the responsibility of bolstering parent resourcefulness and motivation. Bodner-Johnson (1980) sums it up nicely in her comment that the professional must interact and serve in a manner that fosters parent motivation and resolution.

Parents Who Have Not Participated in a Parent-Infant Program

In many cases and for various reasons, children may not come to the attention of professionals until they are 30 months of age or older. Therefore, because of their age, these children are enrolled in the nursery level rather than the parent-infant program, unless of course there is significant overall delay. In these instances, in working with the parents, the nursery teacher is beginning at the same point as in parent-infant programming. For the majority of these parents, the confirmation of hearing loss and/or language delay will require the type of initial approach and goals described in Chapter 7. Giangreco and Giangreco (1976) suggest the following areas of emphasis for parents of children diagnosed as handicapped at nursery age:

- acceptance of the child
- a calm and understanding approach to the child
- recognition of the child's efforts
- consistency and realism in expectations and discipline
- avoidance of overprotection and overindulgence of the child
- encouragement of the child's independence and sense of responsibility
- communication with the child
- care and maintenance of the child's hearing aid if the child is hearing impaired.

These areas represent the basic goals appropriate for parents of nursery-age children. The staff must assist parents in developing resourcefulness in nurturing the progress and development of their child and working cooperatively with the preschool program.

Objectives for Parent Involvement at the Nursery Level

A nursery program will of course develop objectives to be carried out through the curriculum and the experiences of the children enrolled in the program. If parents are to assist in this educational endeavor, objectives must also be specified to meet the individual needs of each family unit. It is vital for preschool staff members and parents to set forth together the goals toward which the family can strive during the enrollment in the nursery-level program.

Horton (1974) notes five general categories that sum up concisely the objectives for parental cooperation with the nursery-school program:

1. to instruct parents in ways in which the auditory environment can be optimized
2. to instruct parents in a manner of communication with their child
3. to familiarize parents with aspects of normal language development and the principles of application regarding their hearing-impaired child

4. to instruct parents in ways of behavior management
5. to provide parents with necessary support in all areas concerning the adaptations of living with a hearing-impaired child

These suggestions are of course general, but they represent basic areas in which parents can grow in independence and resourcefulness in the day-to-day living experience with their child.

Parent Carry-Over of Preschool Programming

Although at the nursery level the child with a language and/or hearing difficulty receives both individual and group instruction designed specifically to enhance development, the total exposure to this setting in the Comprehensive Services Program for full-time enrollment is 12½ hours per week. The majority of time in a preschool child's day is still in the company of the child's family or caretaker. It is therefore of utmost importance that goals and objectives of the nursery program are carried over and receive reinforcement by parents outside the preschool setting.

"Veteran" Parents

Many parents who have been involved intimately in the educational program provided by a parent-infant home program may continue appropriate home stimulation of their child. In this case, cooperation and communication between the parents and the nursery staff becomes a goal in providing continuity in experiences in and out of the preschool class. Depending on personal schedules, parents should be encouraged to observe their child as often as possible, to participate in field trips, class parties, and other such activities, to present topics or activities of interest to the class, or even to create a new and intriguing treat for snack time. (One mother of oriental heritage demonstrated the creation of egg rolls, much to the pleasure of the children and the staff.) In addition, in both the school and the home, visitation conferences should be held regularly. (A total of 10 formal conferences are conducted each year in the Comprehensive Services Program.) If parents transport their children to and from school daily, the staff should be available before and after school hours to answer questions and to provide helpful information concerning the day's progress and activities. Telephone and written communications are also important avenues to share information, answer questions, and instruct and guide parents as to how they might best complement the preschool program for their child.

"Rookie" Parents

Parents who are experiencing professional intervention for the first time by the enrollment of their child in the nursery or prekindergarten may, as mentioned earlier, require a period of adjustment and more individual guidance and attention to assist them in the cooperative education of their hearing- and/or language-impaired child. As Pollack (1970) points out, parents may be surprised or even overwhelmed by the idea that there is need for so much carry-over outside of preschool. They may feel that the education of their child is the school's responsibility, not theirs. This requires much the same support, patience, and guidance that is effective with parents who are beginning parent-infant programs for the first time.

In the Comprehensive Services Program, it is the responsibility of the director to work with such parents until they feel confident and receptive toward the cooperative educational effort. We have found that sitting with parents during observations of classroom procedure and individual therapy, explaining clearly and precisely the purpose of each activity, and providing specific suggestions for carry-over have been extremely beneficial. Another helpful approach is a parent "buddy system," in which veteran parents assist new parents in the initial phases of preschool programming. "Rookie" parents are assigned to other, more experienced parents whose children are similar in age, development, and so forth. Personal suggestions and support are very helpful in assisting in parental adjustment to the educational team.

Parent Groups and Clubs

Parent clubs or groups are an aspect of parental involvement in the educational programs of preschool hearing- and/or language-disordered children. Cain (1976) notes that parents of handicapped children originally formed groups based informally on a common problem they shared. The primary purpose was mutual support of one another in adjusting to such problems. This remains the goal of parent groups.

On a larger scale, parent groups can provide an important resource in the community by sponsoring information services and educating the general public regarding hearing- and language-handicapping conditions. Fallen (1978) suggests that parent groups can be active in securing vital information and statistics regarding handicapped children in the community so that services can be improved.

Parent groups exist in various forms at local, state, and national levels. Parents should be encouraged to lend their support to and participate in such organizations. A listing of national organizations that assist parents of children with hearing and/or language problems is provided in Appendix C.

Difficulties in Organizing a Parent Group

Although parent groups are highly beneficial and to a large degree truly serve the needs of handicapped children, problems can arise in attempting to implement such an organization in association with a preschool program. Although difficulties experienced in the establishment of a successful parent group may be related to a particular geographical setting or population composition and to the distance between the parents, there are general factors that present realistic problems that can hinder the success of any parent organization.

Perhaps the greatest difficulty has been the lack of commonality among the parents. The only mutually shared issue is the presence of at least one preschool child with a hearing loss or language delay. Employment of the parents may range from professional fields in medicine, law, and academia to continuous unemployment. Socioeconomic status may range from upper-middle status to the level of welfare assistance. And education may range from postdoctoral levels to a third-grade schooling. These differences, coupled with factors of distance and time, present hurdles that are often difficult to overcome. Therefore, it has often proved more beneficial to work in small groups or individually with parents.

Alternatives to Parent Organizations

Recital of these difficulties is not meant to constitute a pessimistic portrayal of parent organizations. There are times, however, when certain alternatives may be appropriate.

Organizations associated with public school divisions. One alternative is to encourage parents to join parent organizations that exist in their local school districts. Eventually, the children will be enrolled in the local school program. This association allows parents to become acquainted with others in their community who have hearing-impaired children with similar needs, to provide optimal programming in the schools and improved community awareness or issues peculiar to their area of residence. Another advantage is that parents can interact with families who have hearing-impaired children beyond the preschool level. In many cases, parents of older children are helpful in support of parents with younger handicapped children, by offering information and suggestions that enhance and assist in daily living.

State-wide parent organizations. In many states, large parent groups operate state-wide with chapters in several locations. Parents can be encouraged to participate in these organizations. Many state parent groups are politically active and have managed to exert great pressure toward the improvement of services on a large scale to hearing- and/or language-disordered children. Where local chapters of these groups may deal with problems pertinent to the particular location, the state-wide organization can merge the needs of parents throughout the state. With a large membership, good leadership, and efficient organization, such an organization can often be quite effective in assisting parents and their handicapped children.

Organized family activities. In addition to political, informational, and service activities carried out by various parent groups at all levels, family social events also play an important part. National organizations such as the Alexander Graham Bell Association and the National Association for the Deaf hold national conventions that are open to parents and provide a combination of social and informative activities for families. In addition, state and local groups hold picnics, fairs, and other family social gatherings that allow recreational interaction for families with hearing- and language-handicapped children.

Where a more formal parent organization has not proved successful, such activities might also be implemented through a preschool program. Two or three times in each school term, family picnics or group activities, such as attending the circus, can be organized by the staff and made available to families of children in the program. An emphasis on activities that provide experiences for young children allows the parents to participate for short periods of time in a completely informal situation.

Meeting the needs of parents on an individual basis. If formal parent groups are not conducive to a particular program setting, other avenues are available to assist parents in solving problems individually. As we have frequently noted, communication between the professional and parent is vital for optimal educational intervention. Professionals must serve as providers both of direct information and of the resources for information necessarily obtained from other professionals. A sense of trust and cooperation is of paramount importance in assisting parents to cope with the situation of the handicapped child, regardless of how minimal the problem may be. In some cases, the difficulty may be temporary, as in the case of language delay due to chronic middle-ear disorder. Parents must realize that the prognosis for eventual age-appropriate language and speech may be excellent but that at present certain steps must be taken to guarantee such results. As professionals concerned with optimal intervention of preschool hearing-impaired and language-delayed children, we must never lose sight of the fact that parents are our primary resource.

RECORDS AND REPORTS

One purpose of preschool programs, at both the nursery and prekindergarten levels, is to work cooperatively with public schools and other agencies involved in educational, medical, or social services for hearing- and language-handicapped preschool children. Therefore, it is imperative that complete and accurate records and reports be maintained by both the staff and the administration. However, it is also important that teachers and administrators do not become so bogged down in paperwork that time that could be devoted to educational planning is usurped. A balance of comprehensive reporting and a reasonable time effort must be maintained. Based on feedback from other agencies, parents, and the staff, the Comprehensive Services Program has found the following forms and specifications for information conducive to the records and reporting needs of our own center and of those entities with whom we operate in cooperative efforts.

Intake Information Form

All children serviced by the Speech and Hearing Center in any capacity are required to have a completed information form at the time of initial evaluation. This form, shown in Exhibit 8–1, consists of questions addressed to the history and present disposition of the child.

Release-of-Information Form

Because of the confidentiality of assessment and educational information and the need to share such information with schools, physicians, and other professionals, permission to release such information must be secured from the child's parents (see Exhibit 8–2). The names of the relevant persons or agencies are recorded on the form, subject to parental approval. Parents may also request that reports be sent to certain agencies.

Preschool Emergency and Permission Form

It is important that the preschool staff be informed of any physical limitations that may be medically imposed on a young child's daily activity and participation in preschool experiences. In addition, information is needed regarding medication and dosage a child receives, any allergies that a child may have, the child's reaction to particular substances, and the procedures to be taken if allergic reactions occur.

Due to the young ages of the children, it is vital that a parent or other responsible adult can be reached in case of emergency. This information is required of all children enrolled in either level of the preschool program.

Exhibit 8–1 Intake Information Form

University of Virginia

SPEECH AND HEARING CENTER

Department of Speech Pathology and Audiology

109 New Cabell Hall

Charlottesville, Virginia 22903

CHILDREN'S PRE-EVALUATION INFORMATION

Please fill out this form as fully and accurately as you can and return it as soon as possible. The information you give will enable us to have a better understanding of the problems involved and will expedite the course of the speech and/or hearing evaluation and interviews. All material and information is kept in strict confidence. Following receipt of the completed form, we will schedule an appointment and notify you of the date and hour.

Date ....

Full Name of Person to be Evaluated ....

By what name is he usually called? ....

Address ....

Telephone Number .... Age .... Date of Birth ....

Name and Address of School ....

City, county or private school? .... Grade ....

Principal's Name .... Teacher's Name ....

Father's Name ....

Age .... Education ....

Occupation .... Employer .... Business Phone ....

Mother's Name ....

Age .... Education ....

Occupation .... Employer .... Business Phone ....

Family Doctor or Pediatrician: Name .... Address ....

Shall we send a report to the physician? ☐ Yes ☐ No

Who Referred You To This Center? Name .... Address ....

Other Children in the Family:

Name	Age	Birthdate	Grade	Any Speech or Hearing Problem?

Describe the speech and/or hearing problem of the person to be evaluated:

....

....

Possible cause or causes ....

How does he seem to feel about his speech and/or hearing problem? ....

....

BIRTH HISTORY

A. Pregnancy

Health of mother during pregnancy ....

....

Diseases, accidents, drugs, or X-ray treatment of mother during pregnancy ....

Exposure to any infectious diseases during pregnancy ....

....

Rh factor of mother .... Rh factor of father ....

Exhibit 8–1 continued

B. Birth

1. Delivered in hospital? ....
2. Premature? ....
3. Normal ....
   Caesarean ....
   Breech ....
4. Any instruments used? ....
5. Blue baby? ....
6. Jaundiced? ....
7. Weight at birth ....
8. Length of time from beginning of labor until birth ....

C. Other Birth Complications (convulsions, breathing difficulties, feeding problems, etc.) ....

DEVELOPMENTAL HISTORY

A. Weight of baby at 6 months .... 1 year .... 5 years ....

B. Give age when:

1. First tooth appeared ....
2. First crawled ....
3. First sat without support ....
4. First walked alone ....
5. First fed self with spoon ....
6. First gained control of bladder ....
7. First gained control of bowels ....

C. Does he: (a) prefer the right hand or left hand? ....
(b) fall or lose balance easily? ....
(c) pick up and hold objects readily? ....
(d) seem awkward? ....
(e) walk in a peculiar manner? ....

HEALTH HISTORY

	Age	Severity
Convulsions		
High fever		
Diseases child has had		
Accidents		
Operations		
Nervous trouble		
Visual problems		

EDUCATION

What are his average marks? ....

Did he ever fail a grade? ....

Did he have any serious difficulty in any grade or subject? ....

Has he ever had an intelligence test? .... Explain ....

ENVIRONMENTAL

Does anyone besides the parents and children live in the home? ....

If mother works, who cares for him? .... Where? ....

Is any language other than English spoken in the home? .... If so, what? ....

Does he have contact with anyone having a speech disorder? ....

How does he play with other children? ....

How would you describe his personality?

☐ Friendly ☐ Shy ☐ Talkative ☐ Nervous ☐ Easy-going ☐ Bad-tempered ☐ Quiet

Other: ....

Does he have any nervous habits? ....

Has he ever been a thumb-sucker? ☐ Yes ☐ No At what age? .... How was he broken of this habit? ....

Exhibit 8–1 continued

Has he ever been a bed-wetter? ☐ Yes ☐ No At what age did he stop? ....

Does he sleep and eat well? ....

Has he ever experienced a severe shock or fright? ☐ Yes ☐ No If so, explain: ....

....

SPEECH HISTORY (Give approximate age if not certain):

1. Did he cry normally? ....
2. Did he cry a great deal? .... Very little? ....
3. How much cooing did he do? ☐ A great amount ☐ Moderate amount ☐ Little ☐ None
4. How much babbling did he do? ☐ A great amount ☐ Moderate amount ☐ Little ☐ None
5. At what age did he use his first word meaningfully? ....
6. At what age did he begin to talk in sentences? ....

How did he compare with his brothers and sisters in speech development? ....

....

At what age was his speech and/or hearing difficulty first noticed? ....

....

By whom? .... What was it like? ....

What has been done to overcome the problem? ....

....

Has he had any previous professional help with his speech and/or hearing? ....

Explain: ....

Is there any abnormality in the following?

a. Tongue .... e. Throat ....

b. Jaws .... f. Lips ....

c. Nasal Passages .... g. Teeth ....

d. Palate .... h. Other ....

HEARING HISTORY

Has he ever had painful or running ears? ☐ Yes ☐ No When? ....

Which ear? .... How often? ....Was he examined by a physician? ☐ Yes ☐ No If yes, by whom? ....

Does he respond to: Loud sounds ....; Soft sounds ....; Human voice ....; Telephone ring ....; Airplane ....; Auto horn .... (State yes, no, or sometimes)

Does he seem to hear better in one ear than the other? ☐ Yes ☐ No Which ear? ....

At the present time does his hearing seem to be better, worse, or the same as usual? ....

Is he wearing a hearing aid? .... Make and Model ....

GENERAL

How far do you live from Charlottesville? ....

Is there a speech clinician in your school system? ☐ Yes ☐ No In your area? ☐ Yes ☐ No

If so, please give name and address: ....

May we write to physicians and appropriate agencies you have listed for more detailed information if needed? ....

Name of Person Filling Out Questionnaire: ....

Relationship: ....

Source: University of Virginia, Department of Speech Pathology and Audiology, Speech and Hearing Center. Reprinted by permission.

Exhibit 8–2 Release-of-Information Form

University of Virginia

SPEECH AND HEARING CENTER

Authorization for Release of Information

I hereby authorize the release of information related to the evaluation and/or therapy procedures carried out on

____
(Name)

to the following:

____

____

____

Signature ________________________________

Date ____________________

Source: University of Virginia, Department of Speech Pathology and Audiology, Speech and Hearing Center. Reprinted by permission.

Parental permission is required for various aspects of the preschool program. For example, although field trips are an important experience for young children, the children cannot be taken from the classroom without written parental approval. Because the preschool programs are associated with a teacher training facility, videotaping is often employed for purposes of educational demonstration and supervisory feedback for student teachers. In addition, photographs may be taken for dissemination of information or illustrations may be prepared (as in this text) depicting preschool procedures and environment. Again, parent permission must be secured for these purposes. Combining this information into one form that can be attached to the teacher's copy of each child's folder has proved to be a quick and beneficial means of reference (see Exhibit 8–3).

Exhibit 8–3 Preschool Emergency and Permission Form

UNIVERSITY OF VIRGINIA
PRESCHOOL FOR HEARING-IMPAIRED AND
LANGUAGE-DELAYED CHILDREN

Name ______________________ Date of birth __________

Parent/guardian ______________________________

Address ______________________________

____

Home phone ______________________ Work phone ______

Physician ______________________________

Address ______________________________

Phone ______________________________

Does your child have any allergies? (please list) __________

____

Does your child receive any medication? ____ yes ____ no

Please specify ______________________________

Does your child have any limitations concerning preschool activities participation?

____ yes ____ no Please specify ______________________

Exhibit 8–3 continued

In case of emergency, contact ______________________

Phone ______________________

Address ______________________

I give permission for my child to be taken to the emergency room in case of an accident. ____ yes ____ no

I give permission for my child to participate in class sponsored field trips. I understand I will be notified prior to activities. ____ yes ____ no

I give permission for my child to travel in a parent-driven car for class sponsored field trips. ____ yes ____ no

I give permission for my child to participate in the cooperative Motor Development Clinic (at Memorial Gym). ____ yes ____ no

I give my permission for my child to participate in video taping or photographs for educational and informational purposes. ____ yes ____ no

Signature ______________________ Date ______________

Source: University of Virginia, Department of Speech Pathology and Audiology, Speech and Hearing Center. Reprinted by permission.

Semester Summary Reports

Teacher/clinicians in parent-infant, nursery, and prekindergarten programs are required to complete semester reports on all children, handicapped and normal. These reports summarize the progress the child has made in all phases of the preschool program and present objectives that are appropriate for the following school term. In order to compose detailed and complete semester reports, continuous observations and notes are made by teachers, teacher aides, and the program director on all aspects of the child's development and progress. This includes an ongoing language-speech sample as described in Chapter 6. Examples of two semester summary reports are presented in Exhibits 8–4 and 8–5.

Semester reports are sent to all parents, public schools, and other agencies and professionals who are concerned with the child. Therefore, accu-

Exhibit 8–4 Semester Summary Report: Carl A. Hill

RECORD NUMBER:

University of Virginia
SPEECH AND HEARING CENTER
Charlottesville
SUMMARY FOR SEMESTER (SPRING, 1980)
EVALUATION REPORT

NAME OF PATIENT: HILL, Carl A.
DATE EVALUATED: 10 May 1980
DATE TYPED: 27 May 1980
ADDRESS: Route 1, Box 900, Central, Virginia
TELEPHONE: (804) 555-6176
DATE OF BIRTH: 25 August 1976 **AGE:** 3-9 **SEX:** M F
PARENT OR GUARDIAN: Mr. and Mrs. C. A. Hill, Sr. **INFORMANT(S):**
REFERRED BY:

Background:

Carl is a three year, nine month old hearing impaired child with a bilateral sensori-neural hearing loss in the moderate range. He has attended Comprehensive Services for Hearing Impaired and Delayed Language Children on a three day per week basis in September 1979. Previously Carl was enrolled in the Parent-Infant Program.

Carl's attendance this semester has been good, and his progress satisfactory.

The following report indicates progress in the specified content areas:

I. Language-Cognition and Comprehension
THE CONCEPTS ANALYSIS PROFILE will be administered during the summer session, 1980.

Carl understands and recognizes in context the following concepts:

numbers one, two, three, no more
shapes - circle, triangle,s quare, long, round, tall
fast, slow, stop, go
empty

Carl is able to understand via audition and speechreading word representing the following objects or pictures of objects from the preschool units:

clothing - pants, shirt, socks, shoes, coat, hat, mittens, boots

Transportation - car, airplane, bus, train, boat, bicycle

Face and Body Parts - eyes, ears, nose, mouth, hair, head, arms, legs, hands, feet, fingers, toes

Animals - dog, cat, horse, chicken, bug, bird, worm

Circus - lion/tiger, elephant, bear, monkey clown

Easter - rabbit, basket, egg

Carl is able to match all colors accurately and comprehend the words representing the colors red and blue.

Carl recognizes sameness for objects and pictures and is able to recognize "different" in objects as well as mark out "different" in pictures.

Exhibit 8–4 continued

Carl understands the words representing familiar places in his experience home, school, gym, outside.

II. Language Communication

Carl is scheduled for formal language analysis on May 25. Please refer to that report for more complete information

Two - word utterances

/tu i/	two eyes
/baI kIm/	Bye, Kim
/hIt da n/	Sit down
/ku mi/	Excuse me
/wʌ t nʌ mʌ /	What number?
/ju taiɚ /	You tired?
/dɔ r lakd/	Door locked

Three - word utterances

/ð ae t ravn/	That's round
/aI ge mɔ /	I get more
/bI ta wʌ n/	big tall one
/aI laI dae/	I like that
/aI wʌ n dʒ u/	I want juice
/ju maI kukiz/	You make cookies?
/ubi did I /	Ruby did it
/ai nid hɛ p/	I need help
/ ðae bI tep/	That big step
/aI lai blu/	I like blue
/hI daʊ naʊ /	Sit down now

Four - word utterances

/aI wʌ mɔ dʒ u/	I want more juice.
/mɑ mI meI ðae kukI/	Mommy make that cookie
/pʊ I raI ðɚ /	Put it right there.
/aI pʊ I əweI/	I put it away
/aI wʌ n ə hi/	I want a seed.
/taIm a go ho/	Time to go home.

Five-word utterances

/bɝ go ʌ In saI/	bird go up in sky.
/Lə gI I tu mi/	Laura, give it to me.

III. Speech

A. Pre-speech

Carl's program emphasis centered about development of correct syllabification for two and three syllable words. Ability in this area increased greatly and is exemplified in production of words such as:

Exhibit 8–4 continued

/kuki/	cookie
/taI eI l/	triangle
b ʌ ae ʌ /	banana

Carl demonstrates appropriate contrasts of pitch and intonation patterns in communication.

Carl is beginning to demonstrate lingua-alveolar placement for the consonant/l/ in conjunction with vowels.

Carl demonstrates control for sustained vowels long/ae__________/ and short/ae ae ae/ vowel duration in syllable exercises.

B. Speech

The phonemes production in Carl's repetoire are within the expected range as based on his chronological age although his speech is characterized by omissions of consonants in medial and continuant and strident.

Phontactic processes are in evidence and will be presented in the May 25th report. Feature analysis indicates nonuse of stridency and continuant features with respect to consonants.

IV. Auditory Awareness

Carl responds without visual cues to his name from any location within the preschool setting. He is able to understand familiar language vocabulary without visual cues. Carl demonstrates auditory memory for two-step commands. He responds appropriately to directions in action songs sung in group music with some reliance on visual clues, (actions of other children). Carl is beginning to demonstrate accurat e rhythm skills in musical play activities as demonstrated in clapping, movement and marching activities. He is also aware of loud sounds versus quiet sounds.

V. Fine Motor Ability

Carl's abilities in this area are commensurate with his chronological age range. He is able to:

string 1" beads
build a tower of 9 blocks
trace a square
trace simple dotted line figures with fair accuracy
draw a circle, square, horizontal and vertical line and a +
tear paper
draw correctly positioned facial features
fold paper twice with model
make short snips with correctly held scissors
use knife appropriately for cutting and spreading
use hammer and nails with accurate eye-hand coordination.

Small muscle dexterity for finger plays and number imitation is not coordinated.

Exhibit 8–4 continued

Carl puts his hearing aid ear mold in correctly but inconsistently, with the exception of the helix.

VI. Large Muscle Coordination

Carl's motor skills are commensurate with his chronological age. He is able to imitate gross motor movements upon direction. He also demonstrates the following skills:

walks backwards, sideways
walks on balls of feet (attempting tiptoe) 3 yards
able to roll back/back, leaves 1 foot extended for support
able to jump in place, jump forward 2'
attempts to pump self in swing
able to use slide alone
crawls through tunnel
catches large ball using body and hands
throws ball with 2 hands
kicks large ball
throws ball with 2 hands
throws fisbee correctly
runs well, cannot make sharp turns
stands on 1 foot, right, for 3 seconds
walks up stairs, both feet on 1 step

VII. Social - Emotional Development

Self-Image

Carl engages in dramatic play in imitation of adult activities. He can identify himself in a group photograph, and finds pleasure in being able to identify his own printed name. He delights in his own humor, as exhibited by deliberately giving the teacher the wrong answers or objects (with a smile). He is confident in exploring new objects and discovering how they work ow how they are put together.

Self-Reliance

Carl demonstrates an awareness for the school routine and can make predictions as to upcoming events. He can tolerate the disruption of routine easily, and is able to sacrifice his immediate satisfaction when promised later privilege.

Carl is able to dress himself with help, including pants and socks. He uses and understands the function of school materials and tools. Carl requests help with shoes.

Carl uses table utensils correctly and is adept at feeding himself. He requests a tissue when needed and is beginning to inform an adult of toileting needs.

Carl prefers to play by himself or with one other companion. In group activities, he participates eagerly but does not care to be put in the role of performer. He works well in group activities at the table for 15-25 minutes.

Exhibit 8–4 continued

Recommendations:

Carl will continue to progress through skill sequences in the following areas:

I. Language-Cognition and Comprehension

A. Continue to build experiential and conceptual vocabulary related to nursery units.

B. Maintain present rate of growth in semantic, syntactic - morphological and pragmatic understanding.

II. Language Communication

A. Continue to expand sentences

B. Continue to increase expressive vocabulary in relation to experiential and play activities.

C. Increase expression in rhymes, songs and stories

III. Speech

A. Continue to expand abilities in pre-speech, emphasizing tongue control and duration

B. Continue to develop appropriate syllabification and stress for words and words within sentences.

C. Continue to develop continuant and strident features in speech

D. Continue to develop age-appropriate speech sounds commensurate with age level; increase sounds in repetoire to use in medial and final positions.

E. Continue to develop voice control by self monitoring.

F. Continue to develop intensity control

IV. Auditory Awareness

A. Continue to build listening skills for vocabulary, directions and 2-3 step commands.

B. Continue to develop localization skills without reliance on vision.

C. Continue to develop auditory repetoire for environmental sounds, rhythm and music activities.

D. Continue to build listening and monitoring for speech sounds in repetoire.

E. Begin to develop discrimination skills for likenesses and differences in words and phrases.

Exhibit 8–4 continued

V. Fine Motor Ability

A. Continue present rate of growth for fine motor ability commensurate with age level.

B. Increase finger dexterity through small muscle activities and finger plays.

VI. Larger Muscle Coordination

Continue to develop gross motor skills commensurate with age level.

VII. Social - Emotional Development

Continue to develop skills commensurate with age level.

Educational Recommendations:

Chuck will attend the Pre-Kindergarten (afternoon) session five afternoons a week for the summer session, 1980.

Submitted by:
Beverly R. Dicoskey, M.Ed.
Clinical Supervisor

Approved by: M Suzanne Hasenstab
M. Suzanne Hasenstab, Ph.D.
Director, Hearing Impairment

Source: University of Virginia, Department of Speech, Pathology and Audiology, Speech and Hearing Center. Reprinted by permission.

Exhibit 8–5 Semester Summary Report: Pearl Ann Sweet

RECORD NUMBER:

University of Virginia
SPEECH AND HEARING CENTER
Charlottesville
SUMMARY FOR SEMESTER (FALL, 1979)
EVALUATION REPORT

NAME OF PATIENT: SWEET, Pearl Ann | DATE EVALUATED: 5 Dec. 1979
DATE TYPED: 27 Dec. 1979
ADDRESS: General Delivery, Central, Virginia | TELEPHONE: No Phone
DATE OF BIRTH: 19 September 1976 | AGE: 3-3 | SEX: M F
PARENT OR GUARDIAN: Mr. and Mrs. R.J. Sweet | INFORMANT(S): Amanda Connolly, Associate Teacher
REFERRED BY:

BACKGROUND

Pearl Ann is a three year old hearing impaired child with a bilateral sensorineural hearing loss in the profound range. She was fitted with binaural body-level amplification in September, 1978, which she wears and uses satisfactorily.

Pearl Ann was enrolled in the Parent-Infant Program in the Summer of 1978, and received individual instruction at home twice a week. Since January, 1979, she has been enrolled in nursery level which she currently attends on a full time daily basis. She also receives additional individualized speech and language therapy in half hour sessions. Pearl Ann's progress has been continued and satisfactory.

The following report indicates Pearl Ann's progress in the specified content areas:

I. Language/Cognition/Comprehension

A. Personal-Social Awareness

-demonstrates an understanding that expression intonation and body gestures communicate emotions and meaning.

-occasionally responds appropriately to more obvious meanings of warning, anger, pleasure and/or friendly voice or gesture patterns.

-inconsistently responds to the words "no" and "stop" by temporarily ceasing her activity.

-irregularly attends to, listens, or watches the conversations of others.

-is developing and sustaining better eye contact with the speaker, although more work in this area is indicated.

-in general, requires less use of gestures, demonstrating an awareness of contextual cues, both in following directions and in selecting appropriate objects/pictures on command.

-identifies self in photographs by pointing to self and occasionally vocalizing /m/, "me"; associates classmates with their photographs; is beginning to recognize and identify her own printed first name; irregularly responds to her name being called.

-will imitate the actions and facial expressions of others; will imitate the action or facial expression shown in a picture;

Exhibit 8–5 continued

-imitates actions demonstrated by the teacher upon recall;

-imitates a pictured action upon recall.

-matches a doll's facial features, body parts, and articles of clothing to her own and to teacher's.

-correctly responds to the questions "Where is your head/hands/feet/eyes/nose when accompanied by gesture or in imitation of the responses of others; does not yet know these body parts by speechreading alone.

-usually responds appropriately to simple requests or commands related to the immediate situation and accompanied by gestures; lack of response does not seem to indicate lack of understanding, but rather unwillingness to demonstrate the desired action.

-has not yet demonstrated recognition of the names of objects, pictures, or events presented without visual or gestural cues.

-understands simple cause/effect relationships; uses means to attain ends.

-shows clear signs of anticipation of events (fusses when sees familiar person leaving); demonstrates a sense of present time (recognizes cues for snacktime, outdoor play, "later").

B. Visual Discrimination - Matching

-matches: like objects; similar objects; objects to pictures; pictures to pictures; identical shapes; shapes to outlines of shapes; identical colors, both primary and secondary; line drawings; and pictures of objects seen from different perspective

-when shown an object or picture, the child selects that object or picture upon recall.

-demonstrates understanding of the concept "same", when accompanied by the carrier phrase "Find the same;"

-assembles two-part picture puzzles easily; needs help in assembling puzzles with three or more pieces.

C. Object/Picture Interpretation and Classification

-occasionally shows sustained interest in looking at objects or pictures when they are shown or talked about.

-associates conceptual properties with objects (small objects: little; alarm clock or horn: listen); demonstrates association of common household objects with function by performing appropriate actions; consistently sorts and classifies associated objects on some logical basis (foods, toys, furniture; color, shape, function, etc.); classifies objects which are real and not real (e.g. plastic versus real fruits, etc.)

-shows interest in "how" things function, by "requesting" demonstration of the appropriate use of a particular object (e.g. wrench, screwdriver, etc.)

-sorts and classifies associated pictures on some logical basis (foods, toys, furniture, etc.)

Exhibit 8–5 continued

D. Concept Development

-demonstrates understanding of the following concepts with visual and gestural cues given: locatives: under, in ,on, off, over, through, around; size comparisons: big, little; number concepts: one, two, three; more; shapes: round (spontaneously traces round objects in the air as demonstrated previously by the teacher)

-is beginning to develop understanding of the concept "on" through speech cue occasionally accompanied by gesture.

-associates small, medium, and large objects with other small, medium and large objects.

II. Language/Communication

-produces random vocalizations other than crying, frequently a shrill /ɑ/ or /m/ sound; expresses anger or displeasure by gestures and vocal patterns other than crying; vocalizes, showing signs of pleasure such as laughing or chuckling.

-occasionally is stimulated to repeat her own sounds when a familiar person imitates the child's productions; occasionally experiments with vocal sounds, noises, and gestures, often in imitation of the teacher or other children.

-sporadically babbles, vocalizes, and/or gestures to others; occasionally combines vocalizations with gestures in a meaningful way in spontaneous expressive communication with others (i.e. /mʌ mʌ/ "bye-bye" with wave)

-vocalizes spontaneously and consistently to indicate needs or desires often in the form of a fluctuating or high pitched /ɑ/.

-demonstrates appropriate use of some of the prosodic features of speech (pitch, intonation, rhythm) in spontaneous, interactive vocalizations with others.

-consistently expresses "no" by shaking her head; occasionally expresses "yes" by nodding head.

-occasionally gestures "come here", "stay there", "sit here".

-indicates that objects or pictures are the same by pointing to each and nodding head; indicates they are "not the same" by pointing to each and shaking head.

-gestures "little" spontaneously and appropriately when shown a tiny object by placing thumb and forefinger close together and up to her eye.

-indicates that a classmate is absent "not here" by pointing to that child's picture and shaking head.

-gestures "one", "two" and "three" spontaneously and appropriately when given 1, 2, or 3 objects by showing the correct number of fingers; gestures "none" by shrugging shoulders and shaking head.

-indicates need for help in performing certain actions.

-spontaneously places finger to protruded lips for /ʃ/ as in "Shhhh, be quiet." when shown a "sleeping" doll or picture of a person sleeping (as yet, no aspiration).

-spontaneously rubs her tummy and vocalizes prolonged m-- as in "Mmm, good."

- spontaneously waves and vocalizes approximations of "hi" and "bye-bye" on occasion.

Exhibit 8–5 continued

-occasionally points to picture of self vocalizing /mʌ/ for "me".

-spontaneously vocalizes /ɑ/ or /au/ for "ouch" when hurt or feigning injury in play.

-spontaneously and consistently produces /mɔ/ or /mɔr/ for "more?) spontaneously produced /no mɔ/ (observed once) at snack, accompanied by head shake for "no more" (cookies)

-attempts to imitate the sounds and number of syllables in the vocalizations of others in an approximation of meaningful words; spontaneous imitation and vocalization is increasing steadily.

-occasionally attempts to imitate cued speech with mouth formations for certain words, usually without voicing (e.g. "bye-bye", "wash", "push").

Speech

A. Prespeech Skills

1) Blowing

-tends to purse lips during blowing exercises, but is improving in her production of a strong, continuous breath stream.

-blows well through straws and party horns, and occasionally other musical instruments.

2) Tongue Mobility

-demonstrates good tongue mobility, moving tongue in, out, up, down, side to side, and around the lips.

-imitates many tongue and lip positions for both vowels and consonants (/ɑ/ /u/ /i/ /o/ /m/ /b/ /f/ /ʃ/ /θ/ /l/) but inconsistently voices or aspirates these sounds.

3) Control of Oral Mechanism

-needs work on opening mouth on command: tends to hold upper teeth over lower lip.

-demonstrates good lip strength in blowing out cheeks.

-demonstrates good facial mobility for the production of speech sounds.

4) Prosodic Features

-is beginning to vocalize consistently with stimulus of placing a ring up to the side of her mouth and/or touching throat with the other hand; occasionally places hand to cheek while voicing.

-is beginning to be conditioned to lower the pitch of her voice; pitch elevates noticeably when she is not wearing her hearing aids.

-imitates prolonged and repetitive duration of the vowel sound /ɑ/

-attempts to imitate, rhythm for multi-syllabic words, usually producing a repetitive/ ʌmʌm /.

-imitates moderate and loud vocal intensities; has not yet been observed producing a whisper.

Exhibit 8–5 continued

B. Observed Phoneme and Babbling Set Production

-spontaneous random phonemes include: /ɑ/ /ae/ /ʌ/ /k/ /m/ /b/ /ŋ/

-spontaneous babbling sets include: /mɑ mɑ mɑ/ /mʌ mʌ mʌ/

-phonemes produced in imitation include: /u/ /i/ /a/ /au/ /m/ /p/ /b/ /h/ /f/ /v/ /ʃ/ (without aspiration).

-imitative babbling sets include: /mɑ mɑ m / /bʌ bʌ bʌ/ Ibi Ibi Ibi/ /lɑ lɑ lɑ/ (without voicing).

C. Word Approximations in Imitation

/m/ /mʌ/ /mɑ/ /mɔ/ /mɔr/ -	"more"
/m/ /mʌ/ - -	"me"
/ʌbʌ/ /ʌmbə/ /ʌm/ -	"up"
/m/ /mau/ -	"mouth"
/no/; /mo/ -	"no"
/aʊ/ -	"ow"
/ɔ/ /ɔm/-	"on"
/ɑ/ -	"in"
/a/ /aI/ -	"hi"
/ʌmʌmʌ/ /pʌ pʌ/	"bye bye"
/ʌbʌ/ -	"boom"
/bʌbʌbʌ/ /mə mɑ mɑ/ -	"banana"
/pʌ pʌ/ /pʌ/ -	"pear"
/ae/ -	"apple"
/ae/ -	"cracker"
/ae/ -	"can"
/u/ -	"glue"
/u/ -	"spoon"
/f/ /fɔr/ -	"fork"
/aema/ -	"hammer"
/bʌbʌbʌ/ -	"balloon"
/ɔ/ -	"doll"
/ho/ -	"ho"
/b-ae bae b-ae/ -	"bang bang bang"
/ʌm ʌm/ -	"some"
/ɑr/ -	"star"
/ɔ/ /f/, /ɔ/ /v/ /ɔf/ -	"off"
/m/ -	"drum"
/u/ /i/ -	"Ruby"

IV. Auditory Awareness

A. Attention

- responses to loud, inside environmental sounds when her attention is directed to the sound (e.g. blender, vacuum cleaner, alarm clock, etc.)
- responses to meaningful outside environmental sounds such as a car, bus, ambulance or airplane, when her attention is directed to the sound.
- shows an awareness of some environmental sounds (such as the air conditioner or someone knocking at the door) without her attention being directed to the sound.
- upon hearing a sound she localizes toward the source of the stimulus.

Exhibit 8–5 continued

-indicates awareness that musical instruments, such as horns, produce sounds, but has not yet learned to blow them: rather, she puts the instrument to her mouth and vocalizes.

B. Sound Detection

-responds to the presence of low, loud, gross sounds such as a drum by performing the desired activity (clapping, dancing, marching, dropping a block in a can, etc.) with no visual cues; waits to respond to sound.

-responds to the absence of sound by pointing to her earmold and shaking her head "no."

-shows interest upon hearing a stimulus and indicates this by pointing to her ear, nodding and/or smiling.

-inconsistently responds to her name being called from a distance of not more than five feet.

C. Sound Discrimination

1) Speech Sounds

-discriminates prolonged and repetition duration of the vowel /ɑ/.

-cannot yet discriminate loud and quiet sounds.

-is beginning to discriminate and occasionally imitate pitch changes in an adult female voice from normal speaking level to low.

-cannot yet discriminate formant differences in the vowels /ɑ/ /u/ /i/ when unaccompanied by visual cues.

2) Environmental Sounds

-cannot yet discriminate between gross environmental sounds such a horn and drum.

D. Attitudes Towards Amplification

-wears a functioning hearing aid satisfactorily during all waking hours.

-puts on amplification with help; turns on amplification when directed to do so, puts in earmold with help.

-responds immediately to earmold feedback by pushing her earmold into her ear.

E. Attitudes Toward Listening

-participates willingly in listening activities.

-occasionally she requests or selects an activity involving listening (e.g. musical instruments, playing with an alarm clock, etc.)

V. Gross Motor Skills

A. Body Management

1) Static Balance

-stands steadily with feet shoulder - width apart.

Exhibit 8–5 continued

-stands on one foot without help momentarily.

2) Dynamic Balance

-squats in play
-picks up small object from floor without falling
-walks forward on narrow balance beam with hands lightly held
-walks on wider balance beam (6-8") without assistance, demonstrates good balance in both setting and prone position on a moving scotter.

3) Rolling

-rolls over completely on a longitudinal axis

B. Locomotor Skills

1) Crawling

crawls up and down inclines; crawls through tunnel/varrel

2) walking

-can walk rhythmically at an even pace
-walks on tip toes and heels for several feet
-walks up and down inclines
-walks backward several feet
-walks backward several steps

3) running

-runs well, though not fast, with very little falling; cannot make sharp turns
-runs up and down inclines
-gallops

4) jumping

-jumps down off low object with both feet together
-jumps in place with both feet; cannot yet hop on one foot
-jumps off high platform (4') onto mat
-jumps well with both feet on trampoline

5) climbing

-climbs and descends stairs unaided two feet per step
-ascends stairs one foot per step (alternating feet) with hand held
-climbs slide ladder unaided.

C. Dealing with Play Equipment

1) apparatus skills

-uses a slide unassisted
-pumps a child's swing/glider unaided
-uses reciprocal-action equipment (e.g. glider) with another child
-hangs from bar (over-hand grip) for 2-3 seconds

Exhibit 8–5 continued

-pushes and pulls large toys or objects skillfully
-carries large objects without stumbling or dropping them

2) ball skills
-throws small ball overhand with one hand
-throws and catches own balloon
-anticipates and occasionally catches medium-sized ball, stiff arms
-kicks a large ball with one foot

VI. Fine Motor Development

A) Eye-Hand Coordination

-strings large (1") and small (1/2") beads
-laces a sewing card
-turns pages of a book, one at a time.
-folds paper with a definite crease, after demonstration
-cuts short snips in paper following line; has not yet mastered cutting through attempts to hold scissors correctly with one hand
-screws jar lids onto jars
-stacks cardboard neatly in a pile
-accurately hits large nail with hammer on child's workbench
-uses glue appropriately
-assembles formboard puzzles easily; completes Montessori size seriation puzzles easily; sorts variously shaped blocks in shape - sorting box easily.

B) Pre-writing/Writing Skills

-demonstrates variety of scribbling patterns, including loops and spirals; varied and rhythmical strokes in painting
-attempts tracing between lines and/or following dotted lines
-copies the following designs on blockboard:

____, 1, 0, , , + and the numerals 6, 8, 2

C) Manipulative Abilities

-holds large crayon and chalk appropriately using both right and left hands, slight preference given to the right hand
-manipulates tiny objects easily with thumb and forefinger (pincer grasp)
-demonstrates good digital manipulation in using tape, glue, stickers, and other classroom materials
-rolls, pounds, pulls and squeezes clay
-manipulates large screwdriver well
-carries liquids without spelling

D) Self-Help Abilities

1) dressing

-zips and unzips zippers
-attempts tying own shoes
-can pull on socks and pants with help
-removes shoes and socks
-can find arm holes in dressing
-removes pull-down garments (elastic waist)
-washes and dries own hands
-attempts to close snaps

Exhibit 8–5 continued

2) feeding

-eats well with spoon, fork (may be held in fist); feeds self
-stirs well with spoon
-cuts and spreads soft foods with small plastic knife, unassisted
-can pour from pitcher, some assistance given

VII. Social-Emotional Development

- does not yet play cooperatively but is beginning to share and consistently takes turns

- through often withdrawn and quiet upon arrival, participates willingly in most school activities including prespeech exercises, most songs and fingerplays

- readily cleans up, helps out, and knows the proper storage and care of most school materials; knows and appropriately follows school routine.

- discriminates between strangers and familiar people.

- tends to become withdrawn when a large group or new people are present, or when taken into a 1:1 situation with an unfamiliar adult; with familiar persons, responds well to positive reinforcement and approval in the form of verbal praise, clapping, hugs, etc.

-interacts well with the older children in the afternoon class and is beginning to participate in some of their group activities.

-fusses, whines and occasionally cries when the parents of her classmates come for them at noontime.

-laughs in response to laughter of others.

-occasionally initiates own play activities; chooses some experiences for herself.

-enjoys ritual and repetition; occasionally reluctant to explore new materials such as finger paint or clay.

-looks for missing toys.

-sits willingly on potty chair or toilet, but is not yet toilet trained.

Recommendations:

PAS will continue to progress through skill sequences in the following areas:

I. Language/Cognition/Comprehension

A) continue to build experiential concepts and vocabulary
B) continue to maintain previously introduced concepts and vocabulary with decreased visual reliance and increased reliance on audition
C) increase eye contact and visual attention toward the speaker

II. Language/Communication

A) decrease use of gestures and increase vocalization as a means of communication
B) continue to develop meaningful one and two-word utterances from imitation to spontaneous expression

Exhibit 8–5 continued

C) stress imitation of her vocalizations by teachers and parents to increase pleasure in communication

III. Speech

A) continue to develop production of sustained breath stream both with and without voice

B) increase imitation of babbling sets, both of sustained and short, repetitive duration.

C) continue to develop prosodic features of speech in imitation of babbling sets through variation of pitch, duration, and stress

D) develop discrimination ability to change voice intensity from whisper, to normal speaking level, to loud; and pitch from high to normal speaking level, to low

E) continue to develop a consistent repetoire of vowels with increasing emphasis on anterior, coronal, round and tense features

F) continue to expand repetoire of consonants with increasing emphasis on voiced/voiceless, oral/nasal, and continuant/plosive distinctions

G) continue develop speech approximations and rhythm for meaningful 2 and 3 word phrases (e.g. "Put it in" "Tie it" "Open it" etc.).

IV. Auditory Awareness

A) continue to condition to respond to the presence of sound (both environmental and speech sounds.

B) develop discrimination of gross sounds (e.g. drum, horn, bell)

C) develop auditory attention and memory

D) develop localization skills

E) increase auditory rhythm skills through gross motor activities

F) develop ability to monitor hearing aids and maintain volume control

G) continue to wear hearing aids during all waking hours.

V. Gross Motor Coordination

continue to develop skills commensurate with age level

VI. Fine Motor Skills

A) continue to develop fine, motor digital manipulation (e.g. nuts and bolts, cutting, drawing, buttons, lacing, etc.)

B) continue to develop drawing skills to include tracing dotted lines and within boundaries.

C) continue to develop visual discrimination of like objects with increasing difficulty.

Exhibit 8–5 continued

D) continued development in self-help skills such as eating, cutting, cleaning up, washing and dressing self.

VII. Social-Emotional Development

A) development of cooperative play with classmates

B) development of the ability to share

C) encourage imaginary play and domestic mimicry

D) continued development of communicative vocalizations

E) accomplish mastery of toilet training

Submitted by:
Amanda Connolly
Associate Clinician

Approved by: M. Suzanne Hasenstab
M. Suzanne Hasenstab, Ph.D.
Director, Hearing Impairment

Beverly R. DiCoskey
Beverly R. DiCoskey, M. Ed.
Clinical Supervisor
Hearing Impairment

Source: University of Virginia, Department of Speech Pathology and Audiology, Speech and Hearing Center. Reprinted by permission.

racy, clarity, and pertinent information are of paramount importance. Final approval of all reports is the responsibility of the program director.

Individual Therapy and Progress Report

As part of the preschool program at the nursery and prekindergarten levels, each child receives individual therapy in speech, language, and auditory abilities, based on the child's specific needs. Associate clinicians are assigned to each child for a period of at least one 16-week semester and are required to submit lesson plans for each session, a self-evaluation and therapy evaluation for each session, and a summary progress report for the semester. In addition to observing and supervising therapy, teachers or the director critique each plan before implementation. All final reports are subject to the director's approval before dissemination from the center. An example of an individual therapy and progress report involving two lesson plans is presented in Exhibit 8–6.

Exhibit 8–6 Individual Therapy and Progress Report

Lesson 5

Jeremy 10/1/79
UVAPSHILDC Clinician: Donna Zang

I. General objectives

A. Jeremy will increase auditory awareness by responding to the presence of sound.

B. Jeremy will increase language comprehension through vocabulary building.

C. Jeremy will increase speech abilities at the vowel and syllable level using visual and auditory cues.

D. Jeremy will increase facial contact with the clinician.

II. Activities

A. Auditory awareness

1. Specific objective

Jeremy will respond to the presence of the sound of a drum by putting a block in a can.

2. Procedure

a) Clinician will hit the drum and show that she hears the sound by pointing to her ear and saying, "I hear that!" She will then put a block in a can.
b) Clinician will repeat above, and when Jeremy shows that he hears the sound by pointing to his ear, he will be encouraged to put a block in.
c) Once Jeremy understands the procedure, the clinician will go behind Jeremy and hit the drum.
d) Jeremy is to put the block in when he hears it.

3. Materials: drum, blocks, can

B. Language and speech

1. Specific objective

Jeremy will use eye contact with the clinician and imitate production of /i/, /u/, and /a/.

Exhibit 8–6 continued

2. Procedure
   a) Clinician will hold a puzzle piece up to her mouth and say the /i/, /u/, or /a/ sounds.
   b) Jeremy will be told to say the sound, and when he does, he will be given the puzzle piece to put in.
   c) Clinician will concentrate on one sound at a time at first so that Jeremy will not get confused; if he does well, the sounds will be alternated.
3. Materials: puzzle

C. Language comprehension and speech

1. Specific objective

   Jeremy will point to an attempted approximation of "house, Daddy, barn, cow" in imitation of the clinician. He will also attempt imitation of the words "in" and "out" and demonstrate these.
2. Procedure
   a) Clinician will put out a toy house and a barn and will ask Jeremy, "What is this?" If he doesn't respond, they will be named, and he will be encouraged to imitate.
   b) Toy animals and people will be used; Jeremy will be asked to name the cow and the Daddy.
   c) One item at a time will then be given to Jeremy; clinician will tell him to "put the cow *in*." *In* will be emphasized and repeated.
   d) Jeremy is to put the figures in their correct place. He will be encouraged to imitate *in*.
   e) As each figure is taken "out," clinician will say "take ____ *out*" emphasizing and repeating *out* for Jeremy to imitate.
3. Materials: doll house, people, barn, animals

D. Speech

1. Specific objective

   Jeremy will imitate production of /p/ and /pa, pa, pa/.
2. Procedure
   a) Clinician will use a tissue and produce /pa, pa, pa/ so Jeremy can see the tissue move.

Exhibit 8–6 continued

b) Jeremy will be encouraged to do the same.
c) Bubbles will be used; as they pop, clinician will say /pa, pa, pa/.
d) Jeremy will be encouraged to pop bubbles and imitate /pa, pa, pa/.

Alternate activity: using plastic snap-together necklace, as each new bead is popped on, clinician will say "pop." Jeremy will be encouraged to imitate. When he does, he will be given a bead.

3. Materials: tissue, bubbles, snap beads

III Evaluation of session

Jeremy was cooperative throughout; however he seems to get restless after about 20 minutes. I guess this is to be expected for his age. Animals seem to hold his attention for a long time.

IV. Evaluation of child

Positive: Jeremy imitated /u/ and /a/ accurately with little prompting needed. He attempted a response for the word "cow." Though it didn't approximate the word at first, he quickly responded to my cues to produce a closer approximation: /a ʊ /. Jeremy used much vocalization when playing with animals and "little people."

Negative: Though Jeremy appeared to understand the task of putting the block in the can when I hit the drum, he didn't seem to be able to hear the drum (when his back was turned).

V. Evaluation of clinician

Positive: I made an effort to keep my pitch lower. I showed Jeremy the animals at the beginning this time.

Negative: I should have positioned Jeremy catty-cornered to me, and I should have pushed for more approximations of words such as /in/ /out/ /house/ from Jeremy. When Jeremy gave eye contact in task with puzzle, I frustrated him by starting to give him the puzzle piece as reinforcement but then holding on to it till he made the sound.

Exhibit 8–6 continued

Lesson 6

Jeremy 10/5/79
UVAPSHILDC Clinician: Donna Zang

I. General objectives

A. Jeremy will increase speech abilities at the vowel and syllable level using visual, auditory, and tactile cues.

B. Jeremy will increase facial contact with the clinician.

C. Jeremy will increase auditory awareness by responding to the presence of sound.

D. Jeremy will increase language comprehension and cognition through vocabulary building.

II. Activities

A. Auditory awareness and discrimination

1. Specific objective

a) Jeremy will respond to the question, "Where's Jeremy?" by pointing to his picture.

b) Jeremy will imitate /mi/.

2. Procedure

Clinician will place Jeremy's and Eric's pictures on the table and ask in turn, "Where's Jeremy?" and "Where's Eric?" Jeremy will pick up the appropriate picture. Attempts will be made to elicit an imitation of /mi/.

3. Materials: polaroid pictures

B. Speech and language

1. Specific objective

Jeremy will demonstrate eye contact with the clinician.

2. Procedure

a) Clinician will hold toy cow up to face; when Jeremy looks at clinician, he will be given the cow to put in a box.

b) Attempts will be made to have Jeremy approximate /Kau/.

Exhibit 8–6 continued

3. Materials: cow, box
Alternate activity: use ring stack toy or puzzle to elicit same response

C. Speech

1. Specific objective

   Jeremy will imitate production of /pʌ, pʌ, pʌ/ and /pap/ upon imitation of the clinician.

2. Procedure

   a) Clinician will use snap-on beads and, as she snaps two together, say /pap/.
   b) Jeremy will be encouraged to do the same.

   Alternate activities: (1) Clinician will use bubbles to elicit /pap/ as they are broken. (2) Clinician will use boat and move it saying, /pa, pa, pa, pa/.

3. Materials: pop beads, bubbles, boat

D. Auditory awareness

1. Specific objective

   Jeremy will respond to the presence of the sound of a drum by putting a block in a can.

2. Procedure

   a) Clinician will hit the drum and show that she hears the sound by pointing to her ear and saying, "I hear that!" She will then put a block in a can.
   b) Clinician will repeat above, and when Jeremy shows that he hears the sound by pointing to his ear, he will be encouraged to put the block in.
   c) Once Jeremy understands the procedure, clinician will move behind and hit the drum.
   d) Jeremy is to put the block in when he hears the sound.

3. Materials: drum, blocks, can

E. Language comprehension/cognition/speech

1. Specific objective

   Jeremy will demonstrate understanding of /in/ and /out/ by placing items in and taking them out of a container.

Exhibit 8–6 continued

The following words will be introduced: *pumpkin, witch, ghost.*

2. Procedure
   a) The following pictures will be named by clinician, and Jeremy will be encouraged to imitate: "pumpkin," "witch," "ghost" (approximations or attempts).
   b) Clinician will say, "Put it in," and Jeremy will take a picture and put it in a container (plastic pumpkin).
   c) Clinician will then say, "Take it out," as she takes a picture out. She will repeat "take it out," and Jeremy will take a picture out.
   d) Jeremy will imitate words /in/ and /out/.
3. Materials: pictures, container

Source: University of Virginia, Department of Speech Pathology and Audiology, Speech and Hearing Center. Reprinted by permission.

Home Visitation Summary Report

Teachers are required to conduct home conferences five times a year, at the beginning and end of the 16-week fall and spring semesters and once during the 10-week summer session. Home visitation conferences are designed to give teachers a glimpse of a child's home environment and how the child functions in that setting. They also provide parents with teacher contacts in a less professional atmosphere. Though home visits are arranged at times convenient to parents and may therefore involve a teacher's evening or weekend, the staff has found this practice extremely beneficial. The summary reports are filed in the children's permanent records but are not disclosed to other agencies or professionals. A sample of this report form is shown in Exhibit 8–7.

SUMMARY

The nursery level within the Comprehensive Services Program represents the entry of the young hearing-impaired or language-delayed child into the first experience with a group of peers. Although many objectives may be continued from the parent-infant program, these are extended and

Exhibit 8–7 Home Visitation Summary Report

Home Visitation Summary Report
University of Virginia Preschool Program
for
Hearing-Impaired and Language-Delayed
Children

Name:	Date of visitation:
Parents:	Length of visit:
Address:	DOB:
Phone:	

Background information:

Reason for home visitation:

Family members present:

Staff present:

General impression:

Summary:

Follow-up:

Exhibit 8–7 continued

Respectfully submitted:	Approved by:
______________________	______________________
Clinical supervisor	M. Suzanne Hasenstab, Ph.D. Director-Hearing Impaired Program
______________________	
Associate teacher	Date: ______________________
______________________	
Associate teacher	

Source: University of Virginia, Department of Speech Pathology and Audiology, Speech and Hearing Center. Reprinted by permission.

expanded to meet the developmental and maturational changes occurring in the child. The curriculum contains specific areas of development, but each of these components actually functions interrelatedly with all other aspects of the program content. Although children are addressed in a group rather than individually within their home, the program emphasizes the particular abilities and needs of each child, and a specific program is designed and implemented to accommodate the child's profile. Parents remain an integral part of the child's educational program and are included in the preschool program. The parents are responsible for carrying over objectives into the home and other settings outside of the school.

REFERENCES

Bloom, L., *Language development and language disorders*. New York: Wiley, 1978.

Bodner-Johnson, B., Editorial. *Parent Education Network,* 1980, *1,* 1.

Brown, R. *A first language*. Cambridge, Mass.: Harvard University Press, 1973.

Cain, L. Parent groups: Their role in a better life for the handicapped. *Exceptional Children,* 1976, *42,* 432–437.

Clark, E. V. What's in a word: On the child's acquisition of semantics in his language. In T. E. Moore (Ed.), *Cognitive development and the acquisition of language*. New York: Academic Press, 1973.

Cruickshank, W. M. The impact of physical disability on socialization. *Journal of Social Issues*, 1948, *4*, 78–83.
Cruickshank, W. M. *Psychology of exceptional children and youth*. Englewood Cliffs, N.J.: Prentice Hall, 1971.
deVilliers, J. G., & deVilliers, P. A. *Language acquisition*. Cambridge, Mass.: Harvard University Press, 1978.
Fallen, N. T. *Young children with special needs*. Columbus, Ohio: Charles E. Merrill, 1978.
Giangreco, J. C., & Giangreco, M. R. *The education of the hearing impaired*. Springfield, Ill.: Charles C Thomas, 1976.
Hasenstab, M. S. *A comparative study of hearing and hearing impaired infants on toy preference*. Unpublished doctoral dissertation, Kent State University, Kent, Ohio, 1975.
Hewitt, F. M., & Forness, S. R. *Education of exceptional learners*. Boston, Mass.: Allyn and Bacon, 1974.
Horton, K. B. Infant intervention and language learning. In R. L. Schiefilluisch & L. L. Lloyd (Eds.), *Language perspectives—Acquisition, retardation and intervention*. Baltimore, Md.: University Park Press, 1974.
Hurlock, E. *Child development*. New York: McGraw-Hill, 1972.
Ingram, D. Phonological rules in young children. *Journal of Child Language*, 1974, *1*, 49–64.
Ingram, D. *Phonological disability in children*. New York: Elsevier, 1976.
Kirk, S. A. *Educating exceptional children*. Boston, Mass.: Houghton Mifflin, 1972.
Kretschmer, R. R., & Kretschmer, L. W. *Language development and intervention with the hearing impaired*. Baltimore, Md.: University Park Press, 1978.
Lindburg, L. The function of play in early childhood education. *Principal*, 1971, *51*, 68–73.
McCarthy, D. Language development in children. In L. Carmichael (Ed.), *Manual of child psychology* (2nd ed.). New York: Wiley, 1954.
McLean, J. E., & Snyder-McLean, L. K. *A transactional approach to early language training*. Columbus, Ohio: Charles E. Merrill, 1978.
Menyuk, P. *The acquisition and development of language*. Englewood Cliffs, N.J.: Prentice Hall, 1971.
Menyuk, P. *The development of speech*. New York: Bobbs Merrill, 1972.
Miller, A. L., & Lehman, R. *A practical guide in hearing impaired children*. Springfield, Ill.: Charles C Thomas, 1970.
Muma, J. R. *Language handbook: Concepts, assessment, intervention*. Englewood Cliffs, N.J.: Prentice Hall, 1978.
Murphy, L. B. Multiple factors in learning in the day care center. A hop to sit on and much more—Helps for day care workers, *Childhood Education*, 1971, *1*, 41–50.
Nelson, K. Concept, word and sentence: Inter-relations in acquisition and development. *Psychological Review*, 1974, *81*, 267–285.
Northcott, W. (Ed.). *The hearing impaired child in the regular classroom: Preschool, elementary and secondary years*. Washington, D.C.: A.G. Bell Association for the Deaf, 1973.
Northern, J. L., & Downs, M. P. *Hearing in children* (2nd ed.). Baltimore, Md.: Williams & Wilkins, 1978.
Olson, D. Language and thought: Aspects of a cognitive theory of semantics. *Psychological Review*, 1970, *77*, 257–273.
Pollack, D. The crucial year: A time to listen. *International Audiology*, 1967, *6*, 243–247.
Pollack, D. *Educational audiology for the limited hearing infant*. Springfield, Ill.: Charles C Thomas, 1970.
Pollack, D., & Ernst, M. Don't set limits: Expectations for preschool children. In W. H. Northcott (Ed.), *The hearing impaired child in the regular classroom: preschool, primary and secondary years*. Washington, D.C.: A.G. Bell Association for the Deaf, 1973.

Poole, I. Genetic development of articulation of consonant sounds in speech. *Elementary English Review*, 1934, *71*, 159–161.

Safford, P. L. *Teaching young children with special needs*. St. Louis, Mo.: C. V. Mosby, 1978.

Simmons, A. Teaching aural language. *Volta Review*, 1968, *75*, 26–30.

Smith, L. *Comprehensive performance in oral deaf and normal hearing children in three stages of language development*. Unpublished doctoral dissertation, University of Wisconsin, Madison, Wisc., 1972.

Templin, M. *Certain language skills in children: Their development and interrelationships*. Minneapolis: University of Minnesota Press, 1957.

West, J., & Weber, J. A linguistic analysis of the morphemic and syntactic structures of a hard of hearing child. *Language and Speech*, 1974, *17*, 68–79.

Chapter 9

Prekindergarten Level

M. Suzanne Hasenstab

In the present context, the prekindergarten is defined as a planned educational program for children, aged 4 and 5 years, prior to public school kindergarten placement. In the current literature this level is also referred to as nursery school or preschool. We prefer the term prekindergarten because it more closely focuses on our purposes for this intervention level.

In the Comprehensive Services Program, the prekindergarten level serves as the upward extension of the preceding nursery level in the overall program. In this context, its purpose is to provide continuity, extension, and expansion of the basic goals and objectives outlined at the nursery level. In addition, prekindergarten, as the term implies, has the additional function of providing experiences and opportunities that will foster mastery of abilities in all areas of development to enhance the chances of success in the formal education domain once a child enters kindergarten. In this sense, it serves as a preparatory program.

The overall goal of early intervention—mediation in order that the effects of the hearing and/or language impairment may be lessened—heightens in prekindergarten. This level represents the summation of all foregoing experiences in the preschool programming of the child. The very nature of the purpose of prekindergarten, combined with the ever-increasing diversity among the children, constitutes a complex and challenging responsibility to preschool staff members and parents who are cooperatively involved in their children's education.

THE PREKINDERGARTEN EXPERIENCE

Although there is general agreement that the preschool experience is valuable to 4- and 5-year old children before entering the formal educational structure at kindergarten, the question of what this experience should entail has not been resolved. The field of early childhood education presents a wide range of views pertaining to philosophy, methodology, and the school environment (Parker, 1972). During the 1960s and early 1970s, the traditional nursery school concept was the focus of considerable criticism, primarily with regard to the paucity of attention to intellectual development. There emerged a move toward the "cognitive" basis for preschool instruction and curricula, as represented by programs developed by Lavatelli (1966), Englemann (1969), Kamii and Radin (1970), and Weikart et al. (1970). Yet, despite what appears to be a central impetus to these and other such cognitive-oriented programs, there is still no agreement on exactly what this approach should include or how it can best be implemented.

Prekindergarten Settings

Safford (1978) identifies two types of approaches to preschool programs that have been developed for normal children: the traditional or child-centered program, and the Montessori approach. The traditional or child-centered view fosters play as a medium to learning and emphasizes the child as an explorer and discoverer within the child's environment. This preschool approach also emphasizes that the social interaction of children is vital in preschool experience.

The Montessori view differs in that the structured use of formalized materials is pertinent to this program and the emphasis is on the individual rather than the social learning context. The structure is much more rigid than in the traditional setting, and "pure" Montessori schools de-emphasize creative art and musical activity. Much of the value of the Montessori design is in the development of cognitive ability through sensory discovery.

Project Head Start, though originally designed not for handicapped children but for children with potential educational problems, has been mandated since 1973 to provide services for children with handicaps of all types. In compliance with federal regulations, a minimum of 10 percent of the children served in the program must be handicapped. However, the majority of children served by Head Start are designated as normal. Head Start programs actually vary considerably from one setting to another with respect to curriculum, specific objectives, instructional strategies, and activities. Much of this variation is due to the geographical locations of the programs. An urban setting will obviously warrant different content emphasis than a rural setting, based on the resources and background experiences of the children being served.

Finally, programs for various handicapping conditions are available for children of prekindergarten age. These programs may address one handicap specifically, such as mental retardation, or they may be designed to provide services for children with a variety of disabilities. Programs that service children in later preschool years might enroll only children with handicaps or they might operate as integrated settings in which "normal" children are also part of the class group. This concept is different from that of Head Start programs, in which 10 percent of the total enrollment in a class is deemed "handicapped." In the case of an integrated preschool, the normal or model children are in the minority, and the primary thrust of the program is toward the needs of children with disabilities.

The Comprehensive Services Prekindergarten

The design selected for the Comprehensive Services Prekindergarten borrows concepts and ideas from various preschool models. It is child-centered in that the program is constructed around individual child needs. The "whole child" is addressed, as in traditional programs, with experiences related to the fostering of social maturity and group interaction. The Montessori influence is reflected in educational activities, materials, and goals for self-directed discovery and conceptual development. Emphasis on language is necessarily related to cognition and related sensory skills in audition and vision. And of course, because of the population being served, the needs of special children are central in focus. Finally, the prekindergarten, like the nursery level, is an integrated setting, utilizing the presence of normal children as language and social models.

Variation in Abilities

At each advancing level of educational preschool programming, the diversity among children tends to become more acute. Children who were quite homogeneous at age 2 may be extremely different from one another by age 4. A 6-month variance in ability and maturation in infancy may enlarge to a 2-year span by prekindergarten age. The need to relate to the developmental age or level of the child becomes increasingly obvious in the later preschool years. The variation of ability at prekindergarten age is further complicated by the variation of abilities in each child's individual developmental areas, especially with respect to children with disabling conditions such as hearing and/or language impairment. For these children, the developmental areas of cognition, motor growth, and social maturation may be considered to be within normal range, while linguistic sophistication may display a delay of 2 years. It is also possible that the effect of the hearing loss or language delay could affect other areas of development, such as cognition or social skills, even though the child's interests are on a par with what is expected for the child's chronological age. This variation necessitates intensive individualization of programming while still maintaining the valuable group orientation of the preschool setting in all aspects of the preschool experience.

Variation in Program Entry Time

An additional variation among children is seen in those who do not enter educational programs until age 4 or 5 and who may even have remained undiagnosed until that age. For these children, valuable time in the development of auditory and linguistic ability has been lost during infancy and early childhood. The extent of the disability—for example, in the case of a severe or profound hearing loss—may further complicate the situation. Prognosis for the alleviation of the effects of the handicap as it affects future education may be limited, as compared with what could have been possible had the child been diagnosed and served earlier in life. Alternatives such as mainstreaming, either complete or partial, may even be eliminated in the event that the child's language delay is so extensive as to affect the potential for successful placement in such a setting. A realistic assessment of the child's current abilities and limitations and of the expectations of the parents and staff must be undertaken. Goals must be prioritized so that, even though the child has entered the intervention program relatively late, the child may receive maximum benefit based on the current circumstances.

Acquired Hearing Loss in Late Preschool Years

Some children may have developed normally until late preschool years but then have incurred substantial hearing impairment due to illness at age 3 to 5 years. These children have mastered aspects of early linguistic development, auditory facility, and social interactions, yet the interruption caused by hearing impairment can still greatly interfere with future educational success, continued language refinement and expansion, and sophistication in social behavior.

For these children, prekindergarten can serve as a vehicle to maintain the development reflected in different areas and to assist the child in obtaining new strategies to ensure continued learning. Although the child may have an excellent language foundation and demonstrate maturity in linguistic and communication-related areas, unless intervention services are provided, deceleration of growth can easily occur as an effect of acquired hearing loss beyond the mild range.

DEVELOPMENT DURING PREKINDERGARTEN YEARS

Physical and Motor Development

Physical Changes

Between the ages of 4 and 5, a child with normal physical development will double body length at birth and increase birth weight 5 times (Hurlock, 1972). The rounded, top-heavy baby appearance slowly gives way to the proportionately longer arm-and-leg image of school-age children. Even the facial features begin to take on an "older" look. The size of the head begins to fit more proportionately to the child's overall body size, with the once prominent forehead of baby roundness yielding to a more mature, flattened appearance. The tiny button-like nose so obvious at early preschool age begins to develop the cartilage framework that results in the larger and more definite adult shape.

Motor Development

As the child's physical proportions mature at ages 4 to 5, the skeletal and muscular systems undergo changes that allow for more sophisticated motor performance. The skeletal structure exhibits an increased lengthening of arms and legs. The child's legs straighten, eliminating the slightly bowed effect seen in infants and younger children. The adjustment and the gradual lengthening of the legs permit more versatile use and greater mobility when combined with muscular maturity.

Between the ages of 4 and 6, there is a rapid spurt in muscle growth. In fact, at this age, 75 percent of the weight gain is muscle weight. This gives children increased strength and more agility and coordination in the maneuvering of their bodies. Because of this increased muscle growth, a need for muscle activity is evident in children in late preschool years. Preschool staff members can attest that children of prekindergarten age never merely walk, they skip, run, and hop from one place to another.

Fine-Muscle Dexterity

Fine-muscle development most often associated with the hands, is not as quick to develop in a child as teachers or parents might like. The hands increase in size throughout early childhood, but the fingers remain short and chubby, lacking in the mastery of refined muscle coordination. Prekindergarten children begin to accomplish such tasks as cutting with scissors, producing letters, drawing recognizable human and other forms, and connecting a line from one point to another; but they still have difficulty in holding eating utensils correctly, controlling completely pencils and crayons, and performing finely detailed actions with their fingers. Interest in activities that involve fine-muscle use is often seen in childern at this time, but frustration can easily occur if the activities or materials are too complex and difficult.

Often a child will perform satisfactorily in the use of large muscles in the arms and legs and in control of the body in space but demonstrate immaturity in hand dexterity. In some cases, this is reflected in the fine-muscle apparatus of the facial muscles and tongue and results in difficulty with speech. We have noted this in many hearing-impaired children. The consequential difficulty in intelligible spontaneous utterances and imitative attempts can present serious implications for speech work.

Teeth

Another area related to physical maturity at this age may be the loss of baby teeth. This too relates to work with speech. Children begin to lose baby teeth, beginning with their lower central incisors, between the ages of 4 and 6. For a period of time spaces will exist until the permanent replacements move into place. During this time, some children develop a tongue thrust that should be noted and corrected before such use of the tongue becomes habitual. This is especially noticeable in production of /ð/ and /θ/, but it may also occur with /s/ and /z/ attempts.

Linguistic Development

Normal Language

By the time a normal child enters school, the child has acquired an expressive vocabulary of 8,000 to 14,000 words (Carey, 1977). As children with intact hearing mature through the preschool years, in addition to increasing vocabulary, they acquire sophistication as a language user, and this expands throughout all of the linguistic components. Their language and cognitive abilities will continue to increase through the elementary- and middle-school years of formal education (Chomsky, 1969; Lenneberg, 1967); but, for the most part, by age 5 they will have accomplished the major portion of language development.

Discourse

An obvious development is the use of conversational cues and constraints and the ability actually to partake in discourse with an adult or another child. Prekindergarten children utilize social conventions of language interaction and employ rules of turn-taking and of opening, closing, and maintaining conversations. At this stage, the direct demands noted in younger children are replaced by more polite requests.

Semantics

As the child enters the late preschool years, the content of language becomes more versatile. This is closely associated with an increased understanding of concepts, for example those related to time. Although they are not as precise as adults in their time relationships, 4- and 5-year-olds can relate events that have happened in the past as distinct from those that are presently occurring or those that will occur at some future time. "Last week" may mean last week, or it may mean 2 months ago, but the child is aware of events being past and can express them as such. Tense markers are present, although some restrictions may still exist for irregular verb forms.

Children also become increasingly able to represent objects that are not present. They can talk about "Mommy at work" or "Grandma in Pittsburgh" as well as about objects or people present in the immediate environment. DeVilliers and deVilliers (1978) suggest another aspect that is related to the representation of events and objects outside the immediate situation—that of pretending behavior. Children are able to pretend in increasingly complex ways. Initially, a child uses words to refer to a real object; "chair" refers to a real chair. The child is then able to relate picture or miniature representation to the real object depicted. The doll-house kitchen chairs represent larger chairs used at home around the dinner table. Finally, the child can apply a word to a situation or object that is unlike the real thing. A large building block is designated as a chair in a game of pretend: "Let's pretend I'm the Mom and this is my chair."

The increased proficiency in conversation is related to the concurrent development of other linguistic components. Children are better able to express themselves to listeners through their more sophisticated sentence formation, application of morphological markers, clear articulation, and extended word meaning. Cognition and the higher mental activities may still set boundaries, but 4- and 5-year-olds will have already nearly accomplished humans' most amazing feat.

The use of relational words in the development of word meaning in children has been the subject of some interesting studies (Brown, 1973; Clark, 1973; Donaldson & Balfour, 1968; Sinclair-de-Zwart, 1969). Although there are still questions remaining related to the acquisition and use of these words by children, specific observations indicate a growing perfection in their use by children. Contextual standards, such as those related to size, are employed by 4-year-olds but not by children of age 2. An object may be large in one context and small in another, regardless of its "real" size. The use of spatial adjectives—such as big and little rather than more explicit pairs relating specifically to dimensions of length, width, height, and so on—are used by 4- and 5-year-old children. For example, when asked for the opposite of tall or long, the child may reply "small" or "little." By age 8, children no longer display this confusion. A prekindergarten child would not say "small" to mean tall, long, wide, or thick.

The complexity of diectic expressions, which are obvious only when mastery of temporal and spatial concepts is sufficient, is another aspect of semantics that is not completely mastered by late preschool children. There is particular confusion with respect to words related to standards of relative distance when a standard reference point is absent, for example, here/there, this (these)/that (those). Although the children use these words, they may not understand them correctly when they are spoken by another person. Although late preschoolers have indeed acquired a large number of words, they may not use or understand their full or complete meaning. As they meet the words over and over in varying contexts, the wider meaning of the words becomes evident as the children mature cognitively and linguistically. They are then able to restructure the words' meanings.

Syntax

By age 4 to 5, children have not only expanded their sentences from two-word utterances to sentences made up of seven or more words, they have also developed increasingly complex utterances. Their application of syntactic rules for sentence elements and the use of phrase structure allows them greater efficiency and economy in language production. Phrases replace single words and provide qualitative and quantitative information to listeners. "Doggy run" is replaced by such eloquent sentences as "The fuzzy brown dog ran away from that lady over there." However, phrase structure and word order can be confusing to children at this age, and ambiguities are often not perceived.

At around age 3 or 4, children begin to join sentences with "and." At ages 5 to 6, transformations, such as relative clauses, begin to appear. The mastery of transformations continues throughout the child's elementary school years (Chomsky, 1969; deVilliers & deVilliers, 1978). Yet, confusion in the comprehension of high-level transformations is evidenced at this age. Bever's (1970) study and those by deVilliers and deVilliers (1978) illustrate the confusion in comprehension of the passive transformation. For example, "the truck was bumped by the car" is interpreted as "the truck bumped the car." The morphological markers "was" and "by" are not perceived, so the child comprehends only the word order of N + V + N. Relative clauses may also present difficulty for the same reasons, that is, the true subject, the relative pronoun (who, what, etc.) and verb are not observed. Therefore, the object of the relative clause is placed as the main subject and connected to the main-clause verb. "The boy who bought the puppy drank the milk" is interpreted as "the puppy drank the milk."

Chomsky (1969) suggests another consideration related to the comprehension of relative clauses and other aspects of adult syntax. The noun that most closely precedes the verb (or main-clause verb) is interpreted as the subject. Chomsky refers to this as the minimal distance principle (MDP), which is actually an overextension of a more general use. Children must learn the exceptions in order to master totally correct comprehension.

Phonology

A child with normal language development progresses in speech production from the early stages of vocal play in infancy. However, there may still be phonemes in certain positions or in combinations with other phonemes that the child will not articulate correctly. Speech sound such as /s/, /z/, /v/, / ð /, and /zh/ can continue to develop toward perfected articulation until about the age of 8. Also, children in late preschool may substitute another sound for or distort the phonemes /r/, /ng/, /l/, /sh/, /ch/, /j/, and / θ / but still be within a normal range of phonological maturation (Templin, 1957; Wellman, Case, Mengert, & Bradbury, 1931).

Yet, it is possible for a child of 4 or 5 years of age to have mastered speech sound production and to articulate the phonemes correctly in all positions and in all combinations. Preschool staff members must realize that there is a wide variation in the mastery of articulation. Some children may demonstrate flawless spoken language; others may produce speech distinguished by one or two substitutions or sound distortions; while still others may have achieved correct production only of the earlier phonemes /p/, /m/, /h/, /n/, /w/, /b/, /k/, /g/, /d/, /f/, and /y/. Charts that depict normal phonemic development, such as those in Figure 9–1 and Table 9–1, can be helpful in providing prekindergarten personnel with guidelines to normal ranges in children's speech maturation.

It is important to remember that children of late preschool age require good adult models for speech. Although they may incorrectly produce a sound themselves, they can perceive correctness or error in speech of others. For example:

Bobby: Daddy got this twuck for me.
Dr. H.: This twuck?
Bobby: Not twuck—twuck!
Dr. H.: Oh—truck.
Bobby: Yeah (somewhat exasperated).

Figure 9–1 Normal Age Ranges in the Perfection of Sound Articulation

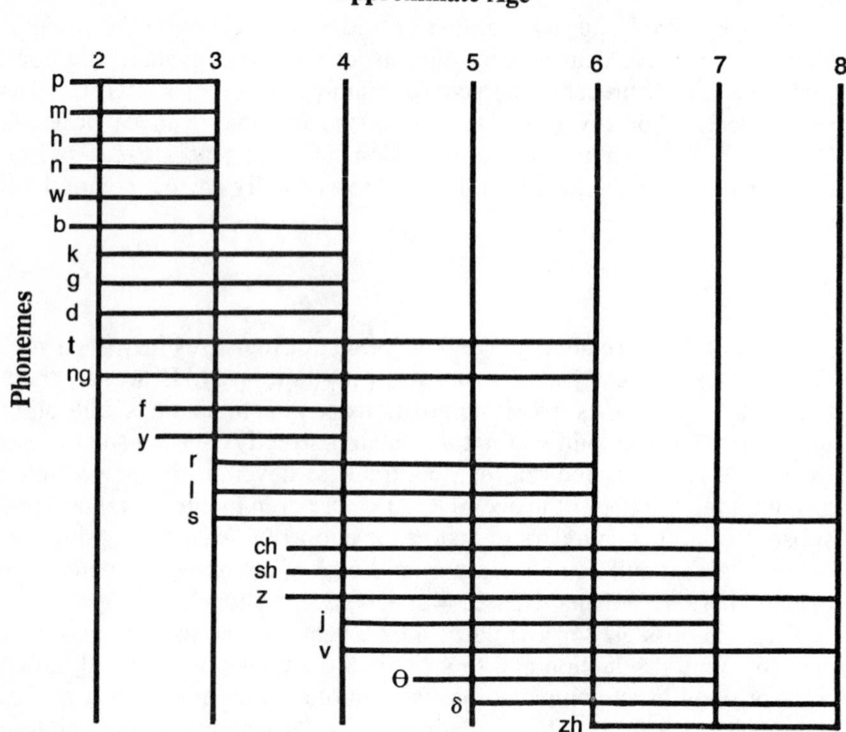

Note: Each line span represents an age range that is considered to be normal in achieving sound articulation. The point of extension of each span to the right indicates the level at which 90 percent of children achieve mastery.

Source: Sander's (1972) adaptation of Templin (1957) and Wellman et al. (1931).

Table 9–1 Development of Speech Elements

Age 2		*Age 3*	
w-	Water	-w-	Flower
m-	Mouth	-m	Comb
-m-	Hammer	-n-	Penny
n-	No	-n	Spoon
h-	Hot	g-	Girl
b-	Boy	-g-	Wagon
-b-	Baby	k-	Cat
p-	Puppy	-k-	Cookie
-p-	Apple	f-	Fish
d-	Dog	-f-	Knife
-d-	Dada	t-	Teeth

Age 4		*Age 5*		*Age 6*	
y-	Yes	-d	Bed	-l	Bell
-ng-	Swinging	r-	Red	-g	Big
-ng-	Ring	-r	Car	-t	Letter
-r-	Carrot	-l-	Yellow	-t	Hat
l-	Light	-b	Bib	ch-	Chair
-mp	Lamp	-ch-	Kitchen	fl-	Flying
j-	Jump	-ch	Watch	th-	There
-f-	Coffee	sh-	Shoe	-th	Nothing
s-	Santa	-sh	Fish	-th	Mouth
		th-	Thumb	-sh-	Fishing

Age 7		*Age 8*	
v-	Vase	-j	Cage
thr-	Three	-v	Stove
z-	Zipper	-th-	Brother
-z-	Scissors	-z	Nose
-s-	Whistle	-z-	Measure
-s	House		
sk-	School		
sl-	Slide		
st-	Stop		
sn-	Snow		

Source: From "Laradon Articulation Scale" by W. Edmonston, in D. Pollack (Ed.), *Educational Audiology for the Limited Hearing Infant,* Springfield, Ill.: Charles C Thomas, 1970.

The suprasegmental features are used most expressively by children in the late preschool years. These children's voice quality is changing from the somewhat delicate voice of younger children to the much stronger and louder voice of school-aged children. A common observation of new graduate students when comparing the nursery children and the prekindergarten group is that the older they get the more active and loud they become.

Accent or stress in certain words or phrases may still occur incorrectly in new words or in utterances the children may not understand. For example, word boundaries may be violated: the song, "Mares eat oats and does eat oats and little lambs eat ivy," is interpreted as, "Marseyotes and doseyotes and little lambsydivey," in this case, "little lambsydivey" is a name. The interpretation of word boundaries thus becomes closely associated not only with how the child articulates the phrase or word but with the meaning applied.

Although children who have been progressing normally through the stages of language acquisition still demonstrate variations from adult language, both receptively and expressively, they are quite able to converse, interact, and manipulate their environment via language. In short, they are well on their way to becoming sophisticated language users. In a rather brief period, the 5-year-old has accomplished the major proportion of man's most impressive ability without any "formal" training. But what about this child's hearing-impaired peer?

Language and Hearing-Impaired Prekindergarteners

Language Development

The hearing-impaired child at age 4 to 5 has the same cognitive and linguistic limitations associated with language development as that child's hearing peer but will, in addition, portray extended deficiency in linguistic components as a function of the hearing loss. Hearing-impaired children of late preschool age are hardly a homogeneous group in regard to language and speech ability. The complexity of variables related to audition, intelligence, general development, intervention, parents, and experience becomes extremely evident by this age. It is therefore impossible to indicate precisely where hearing-impaired prekindergarteners as a group will fall along the continuum of language acquisition. A range of "normal" does not apply here; each hearing-impaired child must be viewed individually, based on the variables we have described.

If the study of the development of language in normal children is a challenge, the study of language acquisition in children with hearing disorders, whether conductive or sensorineural, fluctuating or stable, intensifies the challenge. There is much yet to be discovered in this area. Thus far, however, conclusions can be drawn on certain aspects at least for particular samples studied. The results of research of language in young hearing-impaired children are best summed by Kretschmer and Kretschmer (1978):

1. Spoken language development can be similar to that of normal hearing children, although it is often slower to appear.
2. Development of organized gesture systems . . . in young deaf children . . . seem[s] to be based on symbolic organization distinct from that of spoken English.
3. Manual language acquisition shares many characteristics of spoken language acquisition, but like gesture systems, may come from symbolic bases quite different from spoken English.
4. Hearing children of deaf parents seem to develop manual and spoken language systems that are relatively independent of one another; with regard to some structural issues there may be direct but temporary confounding influences of manual language on spoken language acquisition.
5. Communication competence seems to be poorly developed in preschool hearing impaired children.
6. Parental communication style with their hearing impaired children is noticeably different from interactions with normally hearing children, especially among mothers of deaf children with slow developing language performance. (pp. 104–105)

Of course, as with any generalized statement, there are exceptions to each of these points. The important issue, however, regarding the language of hearing-impaired children is that the child's progress is dependent on the interrelationship of multiple factors in the child's life. The interaction of the factors of early identification, early amplification, early language and speech intervention (whether aural/oral, total communication, or cued speech), and parental cooperation appears to be extremely important in facilitating the child's chances for acquiring competence in linguistic ability (Ling, 1976; Northcott, 1973; Pollack, 1970).

In the prekindergarten, then, may be found hearing-impaired children who are at or very near their normal peers in language comprehension and production, regardless of the degree of their hearing loss or age of onset. There may also be hearing-impaired children with very delayed linguistic abilities, due to a combination of factors. Finally, there will be children at various points in between, again based on their life experiences combined with those aspects related directly to their hearing loss.

Social-Emotional Development

As children develop through the preschool years, they move gradually from adult-child interaction to child-child interaction. In late preschool, children enter into social play that is different from earlier parallel type play, in which they would involve themselves near another child but basically would be centered in themselves and their own interest in other objects or activities. Preference for the company of certain children over others may be obvious in parallel play, but true interaction and cooperative effort do not occur. Piaget (1932) describes this type of play or social interaction between children as rule-regulated and developing gradually from ages 4 through 7. This type of social interchange may depend on the particular child's language facility, since communication is an integral part of this aspect of social development.

Children in late preschool also become less egocentric; though self is still the central focus, they become more oriented toward the group. They become increasingly aware of other children in their own right, and the idea or concept of "friend" is beginning to form. From this age on into elementary school, the peer group will exercise more and more influence on the child's social and emotional attitudes, behavior, and self concept. Children "learn" social and emotional behavior at home and in preschool. They develop a self concept based on various social and emotional interactions with others.

Social and emotional development, as we have seen, are interdependent through the early years. This remains true in late preschool and beyond. As McCandless (1967) notes, emotional interaction interfaces social interaction. Unless overindulged and/or undisciplined, a child by late preschool is learning to express emotion in socially acceptable ways. This is not to say that the age of temper outbursts and pouting is over. But, by assisting the child in understanding emotions, social behavíor, responsibility, and the fact of coexistence, the parents and the preschool staff can aid the child in mastering the ability to interact with others. This also relates to the new influence of other children. Because the children are becoming more aware of one another, they will become increasingly critical and supportive of behavior exhibited by their peers.

The social and emotional maturation of 4- and 5-year-olds represents a blossoming from a prior self-centered point of operation to true interaction and sharing with others. It opens a new horizon of learning experience, although it may not always be pleasant or to the child's liking. A growing facility in language and communication will enhance this area of development and become even more allied with social-emotional maturation than in earlier development.

CURRICULUM

The content of the preschool experience, or more specifically the curriculum, may vary depending on the children served. While in some instances a social experience may suffice, this is not the case with handicapped preschool children. The purpose of early intervention is to mediate in order that the resulting educationally related deficits of a handicapping condition, such as hearing impairment or language delay, may be lessened by the time the child enters formal schooling. The curriculum must therefore reflect this purpose. Kirk (1972) suggests six general areas to consider regarding child experiences at the late preschool level:

1. opportunity for socialization
2. development of communication
3. utilization and training of residual hearing
4. mastery of basic concepts
5. development of early reading ability
6. provision of parent education

These points provide a reasonable framework in which to design and build an appropriate curriculum for the prekindergarten child.

The objectives of development and implementation of the curriculum at the prekindergarten level are, in many respects, the same as those at the nursery level. For example, the continued expansion of basic conceptual understanding and refinement of language ability remain areas of emphasis, even though the children have matured both in age and in these and other aspects of the curriculum. However, in order to have the program remain relevant and effective, specific objectives, activities, and use of instructional materials are altered to provide experiences appropriate to the 4- and 5-year-old child's expanding interests.

Extending the Curriculum from the Nursery Level

In the Comprehensive Services Program, the basic curriculum components at the nursery and prekindergarten levels are the same. As noted in the previous chapter, these basic components are:

- cognition and language comprehension
- language expression
- audition
- motor development

- social and emotional maturation
- self-help skills

The central purpose in each area remains the same throughout the preschool program, but in each area individual goals are altered to match the age abilities (or limitations) and interests of the children. Finger dexterity and eye-hand coordination are objectives at both the nursery and prekindergarten level. Dot-to-dot picture completion may be appropriate for a 4½-year-old, but it is not an activity that finds much success with an early 3-year-old. Therefore, each curriculum area must expand and extend to keep pace with the maturing child. Because of the variation in children we have noted, specific objectives in curriculum areas might very well reflect goals that would be applicable to a younger child. For example, a hearing-impaired child with a profound hearing loss who enters prekindergarten at age 4 without having received prior amplification or educational intervention may have a language production objective of signs and speech at the one-word-utterance level. Although, developmentally, this language level occurs much earlier than age 4, it is where this child is functionally at the present time and is therefore appropriate for him. However, because the child is 4 years of age, words like *potty* or *bottle* would be inappropriate. Signs and words that are more specific to the child's age interests and requirements will be needed.

Curriculum content is best modified through close observation of the child. A keen awareness of what a particular child is able to do, is interested in, and is intent on accomplishing should dictate content, activities, and materials. The concept of ordinal position can be demonstrated just as well by lining up toy trucks along a pretend highway as by indicating a row of stars on a worksheet or by positioning stuffed animals along a counter top. Curriculum areas and objectives can remain intact, but implementing content must be flexible.

An additional goal of the curriculum in prekindergarten is based on the fact that children will soon be passing into the formal educational structure of the public schools. The final years of the preschool experience represent an effort to "ready" the handicapped child for this move. Much of what the child has been able to accomplish (hopefully) during preschool will have an effect on the placement of the child during the elementary school years. This period therefore represents in the curriculum the final tying together of all areas in order that the child can leave the prekindergarten with the best preparation possible, based on factors within the child's particular situation. To this end, prekindergarten curriculum emphasizes or targets two additional areas that were previously present but parts of other areas, such as cognition and language.

Additional Curriculum Areas in Prekindergarten

One purpose of the prekindergarten experience is to provide the older preschool-aged, hearing-impaired or language-delayed child with an opportunity to explore and possibly master prerequisites for academic phases of his future educational career. Since the majority of the children completing the Comprehensive Services Program will be placed in at least a partial mainstream setting for kindergarten, we feel it is imperative that the children be able to operate effectively and successfully in that placement. Therefore, a large component of the prekindergarten experience relates both formally and informally to the academic areas of early reading and mathematics. Although these two additional curriculum components are specific components at this level, they are also still closely interrelated with all other curriculum areas. For example, cognition and language comprehension now include more specific orientation toward mathematics-related concepts of quantity, size, and so forth, and story time becomes an important social experience.

Early Reading

An orientation to reading for hearing-impaired children at the preschool level is not a novel idea. Informal use of the printed word with young hearing-impaired children has been encouraged by Hart (1963) through the use of experience stories, printed labels, and the building of basic sight vocabulary. She also emphasizes the fostering of favorable attitudes toward reading and recognition of its purpose. Language has been visually enhanced and taught to young hearing-impaired children through exposure to the printed word and by encouraging early motivational strides toward reading and books. This approach has been used in several curricula for the hearing impaired, such as those in the Clark School (1972) and the Lexington School (Hart, 1963, 1978) programs for young children.

Reading at the prekindergarten level in the Comprehensive Services Program is not viewed as a set of discrete skills, such as left-right progression or grapheme-phoneme interpretation, but as a linguistic form. Reading is defined as printed language. Although not identical in form to spoken language, it has the same purpose of communication: derivation of meaning. Since it has been shown that a school-age child with a reading problem is a child with a language problem (Goodman, 1973; Smith, 1975), this area is considered a necessary aspect of the curriculum at the late preschool level.

The central purpose of the early reading program is to provide a foundation to enable the children to attain success in the formalized reading instruction of the primary grades. Specifically, the program's objectives may be summarized as follows:

- to provide a wide exposure to various reading materials: books, magazines, newspapers
- to promote concepts for the various uses and purposes of reading: pleasure, function, information
- to foster a desire to read and an interest in reading
- to develop a personal sight vocabulary
- to encourage independent reading if the child demonstrates the requisite ability

The reading component in the curriculum is not a separate "lesson" time set aside, except perhaps for the story telling time when teachers or aides read to the children. It involves coordinated activities with the other curriculum components (it is of course also a popular free-time activity). Books and other reading materials are used as instructional materials, and informal presentation of the printed form is used in a variety of activities, from a word-picture listing of what foods will go on a picnic to short sentences explaining "job" responsibilities in the classroom. Although the reading program is informal, it requires specific, in-depth planning on the part of the staff. Truax (1978) and, earlier, Hart (1963) have indicated three types of reading: recreational, functional, and informational or instructional. The first two types are emphasized in the prekindergarten program. Since motivation and enjoyment related to printed language are objectives, the children are presented with extensive opportunities to discover and explore reading materials. Functional reading from names to safety signs to simple directions provide graduated experiences in the purposeful aspects of reading. Informational reading is related to later reading mastery, such as that in academic subject areas in elementary school, and is therefore somewhat advanced for preschool children.

Although exposure to books, storytelling, and other reading-related activities is part of the programming for children from infancy, it is at the prekindergarten level that intensive emphasis is placed on this aspect. Teachers must be aware of each child's linguistic ability and must develop objectives in reading that will coincide and enhance the child's language base.

Mathematics

The second supplementary curriculum area that receives specific emphasis in prekindergarten is mathematics. Otto and Smith (1980) highlight two important facts to support attention to mathematics at the late preschool level: (1) Programs in modern mathematics now used in schools require comprehension of a wide range of concepts and processes. (2) Students who enter an educational program with a strong foundation in fundamental mathematics tend to do better than those who do not have such a foundation. Indeed, mathematics is related to intuitive and inductive thinking as well as to deductive reasoning. Mathematical concepts are also part of language and cognitive understanding. Since these latter areas are already addressed in preschool objectives, mathematics is a logical and necessary supplement.

As in the early reading program, mathematics instruction is designed to be integrated with other aspects of the curriculum. It is therefore termed an informal aspect, although this does not infer a haphazard approach. Emphasis is on the functional use of mathematics in daily living and on opportunities for problem solving and exercising logical thought processes.

Activities in mathematics involve counting, combining quantities, recognition of printed numerals and numbered names, as well as planned experiences with mathematical concepts and language appropriate to the child's linguistic and cognitive functioning levels. Previously targeted concepts, such as size, shape, and position that relate to mathematics, are also expanded, together with the vocabulary associated with the extended meanings.

Summary

The two additional curriculum areas of reading and mathematics, together with the other curriculum components that are extended and expanded from the nursery level, are coordinated and interrelated in support of one another. This, combined with a high degree of individualized attention to the abilities and deficits of individual children, makes the curriculum appropriate, flexible, and purposeful. In this context, parents are encouraged to apply curriculum goals outside of the school setting so that transfer of learning can occur and the relevancy of gains in one situation will generalize to other areas of the child's life.

PARENTS AND PREKINDERGARTEN

Parents and families of children enrolled in the Comprehensive Services Prekindergarten are, as we have noted, an integral part of the child's educational experience. "Rookie" parents must be guided and supported, and "veteran" parents must continue to aid in the cooperative effort of the program.

A new issue arises for parents when their children complete the preschool experience and enter the formal educational placement of kindergarten. Where the child will attend school, what type of classroom will be most conducive to the child's needs, what support services will be available—these are important concerns that must be addressed. Parents as well as children must "graduate" from preschool. They will no longer be part of a small select group but only one of many groups in a school system. This prospect is often overwhelming, even though the local school district has most likely already been involved and is familiar with the parent and child. Change in itself shakes security. Thus, preschool personnel must be keenly aware of parental feelings in this matter.

It is the responsibility of the preschool staff to ensure that the transition from preschool to elementary school is accomplished smoothly. Parents and representatives from the preschool and local education agency should discuss exactly what program the child will receive and should finalize plans within the year prior to formal entry. If such educational provisions are not made, the parents have recourse to due process procedures as outlined by their state department of education. Although this process can be a long and difficult procedure, fraught with much compromise, parents should be informed of their rights and the rights of their children. Preschool professionals must be responsible for providing necessary information to the parents before their children move into the formal academic process.

BEYOND PREKINDERGARTEN

In most instances, the preschool experience is completed between the child's 5th and 6th birthdays, although in some cases children remain in the Comprehensive Services Program for one additional year if the local educational agency and preschool staff deem that placement most appropriate at the time. Attention must now be directed to the educational alternatives available, specifically to those that will best serve the child's particular needs upon completion of the preschool program. During the late preschool period, the parents and preschool staff must cooperatively interact with local school personnel regarding the educational needs and requisite provisions once the child enters kindergarten.

Placement

The educational alternatives that are available to a hearing-impaired and/or language-delayed child upon completion of preschool will depend on the particular circumstances. Public Law 94–142, the Education of All Handicapped Children Act of 1975, states that such children must receive "appropriate" education within the "least restrictive environment." Though such placement is not always realized, the purpose of the act is to ensure that the educational and support needs of children who are deemed handicapped are met effectively and appropriately. Placement according to Fallen (1978) is governed by the child's needs related to the disability and also to the service alternatives available in the geographical area. Options for placement may therefore be limited, depending on the facilities within the region.

Program Alternatives for Children with Language Delay

Program placement for children who have been enrolled in the preschool due to a specified delay in language development will depend on the extent of the delay still present at the completion of prekindergarten and on the associated cause of the delay itself. The majority of the children who exhibit delays in language in the Comprehensive Services Program displays recurrent otitis media sufficient to interrupt the natural flow of normal linguistic development. By the time prekindergarten is completed, this difficulty has most often been controlled and the children have progressed to achieve normal or near-normal language levels. These children enter a regular kindergarten class, but their hearing continues to be monitored closely. Language and speech services will continue, if that is determined to be necessary, but these will now be assumed by the school's speech pathologist.

Language delay that is secondary to mental retardation or learning disability (usually related to auditory processing problems) may require an additional year in prekindergarten, although such students do not remain much beyond the age of 6. Other alternatives include placement in a regular kindergarten with supportive speech and language services through the public school speech personnel, resource room placement with partial mainstreaming into a kindergarten class, or placement in a primary classroom for moderately retarded or learning-disabled students. Each of these alternatives must be carefully examined by parents, public school personnel, and the preschool staff, and the one best suited to optimize continued growth should be selected. This becomes a joint responsibility of all concerned with the child's educational future. All aspects of the child should be examined carefully, including progress to date, rate of progress, extent of handicap on all areas of development, personality, and so on. Medical labels assigned early in life should not be automatically applied as educational labels.

Program Alternatives for Hearing-Impaired Children

In its surveys of programs and services for the hearing-impaired, the Office of Demographic Studies at Gallaudet College in Washington, D.C.

listed the following six classes of program alternatives available for school-aged, hearing-impaired students (Rawlings & Trybus, 1978).

Residential Schools for the Hearing Impaired

This type of educational facility, designed specifically for the hearing impaired, includes state residential schools and privately funded and operated residential programs. Moores (1978) reports a total of 79 residential-type programs for school-aged, hearing-impaired students, 63 of which are public and 16 of which are private. In most cases, their scholastic programs extend from the primary level through high school. As the term implies, the students attending these schools are housed in dormitories or cottages within the facility environment. Some residential programs accept day students living in the near geographical area, but the majority of those enrolled resides full-time on campus. In the Office of Demographic Studies' 1975 survey of programs with a residential setting, 69 or 87 percent responded. The responses indicated that 19,521 students or 32 percent of the hearing-impaired school population were enrolled in residential programs for the hearing impaired (Rawlings & Trybus, 1978). For the 978–1979 school year, Schildroth (1980) reports that the public residential schools enrolled a total of 16,504 hearing-impaired students. Although this represents a decline in student numbers, Schildroth attributes the reduction to a decrease in the population of school-age children in general.

Residential Schools for the Multihandicapped

Like residential school programs for the hearing impaired, residential schools for the multihandicapped may be state or private, and the enrolled students reside on campus. However, in these schools, the program emphasis is on serving children who are diagnosed as multihandicapped. Thus, hearing loss is only one aspect to be considered in these schools' programming. The 1975 survey indicated that 2,435 hearing-impaired students were enrolled in this type of service facility. This constitutes about 4 percent of the school-age hearing-impaired population. Schildroth (1980) reports a 3.3 percent increase in the enrollments of multihandicapped students nationally between 1970 and 1977. This includes not only residential facilities but also day schools, which are discussed in the following sections. This increase may be due to better child-find programs as well as more accurate diagnosis of handicapping conditions.

Programs in an institutionalized setting are recognized by Public Law 94–142 as legitimate placement settings for children who are severely or profoundly handicapped and may therefore require services in a more restrictive environment than that provided in a public school setting. In most cases, children with hearing impairment and language delay do not fall into this category unless additional disabilities are also present, such as mental retardation or blindness. In such instances, the children are actually multihandicapped and may indeed benefit from specialized services in other settings. For the majority of children with hearing and/or language difficulties, however, placement in local day programs is most often preferable. If such local programs are not available, the child may be enrolled in a residential setting, even though the child's specific needs might be better met in a different placement setting.

Day Schools for the Hearing Impaired

Programs that are housed in a facility specifically for hearing-impaired students but do not offer a residential setting are referred to as day schools. This type of educational placement is most often found in urban areas that support a large population; and they may be part of a city, county, or regional special education service administration. Although, historically, most day schools have been privately operated, this is not presently the case. Oyer (1976) found a total of 65 day schools under public education and only 22 operating as private programs. Scholastic programs in day schools may serve only the elementary grades (1–6 or 1–8), or they may offer a complete curriculum through high school levels. The 1975 survey of the Office of Demographic Studies found that 85 percent of the day schools that responded to its questionnaire had an enrollment of 7,513 students or 12 percent of the school-age, hearing-impaired population (Rawlings & Trybus, 1978).

Day Schools for the Multihandicapped

Another program alternative is provided by day school programs for multihandicapped students that offer a specific orientation for the hearing impaired. These day schools may operate as either public or private educational services, but the children do not reside on campus. As with the residential programs for the multihandicapped, only 4 percent of the school-age, hearing-impaired population was reported to be enrolled in this type of setting.

Day Classes for the Hearing Impaired

In their attempt to classify services offered by local educational agencies, Rawlings and Trybus (1978) indicate two basic categories. The first is full-time, self-contained classes for the hearing impaired. In this setting, a class or classes offer educational services to hearing-impaired students within a school for normally hearing children. Day classes may be held in one centralized location within a city, county, or regionalized district, or they may be located in various school buildings throughout a program locality. Day classes usually infer total self-contained instruction by a teacher of the hearing impaired, but they may include mainstreaming during lunch, recess, and/or in nonacademic offerings such as physical education or art. Although the classes may be housed in a school for normal children, the self-contained day class may be quite isolated from regular school interactions. Rawlings and Trybus differentiate between local school systems that offer enrollment in full-time day classes and those offering other support services. They report that the 1975 survey of the Office of Demographic Studies indicated that 7 percent of the total school-age, hearing-impaired population, or 4,365 children, attended such full-time day class settings.

Part-time Classes and Services for the Hearing Impaired

The final category of program alternatives listed by the Office of Demographic Studies consists of services offered by local education agencies aside from self-contained day classes. This includes the resource room setting, itinerant programs, or other part-time instruction received from a teacher of the hearing-impaired (Karchmer & Trybus, 1977). These services are considered part-time in that the hearing-impaired student attends regular classrooms for academic and nonacademic instruction to the extent that the student is able to function successfully. In the resource setting, a teacher of the hearing impaired offers specific instruction in needed areas to all hearing-impaired students in the school. The teacher may, for example, instruct in reading and language arts and mainstream the students for other subjects. Instruction is usually individual or in small groups. The itinerant teacher of the hearing impaired serves hearing-handicapped children enrolled in "neighborhood" schools and travels throughout a district. Children in this type of program attend regular classes on a full-time basis but receive specific instruction from the itinerant teacher, much as in a tutorial program. The 1975 survey indicated that 24,138 children or 40 percent of the total school-age, hearing-impaired population receive services in this category. Oyer (1976) reports that there are approximately 525 such programs in the public school systems.

Figure 9–2 shows enrollments of hearing-impaired students in various educational settings based on the degree of hearing loss. Figure 9–3 shows percentages of children in integrated or mainstreamed settings based on the degree of hearing loss. These figures indicate that the largest percentage of profoundly hearing-impaired students is in residential schools, followed by day schools and day classes, with the smallest percentage in mainstreamed alternatives. The reverse is true for children with mild and

Figure 9–2 Distribution of Hearing-Impaired Children by Type of Loss (Degree) and Educational Facility

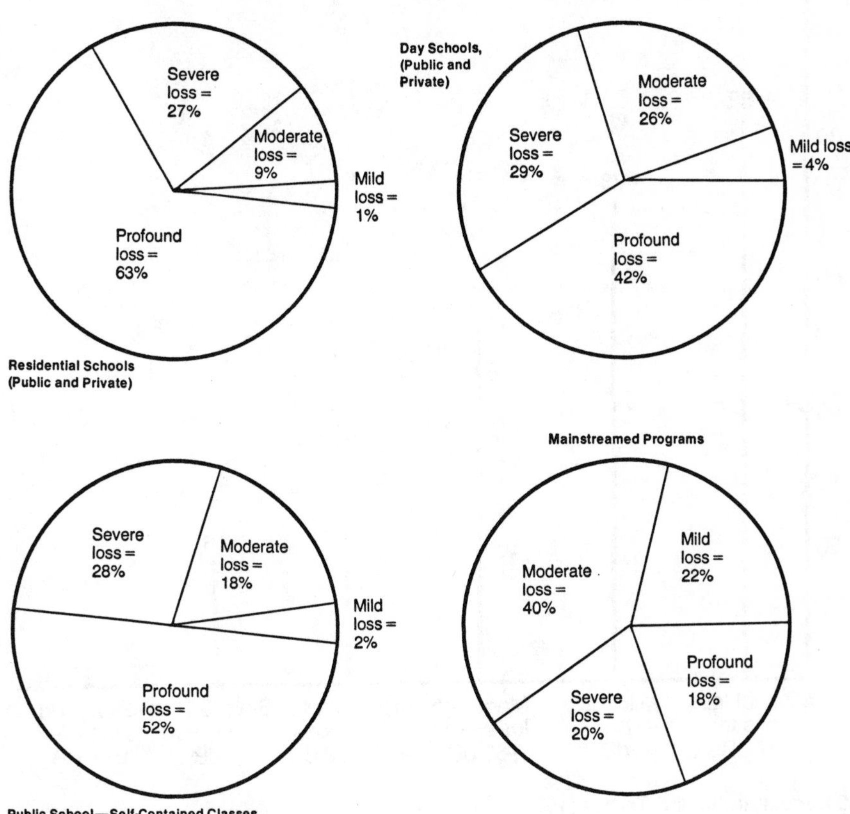

Source: Karchmer & Trybus (1977).

Figure 9–3 Percentages of Children in Mainstreamed Programs by Degrees of Hearing Loss

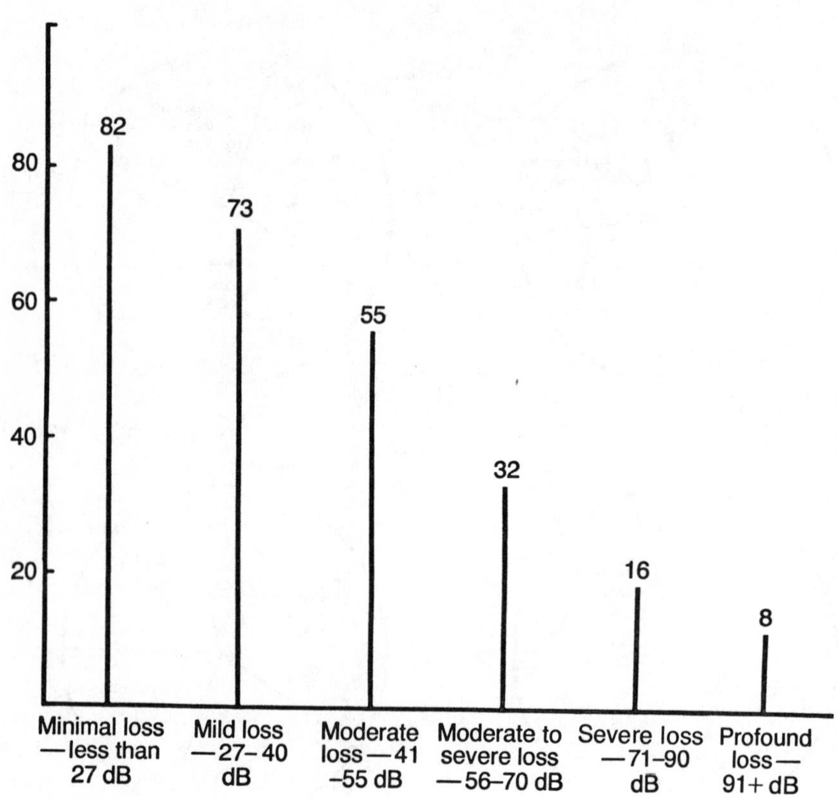

Source: Karchmer & Trybus (1977).

moderate impairment. Children classified as having severe hearing losses are nearly equally represented in all settings, with slightly lower enrollments in mainstreamed alternatives.

This information is helpful, yet placement cannot be determined based only on the degree of hearing loss. Factors relating to age of onset, hearing age, cause of hearing loss, preschool experiences, cognitive abilities, linguistic and communication level and facility, social and emotional development, motor ability, personality, self concept, parents, and other personal and sociological aspects must all be considered in determining the optimal placement of a child.

Other Alternatives

In addition to these program settings, there are other service possibilities or service combinations that may suit the individual needs of some hearing-impaired children entering formal education. By age 6, many children have outgrown extensive problems with bouts of otitis media. If they have received preschool services and their hearing is functioning at a stable, normal level, they will not usually be classified as hearing impaired, but they may still require language and/or speech therapy to bring production and usage to appropriate levels. Children with sensory neural impairment in the mild or moderate range who have benefited from early amplification and education may also succeed with the help of language and/or speech therapy and the additional support of an itinerant or resource room teacher.

The placement alternatives for children with severe or profound losses will vary depending on their preschool and present functioning levels. The alternative may be speech therapy and itinerant services or a resource-room setting supplemented by speech work. The amount of mainstreaming that is possible will depend on individual capabilities and limitations.

It is possible that some children will require an intensive primary self-contained class setting when first entering public school programming. In these instances, mainstreaming is often arranged for nonacademic areas. Frequently, the children are initially enrolled in a self-contained program in the primary grades and gradually mainstreamed to extended degrees throughout their elementary experience.

Placement Concerns

Our examination of educational alternatives indicates quite an array of available services. Each option has its own rationale and philosophy to support its existence and services. Given this broad range of considerations, certain issues, discussed below, should be of prime concern to the teachers and parents of preschool children.

Availability of Alternatives

If all of the placement options we have examined were available to all children with hearing loss, appropriate placement would be a relatively simple matter. As we have noted, however, this is not usually the case. A child may attend a residential school or a day school for the hearing impaired because there is nothing else available, not because the child requires that particular type of programming. Another child may receive only speech services or itinerant programming even though more intensive educational support is required, simply because such programming is all there is in the child's school system. Indeed, for many children, there is only one option, and that option may not be the most "appropriate" nor represent the "least restrictive environment." Hearing-impaired children who live in rural areas or smaller cities or in areas without regionalized programs may be especially affected by this lack of alternatives. Generally, more heavily populated areas can, in theory at least, present a wider continuum of services.

Quality of Programming

A second concern involves the quality of the programs available. Among the alternatives presented, there is a wide variation across programs with regard to quality in teachers, curriculum, instruction, and support services, as, for example, in speech therapy, psychological and audiological assistance, and personnel. This means that teacher training institutions, state certification standards, and public school requirements must be maintained to employ quality educators and support personnel who are current in their knowledge of hearing impairment and language and in their ability to apply this knowledge to an academic program. Speech therapists and school psychologists need specific training and experience with a variety of hearing-impaired students in order to provide effective services.

Mainstreaming

A third concern is with the definition of "mainstreaming" (Vernon & Prickett, 1976). Integrated programs for hearing-impaired children must not merely place students in a classroom for hearing children and then abandon them. The failure of past mainstreaming efforts is due, in part, to the lack of support services provided such children who are placed in regular instructional settings. The need of the regular classroom teacher for information on how the classroom can be made optimally effective for the hearing-impaired student is both an aspect of support service and a definition of mainstreaming. In-service—in the form of workshops, presentations, discussions, and conference time available with resident experts in hearing impairment—is vital in the provision of an appropriate mainstreamed placement.

It is important for parents to be aware of these issues concerning the continued education of their child. A well-designed and implemented program for hearing-impaired students in any educational alternative, but especially in a mainstreamed environment, requires foresight, planning, and continuous monitoring in order to achieve progress and effectiveness. Preschool interventionists share in this responsibility. They must ensure that parents and children enter the formal education experience not only with an excellent preschool program on which to build new knowledge and growth but also with information and a sense of realism as to the future educational needs of the children.

SUMMARY

The prekindergarten level in the Comprehensive Services Program may be regarded as an important transition period from the early foundation of child development through the parent-infant and nursery levels to the "real school" orientation, which begins at about age 6 with entry into kindergarten or perhaps the first grade. Curriculum objectives and activities are expanded and extended to accommodate the enlarging abilities of the children, but they must still concentrate on individualization for each child and in each area of development within that child's growth profile. By assisting in the selection and perhaps securing, of an appropriate placement that will optimize the child's learning throughout the school years, prekindergarten can serve to prepare parents for the entry of their children into formal education careers.

REFERENCES

Brown, R. *A first language*. Cambridge, Mass.: Harvard University Press, 1973.

Carey, S. The child as a word learner. In M. Halle, J. Brisman, & G. A. Miller (Eds.), *Linguistic theory and psychological reality*. Cambridge, Mass.: MIT Press, 1977.

Chomsky, C. *The acquisition of syntax in children from 5 to 10* (Research monograph No. 57). Cambridge, Mass.: MIT Press, 1969.

Clark, E. *The acquisition of semantics.* A short course presented at the convention of the American Speech and Hearing Association, Detroit, Mich., 1973.

Clark School for the Deaf. Reading. Northampton, Mass.: Clark School for the Deaf, 1972.

deVilliers, J. G., & deVilliers, P. A. *Language acquisition.* Cambridge, Mass.: Harvard University Press, 1978.

Donaldson, M., & Balfour, G. Less is more: A study of language comprehension in children. *British Journal of Psychology,* 1968, *54,* 461–472.

Englemann, S. *Preventing failure in the primary grades.* Chicago, Ill.: Science Research Associates, 1969.

Fallen, N. *Young children with special needs.* Columbus, Ohio: Charles E. Merrill, 1978.

Goodman, K. Analysis of oral reading miscues: Applied psycholinguistics. In F. Smith (Ed.), *Psycholinguistics and reading.* New York: Holt, Rinehart, and Winston, 1973.

Hart, B. D. *Teaching reading to deaf children.* Washington, D.C.: A. G. Bell Association for the Deaf, 1963.

Hart, B. D. *Teaching reading to deaf children* (rev. ed.). Washington, D.C.: A.G. Bell Assoc. for the Deaf, 1978.

Hurlock, E. B. *Child development* (5th ed.). New York: McGraw Hill, 1972

Kamii, C., & Radin, N. A. A framework for preschool curriculum based on Piagetian concepts. In I. J. Athey & D. O. Rubadeau (Eds.), *Educational implications of Piaget's theory.* Waltham, Mass.: Ginn-Blaisdell, 1970.

Karchmer, M. A. and Trybus, R. J. *Who are the deaf children in mainstream programs?* (Series R, No. 4). Washington, D.C.: Gallaudet College, Office of Demographic Studies, October 1977.

Kirk, S. A. *Educating exceptional children.* Boston, Mass.: Houghton Mifflin, 1972.

Kretschmer, R. R., & Kretschmer, L. W. *Language development and intervention with the hearing impaired.* Baltimore, Md.: University Park Press, 1978.

Lavatelli, C. S. A Piaget derived model for compensatory preschool education. In J. L. Frost (Ed.), *Early childhood education rediscovered.* New York: Holt, Rinehart, and Winston, 1968.

Lenneberg, E. H. *Biological foundations of language.* New York: John Wiley & Sons, 1967.

Ling, D. *Speech and the hearing impaired child.* Washington, D.C.: A. G. Bell Association for the Deaf, 1976.

McCandless, B. R. *Children behavior and development* (2nd ed.). New York: Holt, Rinehart, and Winston, 1967.

Moores, D. F. *Educating the deaf—psychology, principles and practices.* Boston, Mass.: Houghton Mifflin, 1978.

Northcott, W. H. *The hearing impaired child in a regular classroom: Preschool, primary and secondary years,* Washington, D.C.: A. G. Bell Association for the Deaf, 1973.

Otto, W., & Smith, R, J. *Corrective and remedial teaching.* Boston, Mass.: Houghton Mifflin, 1980.

Oyer, H. J. *Communication for the hearing handicapped—an international perspective.* Baltimore, Md.: University Park Press, 1976.

Parker, R. K. *The preschool in action—exploring early childhood programs.* Boston, Mass.: Allyn & Bacon, 1972.

Piaget, J. *The moral judgment of the child.* London: Kegan Paul, 1932.

Pollack, D. *Educational audiology for the limited hearing infant.* Springfield, Ill.: Charles C Thomas, 1970.

Rawlings, B. W., & Trybus, R. J. Personnel, facilities, and services available in schools and classes for hearing impaired children in the United States. *American Annals of the Deaf,* 1978, *123,* 98–114.

Safford, P. L. *Teaching young children with special needs.* St. Louis, Mo.: C. V. Mosby, 1978.

Sander, E. K. When are speech sounds learned? *Journal of Speech and Hearing Disorders,* 1972, *37,* 55–63.

Schildroth, A. N. Public residential schools for deaf students in the United States, 1970–1978. *American Annals of the Deaf,* 1980, *125,* 80–91.

Sinclair-de-Zwart, H. Developmental psycholinguistics. In D. Elkind & J. H. Flavell (Eds.), *Studies in cognitive development.* New York: Oxford University Press, 1969.

Smith, F. *Comprehension and learning.* New York: Holt, Rinehart, and Winston, 1975.

Templin, M. *Certain language skills in children.* Minneapolis: University of Minnesota Press, 1957.

Truax, R. R. Reading and language. In R. R. Kretschmer & L. W. Kretschmer (Eds.), *Language development and intervention with the hearing impaired.* Baltimore, Md.: University Park Press, 1978.

Vernon, M., & Prickett, H. Mainstreaming, past and present: Some issues and a model plan. *Audiology and Hearing Education,* 1976, *2,* 5–11.

Weikart, D., Rogers, L., Adcock, C., & McClelland, D. *The cognitively oriented curriculum: A framework for preschool teachers.* Washington, D.C.: National Association for the Education of Young Children, 1970.

Wellman, B., Case, I., Mengert, I., & Bradbury, D. Speech sounds of young children. *University of Iowa Studies in Child Welfare,* 1931, 5, 1–82.

Appendix A

Definitions of Semantic Cases

Noun Cases	Definitions/Examples
1. Agent	One who produces action on an object. "*Tom* hit the boy."
2. Mover	Person or object that produces action on itself. "The *cow* ran away."
3. Patient	Object that receives the action. "I tore up the *picture*."
4. Experiencer	Object that has internal feeling. "*Eric* loved Marian." (Has a process verb)
5. Complement	Object that results from action itself. "I painted a *picture*." (The end result)
6. Recipient	Person who gets the "fall out" of the action—tends to reap the benefit of the action. "I gave the ball to *Mommy*."
7. Possessor	Person who has temporary or permanent ownership of an object. "*Jimmy* has a ball." (*Jimmy's* ball)
8. Entity	Object that exists, and is not acted upon. Only used with stative verbs. "There is a *ball*."
9. Part	(Part to whole)—Part of the whole. "He has *eyes*." (As opposed to "he has a car")
10. Content	(Subject matter)—What an entity is about or made up of. "This story is about *Cinderella*." (Cued by "about")
11. Phenomenon	Byproduct of a recognized action when the action itself or the end result is not seen. "The boy heard the *footsteps*."
12. Vocative	Attention getting device—a summons. "*Mommy*!"

13. Entity-Equivalent	Two nouns are equivalent. "*Mary* is *president*." (A predicate nominative sentence)
Verb Cases	**Definitions/Examples**
14. Action-Causative	External action produced by agent on a patient. "Jack *hit* Robert." "Robert *was hit* by Jack." (Passive voice)
15. Action-Affective	Action produced by a mover. "The cow *ran* away." (No direct object)
16. Process-Causative	Process results in a complement or an action on a patient. "I *thought* up the idea." "Dominic *thought* about school." (Cued by "up")
17. Process-Affective	An internal action where effect is on self (this does not take a direct object). "David *slept*."
18. Ambient Action	Natural phenomenon where the pronoun does not stand for anything. "It *is* raining."
19. Ambient/Stative	A surrounding condition. "It *was* fun."
20. Stative-Static	It is; it exists. "The apple *is* red."
21. Stative-Dynamic	It is, and it got to be that way as a result of a process over time. "The fire *is* hot." (The fire became hot)
Modifier Cases	
22. Existence	That is. "I see *that* ball."
23. Nonexistence	Does not exist. "There are no bananas."
24. Recurrence	More of the same; recurrence or reappearance. "I want *more* milk." "I want *another* cookie."
25. Disappearance	Was there, but not anymore. "The milk is *all gone*."
26. Denial	Refusal to believe or agree with the proposition. "I did *not* spill the milk."
27. Size	"I see a *little* boy."
28. Condition	"I have a torn shirt." "Jerry is *happy*."
29. Shape	"The moon is *round*."
30. Quality	"The cloth is *rough*."
31. Age	"John is an *old* man."
32. Color	"Elinor has a *red* dress."
33. Cardinal	"I see *ten* boys."
34. Ordinal	"I want the *fifth* apple."

Adverbial Cases	Definitions/Examples
35. Instrument	The object the agent used to accomplish an action. "I cut myself with a *knife*."
36. Reason	The "why" for doing it. "I made some cookies for the *party*." (Cued by "for")
37. Locative-Action	Place or end point of the action. "I hit Mary at *school*."
38. Locative-Stative	Where something is. "The book is on the *table*."
39. Locative-Goal	Place or end point of the action. "Jim walked to the *hospital*."
40. Locative-Source	Point where action began. "Ted walked home from *school*."
41. Time-Action	Time when action occurred (must carry action verb). "The class went on *Tuesday*." (when?)
42. Time-Duration	The length of time something occurs. "Harry worked *all week*." (How long?)
43. Time-Source	The beginning. "He began at *one o'clock*."
44. Time-End	The goal, when finished. "He finished at *two o'clock*."
45. Time-Frequency	A series of points in time. "He goes to church every *Sunday*." (Cued by "every," "each," and "several")
46. Time-Manner	How? "The rabbit runs *quickly*."
47. Intensifier	Adverbs of intensity, such as "too," "very," and "so." "He ran too *fast*."
48. Inclusion	Thing is part of a group. "I want to go *too*."
49. Comparison	Comparing one thing to another. "He runs *like* a rabbit." (Cued by "like" and "as")

Appendix B

Suggested Language Goals, Objectives and Activities for Hearing-Impaired and Language-Delayed Preschool Children

SUGGESTED GOALS AND OBJECTIVES

A. Receptive Language/Cognition

Goal 1.
a. Development of concepts pertinent to the child's environment and functioning
b. Association of words with referent: understanding of familiar objects and names through the use of speech reading and audition

Subskills:

1. Recognition of child's own name and names of family members
2. Learning names of body parts and facial features
3. Learning the personal pronouns "me" and "you"
4. Developing the concept of ownership
5. Dramatizing feelings/emotions
6. Learning "no"
7. Learning "hi" and "bye-bye"
8. Developing concepts related to toys
9. Developing concepts related to food
10. Learning clothing names
11. Developing concepts related to animals
12. Developing the concepts clean/dirty, wet/dry, hot/cold, etc.
13. Learning common nouns
14. Developing number concepts
15. Developing categorization skills (for the older child)

Goal 2. Development of visual attention combined with listening activity

Goal 3. a. Recognition of similarities in shapes and familiar objects: matching

b. Awareness of size perception differences and color concepts

Subskills:

1. Matching identical objects
2. Matching pictures to real objects
3. Developing the concept "same"
4. Developing color concepts
5. Developing the concept of size differences
6. Developing the concept "round"
7. Matching objects by feeling
8. Reproducing a sequence (for the older child)
9. Developing the concept "different" (for the older child)

Goal 4. Understanding of simple locative concepts and words

Subskills:

1. Learning "in" and "out"
2. Learning "off" and "on"
3. Learning "up" and "down"
4. Learning "under" and "behind" (for the older child)

Goal 5. Understanding of simple commands and carry-through with appropriate behavior

Subskills:

1. Conditioned response to voice
2. Imitation of body movements
3. Learning "no" with cessation of activity
4. Learning "come here"
5. Learning "stand up" and "sit down"
6. Learning "open"
7. Learning "push" or similar action verb
8. Learning "point to," "show me," "give me," etc.
9. Imitating actions in pictures (for the older child)

Goal 6. Comprehension of simple question forms

B. Expressive Language

Goal 1. Control of tongue, lip, and facial muscles

Subskills:

1. Control of tongue
2. Control of lip and facial muscles

Goal 2. Control of breath stream and blowing

Subskills:

1. Production of breath stream
2. Control of breath stream

Goal 3. Imitation of meaningful gestures and actions

Goal 4. Vocalization through imitation and spontaneity

Subskills:

1. Imitation of vowels
2. Imitation of babbling sets (consonant-vowel combinations)
3. Vocalization for expression of needs
4. Production, through imitation and spontaneity, of babbling sets that will lead to one-word utterances
5. Imitation of prosodic features (i.e., stress, pitch, timing, rhythm, duration)

Goal 5. Vocalization of meaningful words

Subskills:

1. Production of "more"
2. Production of "no"
3. Production of "hi" and "bye-bye"

SUGGESTED COORDINATING ACTIVITIES

A. Receptive Language/Cognition

Goal 1. a. Development of concepts pertinent to the child's environment and functioning

b. Association of word with referent: understanding of familiar objects and names through the use of speech reading and audition

(Note: the following subskills are *not* listed in strict developmental order)

Subskill 1: Recognition of child's own name and names of family members

Activities:

- Teach child's name through natural usage. Call the child's name each time you enter his room or want his attention. When the child looks up, say, "Yes, I called (Ricky)," and provide social reinforcement by smiling or nodding.

- Use a mirror and ask, "Where's (Mary)?" "There's (Mary)," while pointing to the child. Encourage the child to point to herself.
- Use a puppet to talk to the child; call his name often. "Hi (Billy)." "Where's (Billy)?" "There's (Billy)," while pointing to the child. Again, encourage him to point to himself.
- Use the child's name frequently during bathtime while naming body parts. "Let's wash (Sally's) feet." "Here's (Sally's) nose," etc.
- Play hide-and-seek. Hide your face or hide behind a chair. Say, "Where's (Johnny)?" Peek out and look at the child, saying, "There's (Johnny)," and point to the child. Reverse roles. Pretend you are looking for the child, saying, "Where's (Johnny)?" Repeat this question often until you "find" the child. "Oh! There's (Johnny)!"
- Teach names of family members through general usage by talking about Mommy, Daddy, or siblings, and directing the child's attention to that person.
- Paste pictures of family members in a scrapbook and talk about them. You may also use an existing family photo album. Have the mother paperclip pages of family members that the child frequently comes in contact with. Go through the pictures, continually naming the family members in the pictures (Mommy, Daddy, Grandma, Grandpa, etc.). Be sure the child can see your face as you point to and name the people in the pictures. (You may change the wording around, but always use the person's name.) At first, select only one or two family members to name at a time. You may want to use several pictures of these people to ensure the child's understanding that the name and the picture go together.
- Take one picture of each of the persons named and place it in front of the child. Ask the child "Where's (Grandma)?" "Point to (Grandma)" or "Show me (Grandma)." Direct the child as necessary.
- Have family members play "Come to (Daddy)." Child is rewarded when he/she goes to (Daddy) by a hug or by being picked up.
- Encourage the child to look at various members of the family by asking "Where's (Sis)?"
- Have family members seated around the room. Tell the child to "Go find (Daddy)" or "Take this to (Daddy)." Reinforce appropriately.
- One family member hides in the room. Others ask the child to find that person. The name of that person is repeated often until he or she is found.
- The child is given an object such as a piece of fruit or a toy. He is told "This is for (Mommy)" and is guided in giving that piece out appro-

priately. Then he is told, "This is for (child's name)," and the child keeps that particular piece. This procedure is repeated until all items are distributed. Later, child is expected to complete the task independently. Vary appropriately when teaching pronouns such as "you" and "me."

Subskill 2: Learning names of body parts and facial features

Activities:

- Use a mirror. Position yourself behind the child with the mirror in front of both of you. Point to your (nose) and say, "Here's (Mommy's) (nose)." Point to the child's (nose) and say, "Here's (Steven's) (nose)." Encourage imitation. Repeat this activity with other body parts.
- Ask the child,, "Where are (Mommy's) (eyes)?" Use his finger to point to your (eyes). Ask him, "Where are (Bobby's) (eyes)?" Help him to point to his own (eyes). Repeat for other body parts.
- During bathtime, play a guessing game. "Where's (Susie's) (foot)?" "Here's your (foot). It's under the water." Encourage the child to find her body part on request.
- Use a doll with real-life features and again ask the child to point to various body parts. Guide his fingers to the appropriate place on the doll.
- Give the doll a bath. Talk to the child about the doll's body parts. "Let's wash the doll's (feet)." Ask the child to find the doll's (feet).
- Have the child lie down on a large sheet of butcher paper. Trace the child's feet and talk about the child's arms, feet, head, etc.
- Spray Windex or shaving cream on a mirror. Draw a face and talk about the facial features you are drawing. "Look at the (eyes). I'm drawing (eyes)." Point to your (eyes) and say, "Here are (Mommy's) (eyes)." Point to the child's (eyes) and say, "Here are (Cindy's) (eyes)." Do this several times with the rest of the facial features. Encourage imitation.
- Cut a round face out of construction paper and draw some hair. Cut out eyes, ears, a mouth, and a nose. Show the child the eyes and hold them up to your eyes, saying, "These are eyes" or "Here are some eyes." Help the child to paste the eyes onto the face. Repeat with the rest of the facial features.
- Use Mr. Potato Head or other comparable toy. Place the eyes, nose, mouth, and ears out in front of the child. Wait for eye contact, then tell him what facial features you are putting on. "Let's put the (eyes) on." Hold the (eyes) up by your (eyes). "See the (eyes)?" Then place

them on the Mr. Potato Head. Repeat with the remaining pieces. After all the features have been placed on Mr. Potato Head, take them off and place them back down in front of the child. Ask him to put the eyes) on. (So as not to overwhelm the child, you may wish to use only one or two facial features in a session.) Repeat with the other facial features.

- Look in books or magazines for pictures of certain body parts (e.g., feet). Show them to the child and talk about them.
- For the older child, look through magazines for pictures of faces. Cut some up and ask the child to find the various parts. Then have him point to the corresponding parts on a whole face.
- Sing rhyming songs about the face and body parts. "Where is your nose?" "Touch your nose," etc.

Subskill 3: Learning the personal pronouns "me" and "you"

Activities:

- Using a family scrapbook or photo album, go through pictures of family members, saying, "That's not you," "That's not you," "That's you!" pointing to the child and to his picture.
- Using two sets of identical items, or items different in one characteristic such as color, distribute the materials equally, saying, "This is for me," "This is for you," etc., repeating until all objects have been sorted.
- The child is given a piece of fruit. He is told, "This is for me," (mother/clinician) and is guided in giving that piece out appropriately. Then he is told, "This is for you," and he keeps that particular piece. Again, this procedure is repeated until all items are distributed.
- Teach these pronouns incidentally through such everyday phrases as "I see you" or "I hear you," pointing to the child, or "Give it to me," "Show me," etc.

Subskill 4: Developing the concept of ownership

Activities:

- Ask one or two family members to join in and sit in a circle. Have everyone remove their shoes and place them in the middle of the circle. Depending on whether possessive pronouns ("mine," "yours") or proper nouns are being stressed, have everyone ask, "Where are (person's name)'s shoes?" or "Where are my shoes?"

After asking this several times, have the person retrieve his or her shoes. Guide the child in doing this as well.

- Teach ownership incidentally in the home while sorting laundry. Have the child help sort the clothes according to ownership and put in the owner's drawer or room.

Subskill 5: Dramatizing feelings/emotions

Activities:

- Whenever the child displays an emotion such as delight, sadness, fear, or anger during his normal activities, put his feelings into words: "You're mad," "You look happy," etc.
- Select pictures in magazines or books that depict clearly defined moods or feelings. Show the child the picture and describe it. "Look, the baby's crying. He's sad." Act it out and encourage the child to join in. (Adult expresses verbally the feeling associated with the mood.)
- You may use flannel board cut outs, puppets, home made props, or large pictures to dramatize simple stories or fairy tales, such as the Three Bears or Billy Goats Gruff. Emphasize or dramatize the emotions portrayed in these stories, using lively but natural gestures and facial expressions.

Subskill 6: Learning "no"

Activities:

- Say the word "no" firmly while shaking your head or finger to indicate "no" when undesirable behavior or dangerous situations occur.
- Remove the child from an undesirable situation, saying "no" and shaking your head, and provide a distraction to change her focus of attention.

Subskill 7: Learning "hi" and "bye-bye"

Activities:

- Teach through natural usage whenever the child is arriving or leaving or people are coming to or leaving the child. Simultaneously wave and say "hi" or "bye-bye." Encourage imitation.
- Use a doll house and dolls, and have the dolls walk in and out of the front door. Wave and say "hi" as they enter the house; wave and say "bye-bye" as they leave the house.

- Dress a doll in a coat; have the doll wave "bye-bye" to the child and take the doll out of the room.
- Use puppets to say "hi" to everyone in the room. Have the puppets say and wave "bye-bye" as they are taken away. Encourage the child to imitate.
- Play a game where the child stands at a door in the house waiting for you to knock on it. Knock at the door. Wave and say "hi" as the child opens the door. Leave again, waving and saying "bye-bye" as you go out the door. Repeat several times and encourage the child to imitate. You may wish to first demonstrate this activity with another adult or older child.
- Pick up a toy telephone. Say "hi" as you answer it. Say "bye-bye" as you hang up.

Subskill 8: Developing concepts related to toys

Activities:

- During ball play, name and perform for the child several different actions. Encourage the child to perform (or imitate) the action on verbal cue (e.g., "Roll it"). Actions: roll, push, bounce, throw, catch, kick, hide under blanket or behind furniture.
- Toy car (same as above): push, push down incline; put one car in each of several bags, have the child open one bag at a time and find the car.
- Playdough or clay (same as above): roll, squeeze, pat.
- Doll (same as above): dress, wash, feed, put to bed, hide under a blanket.
- Toy animals (same as above): make animals run, jump, eat, sleep, go into a barn, etc.

Subskill 9: Developing concepts related to food

Activities:

- Egg nog: Get out milk, bowl, glass, beaters, honey, eggs, vanilla, etc. Talk about all the foods and stages of preparation while the child watches and helps. "Crack the egg," "Turn the beater," "Its foamy," "Open the milk carton," "Stir it," "The honey is sweet."
- Make fresh orange juice. Go through the process of cutting the orange, squeezing the orange, and drinking the juice. Talk about each stage, letting the child participate, smell, and taste whenever possible.

- Bake cookies with the child. Possible language: "The cookies are hot." "Do you want a cookie?" "You have two cookies." "Mmm . . . they're good." "You want some more?" "This cookie is big."
- Cheese and crackers: "Smell the cheese." "The crackers are salty." "Cut the cheese."
- Use foods with distinctive odors, such as oranges, bananas, cheese, freshly baked bread, cookies, peanut butter, and chocolate. Name the foods as you use them, and let the child smell, taste, and possibly feel them (e.g., honey, fruits, etc.
- Discuss the qualities of sweet, salty, and sour as you give the child samples of each. Honey, cookies, and certain fruits may be labeled as sweet, lemons and vinegar as sour, and pretzels or potato chips as salty.
- Encourage the child to taste and smell all types of food.
- Look through magazines for a given food item; compare with the real object, emphasizing "sameness."
- Make up a very simple shopping list, cutting out and pasting on index cards pictures of certain food items, e.g., bread, fruit, eggs, canned goods, etc. Take the child and the cards to the store and help him "find" the items, comparing them with the pictures.
- Let the child smell things she cannot taste to develop her sense of smell and to further develop her concepts of these objects. Good "smelly" items include: flowers, grass, perfume, shaving lotion, and baby powder. Explain that these things smell good, but are not to be eaten. (Pay particular attention to the younger child who may be inclined to put everything into his or her mouth.)

Subskill 10: Learning clothing names

Activities:

- Teach through natural usage, naming clothing items as you dress the child.
- While sorting laundry, put out all the (socks, shirts, or pants) if one particular item is being taught.
- Dress a doll or flannel-board figure. Cut a boy or girl figure out of flannel. Make flannel clothes to stick to the figure.
- Play with dress-up clothes.
- Trace the child's body on a large sheet of butcher paper. Cut out various pieces of clothing from sheets of construction paper (i.e., pants, shirts, shoes, socks, mittens, etc.), and help the child place the clothing on the paper doll. Talk about the corresponding body parts. "Let's put the socks on the feet," "Put the mittens on his hands."

- Look for and cut out given articles of clothing from catalogues or magazines.
- During laundry time, for general language development, discuss all items as they are pulled from the laundry basket and folded.

Subskill 11: Developing concepts related to animals

Activities:

Note: It is always a good idea to expose the child to real objects, if possible, before exposing him to toys or pictures. Otherwise, the child may develop an incorrect concept about the animal.

- Teach names of animals incidentally as you walk around the neighborhood. "Look, there's a dog." "What a nice dog." "Pat the dog." "He says 'woof, woof.' "
- Visit a pet shop, animal shelter, farm, or zoo (for exposure to animals, rather than the teaching of specific animals at this stage).
- Show the child a realistic animal toy. Name the animal, and make the sound the animal makes (woof, woof; meow, moo, etc.). Encourage imitation.
- Demonstrate the toy animals running, jumping, eating, etc.
- Set up a toy farm or a toy house and show the child where the animal lives.
- Show the child a picture of the animal. Show him that the picture and the (toy) animal are the same.

Subskill 12: Developing the concepts clean/dirty, wet/dry, hot/cold, etc.

Activities:

Note: these kinds of concepts are best taught incidentally. Supplement the following suggestions with your own ideas; there are many occasions during the day when these modifiers may come up.

- Talk about dirty objects, such as dishes, clothing, the child's hands or face, etc.; wash, and compare the clean with the dirty objects.
- Play outside in the dirt. Talk about toys and clothing getting dirty.
- Let the child help dust furniture; talk about the dirt that appears on the rag.
- Talk about wet and dry as you bathe and dry the child; do this with dolls as well.
- Talk about the baby's diapers as being wet or dry, clean or dirty.

- Talk about certain foods as being hot or cold (e.g., warm, freshly baked cookies or cold ice cream).
- Using caution, let the child see and feel that certain household appliances may be very hot (e.g., stove, oven, toaster). Others, like the refrigerator, are cold.
- Discuss the temperature outside as you dress the child appropriately. "Its cold outside," "Put your mittens on," etc.

Subskill 13: Learning common nouns

Activities:

Note: Children differ as to how long it takes them to learn to recognize their first word. It may take months of repetition and work. However, once the child realizes that a particular object has a referent or name, the first major step has been taken, and learning new words will be easier all the time. At first, as you use a word you should expect absolutely nothing in the way of a response. The child has to see this first word on your lips dozens, hundreds, maybe thousands of times before he can recognize it. You continually bombard him with the word and fill his environment with the object it represents. He has to see the particular lip movements that go into saying (ball) and has to see them in direct association with (some kind of ball) until he can always recognize them. Be patient. It does take time.

- Child and adult each have a sack containing identical objects. Adult looks into her sack and says "I have a (ball)." ["You find a (ball)."] Adult may initially help the child find his (ball). When first teaching nouns, have nothing but three or four (balls) in each bag. When the child knows several nouns, use several of each of two items (e.g., four shoes and four books in each bag). "Find a shoe." "That's not a shoe. That's a shoe. You found a shoe, etc." Progress to one only of many different items in each sack as the child learns more nouns.
- Ask the child, "What's that?" while pointing to or showing him something. Then say "It's (an airplane)."
- When she is holding a (ball), ask the child "Where is your (ball)?" If she looks at it, raises it, or hands it to you, praise her. If not, point to it and say, "Here it is. . . . Here's your (ball)."
- When the toy is nearby, ask the child "Where is your (teddy bear)?" If he looks or points to it, reward him. If not, get the toy and say, "Here it is . . . . Here's the (teddy bear)."
- Turn slowly through a book with large, clear pictures. Choose a book that has pictures of objects you think would be interesting to the child.

Point to specific pictures and name them. (You may change your wording around, but always use the object's name. Don't call it "it.") Begin this activity with only a couple of pictures at first. Be sure the child can see your face. Ask the child "Where's the (boy)?" or "Show me the (boy)." Encourage her to point. If she does not respond, show her. "Here he is, here's the boy," and guide her hand to the picture.

- Place one kind of object (e.g., five or six cars) in a corner of the room and a second kind of object (e.g., five or six dolls) in another area. Wait for eye contact. Ask the child to "Go get a (car)." If the child returns with the correct object, reward him.
- Place two or three objects commonly used by the child throughout the day in front of her. Wait for eye contact and then name the different objects. Demonstrate their use (e.g., if the child has a particular spoon she likes to use, pretend to eat with it, telling her, "We eat with the spoon."). Let her play with the (spoon). Do this with the other object(s), continually naming and talking about them. Later, place the objects in front of her, several inches apart, wait for eye contact, and ask her to show you a particular one. The child may indicate understanding by looking at, pointing to, or touching the object.

Subskill 14: Developing number concepts

Activities:

- Use opportunities throughout the day to count for the child. Count his fingers, toes, buttons on his clothing, crackers, etc., so that he gets exposed to numbers being applied to certain things.
- Introduce "one" as a modifier to describe a familiar thing. You may also use (one) of your fingers to indicate the appropriate number (one). Encourage imitation.
- Ask the child to give you one (book). Gently correct her if she brings more than one. "I need only one." And put the extra books away.

Subskill 15: Developing categorization skills (for the older child)

Activities:

- Give the child a group of objects. Allow him to explore and look at them. Ask him, "What do we eat with?" If he does not identify the spoon (and don't expect a response), begin eliminating objects, saying, "Do we eat with a (book)?" pointing to the (book). "No." Repeat this until you come to the spoon. "We eat with the spoon," and pretend to eat with the spoon. Continue asking for other objects in the same way to expose the child to hearing the function of an object as well as its name.

- Cut pictures of commonly known objects out of magazines or catalogues. Divide pictures into categories (e.g., clothing, food, animals). Talk about the pictures and let the child watch and help as you paste each category on a large piece of paper or in a given section of a scrapbook.
- Mix up two or three groups of objects in a large, shallow box (e.g., three toy cars, three balls, and three toy animals). (The objects in any one category should not be identical.) Sort these objects into three smaller boxes. Talk about the (cars), (balls), and (animals). Encourage the child to imitate. Start to repeat this activity. Have the child finish sorting/categorizing.
- The above activity may also be done using two or three sets of pictures showing different kinds of the same object (e.g., a variety of hat pictures; a set of dog pictures showing different breeds, colors, and sizes; or a set of tree pictures, showing different sizes and species). If necessary, aid the child to sort them into different piles. Encourage spontaneous sorting.

Goal 2. Development of visual attention combined with listening activity

Activities:

- Talk to the child during the day in a face-to-face, eye level manner. Try to establish good eye contact with the child.
- Encourage parents, siblings, and family friends to talk or sing to the child while feeding, clothing, bathing, or playing with her. When the child shows awareness of voice by looking at the speaker, she is given social reinforcement.

Goal 3. a. Recognition of similarities in shapes and familiar objects: matching
b. Awareness of size perception differences and color concepts

Subskill 1: Matching identical objects

Activities:

- Child and adult each have a sack containing identical objects. Adult looks in his sack, pulls out an object and says "I have a (ball). You find a (ball)." The adult may, if necessary, help the child find his (ball). "You found a (ball). They're the same." When initially introducing the skill of matching, put nothing but three or four (balls) in each bag. After the child becomes thoroughly acquainted with this procedure, use several of each of two items (e.g., four balls and four shoes) in each bag. "I found a shoe. You find a shoe. That's not a shoe. That's a shoe! You found a shoe. They're the same." Progress to only one of several different items in each sack as the child develops his matching ability.

- Another way to introduce matching is to put two sets of matched objects in a box. As the child watches, say something about one of the objects (e.g., "I'll get a spoon"). Take it out and let the child play with it. Say, "I'll get another (spoon)." Take it out and compare it to the first object. Talk about the objects being the same. Follow this same basic procedure for the other sets of objects. Pair these objects together on the table.
- Give the child several sets of matching objects. Allow her to play with them. If she arranges them in pairs, talk about their "sameness."
- Distribute three or four sets of identical objects between you and the child. Let the child explore them while you name and talk about them (remember to establish or wait for eye contact before you speak). Hold up one of the objects and ask the child to find one in his pile that's the same. If necessary, help him to find the matching object. Set them down on the table as a pair and reemphasize that they are the same.

Subskill 2: Matching pictures of real objects

Activities:

- Cut pictures of common household items out of magazines or catalogues. Talk about the pictures and let the child match pictures with the actual item. He or she can go around the house and tape pictures to the real objects.
- Put two kinds of objects in a sack (e.g., apples and bananas) and pictures of those two objects on the table in front of the child. Take a (banana) out of the sack and have the child match it to its corresponding picture. Gradually increase the number of different items and pictures. (This activity may be repeated using many different kinds of objects and pictures.)

Subskill 3: Developing the concept "same"

Activities:

- Line up differently colored blocks about 2 inches apart in a row in front of the child. Keep their "mates" in your hands. Demonstrate matching the blocks by placing your (red) block on the (red) block in the child's row. Emphasize the fact that the blocks are the same. Hand her a colored block and ask her to match it. (If the child is having difficulty, you may go through each unmatched block and ask the child if the one she is trying to match goes with it. Encourage her to respond "no" or shake her head.)
- Cut out circles, squares, and triangles from construction paper. Make sure each group of shapes is the same color. (e.g., red circles, yellow squares, and blue triangles). Help the child sort the shapes into three piles. Show him that they are the same. Encourage him to feel around the edge of the shape. When he is able to sort these shapes without trial and error, present a group of squares, circles, and triangles that are the same color. Help him to match one shape, then allow him to proceed, matching all the shapes. (Here, the child will be matching by shape cues alone.)
- Gradually add various types of shapes (diamonds, rectangles, half-moons, etc.) and repeat the above activities.
- Cut two 2″ circles of any fabric remnants you can find. Glue these to 2″ circles of tagboard for strength. Have the child match these fabric "chips." Here, the child is matching, not by shape, but by color and texture. Emphasize the concept "same" throughout these activities.
- Using shapes the child is familiar with, give the child a set of cards with the shape outline on it. Help the child match his card to a set which you have put in front of him on the table.
- Shapes should also be taught incidentally, pointing out to the child that certain household items (such as a clock) possess certain shapes (e.g., circle). Use these shape names.
- For the older child, make two sets of identical flashcard pictures (e.g., two with yellow circles, two with blue squares, etc.) or glue two sets of identical pictures or stickers onto index cards. Start with two or three sets of cards, placing them all face down on the table. Have the child turn over two cards. If they are the same, the child may keep them. If they are different, have the child put them back, face down on the table. Adult and child take turns trying to match pairs. Increase the number of cards as the child becomes more proficient (similar to the game *Concentration*).

Subskill 4: Developing color concepts

Activities:

Note: It is expected that the child will progress through stages of matching colors, knowing color names receptively, and finally using the names of colors correctly.

- Teach incidentally, using color words to describe the child's clothing as you dress her, to describe the child's toys or various household objects, etc.
- Give the child a tin of wooden blocks with two or three different colors. Help him to sort according to color by dropping the blocks in smaller, appropriately painted boxes. Encourage spontaneous sorting, as you name and repeat the colors for the child.
- Separate different colored beads or buttons into groups according to color. You may wish to use something like a muffin tin, in which you have "papered" the cups with the appropriate colors, for the child to drop the beads or buttons into.
- Paint a picture using one color only. Talk about the color.
- Have the child go around the room finding all items of a given color.

Subskill 5: Developing the concept of size differences

Activities:

- Teach incidentally (e.g., by comparing your body or clothing size with that of the child; comparing portions of food— "I have a big cookie, You have a little cookie," etc.). Expect understanding of "largeness" or "bigness" to come before understanding of "smallness." While doing structured activities, generally concentrate on the larger concept or item first.
- Gather together several large objects (e.g., beach balls, large dolls) and corresponding small objects (e.g., tennis balls, small dolls). Separate small objects from large ones and encourage sorting by the child.
- Use a variety of buttons or beads (preferably similar or identical in all features but size) and help the child sort according to size.
- Make bubbles with large and small rings (both sets are available in many dime stores).
- Cut out large and small paper fish and attach a magnet to their backs. "Fishing poles" can be made with a piece of string and paper clips for hooks. Mix the fish together in a basket. Using the fishing pole, help the child pull the magnetized fish out. Separate large fish from small fish and talk about each. (This game may also be adapted for teaching colors and shapes.)

- Using blocks, buttons, dolls, toy cars, or cut-out shapes with obvious size differences, give two or three items to the child. Ask her to give you the (big) one, using gestures if necessary.
- Decrease the size differences by giving the child a series of objects such as nesting cups, measuring spoons, or cut-out shapes with less obvious differences. Ask the child to give you the (big) one from a group of two or three. If the child selects the wrong one, help him compare the one he gave you with the one that is biggest.
- Blow up a balloon and talk about the size relationships. The balloon gets bigger as you blow it up and smaller as you let the air out.

Subskill 6: Developing the concept "round"

Activities:

- Form a circle, holding hands. Circle, singing "round, round, round, round, all fall down." Stand up and repeat.
- When stirring food or beverages, talk about stirring round and round.
- Draw round circles (you may have to aid the child, depending upon the age).
- Make wheels turn round and round.
- Move a train around a circular track.

Subskill 7: Matching objects by feeling

Activities:

- Collect two sets of objects such as wooden spools, Ping Pong balls, wooden blocks, large safety pins, cotton balls, pieces of sandpaper, etc. Put one set of these objects on the table in front of the child and the set of matching objects in a sack (you could put the objects in one at a time). Have the child reach into the sack and identify the object that she is feeling. Pull the item out of the sack and compare. For the younger child, let her feel the object in the sack, take it out, and match it to the identical object on the table. For the older child, encourage her to identify the object in the sack by tactile cues alone.

Subskill 8: Reproducing a sequence (for the older child)

Activities:

- Use different colored blocks or shapes cut from construction paper. Set them out in a row. Tell the child to make a row like yours underneath or beside yours. Start with only two or three blocks and increase the number as the child gains proficiency.

- Repeat, using colored pegs. Let the child make a row underneath yours first; then, using a second pegboard, have him repeat the task. Help the child select the appropriate peg by checking back and matching his peg to yours.
- String wooden beads. Let the child make her own pattern of various colors and have her reproduce her pattern in a second row. Again, begin this activity having the child reproduce a sequence of only two or three beads.

Subskill 9: Developing the concept "different" (for the older child)

Activities:

- On several squares of paper affix sets of three identical stickers and one different sticker. Show papers one at a time. Talk about the fact that one sticker is different. Repeat with series of papers. Later, ask the child, "Which one is different?" Help the child choose the correct answer.
- Give the child all the materials and let him arrange them. Talk about those that are the same and point out which one is different.

Goal 4. Understanding of simple locative concepts and words

Subskill 1: Learning "in" and "out"

Activities:

- When taking toys out of a box or a bag for certain activities, tell the child, "I took it out," or "You take it out." Similarly, when putting the toys away after an activity, have the child put the toy back in the box or bag. Tell her, "Put it in. You put it in."
- Use all possible incidental situations that come up during the day to stress "in" and "out."
  —Talk about putting dolls "in" a house and taking them "out."
  —Put toy animals "in" a barn and take them "out."
  —Put chips "in" a container and dump them "out."
  —Put puzzle pieces "in" a formboard and take them "out."

—Put pop-beads together. Tell the child to "push it 'in'" and "pull it 'out.'"

—Put a doll "in" the bathtub. Take it "out."

You will find that these concepts can be stressed frequently without necessarily developing specific activities for this purpose.

- Parents can talk frequently about "in" and "out" during the day:
  - —Put dishes "in" the dishwasher and take them "out."
  - —Put dishes away "in" the cupboard or take them "out."
  - —Put silverware "in" the drawer or take it "out."
  - —Put clothes "in" the washing machine or take them "out."
  - —Put the child "in" the bathtub and take him "out."

Gestures may initially be used to develop the child's understanding of these concepts.

Subskill 2: Learning "off" and "on"

Activities:

- When child is watching, adult says "Pull it off" "Take it off" or "Turn it off" and does one of the following:
  - —Takes strips of tape off the table.
  - —Pulls stickers off paper.
  - —Takes clothes off a doll.
  - —Wipes chalk marks off a blackboard.
  - —Takes magnets off metal.
  - —Turns a light or flashlight off.
  - —Takes lids or covers off containers.
- To encourage expressive language development, encourage the child to vocalize or attempt to say "off" before the action occurs.
- When teaching "on," follow the general procedures outlined above:
  - —Turn a lamp or flashlight on.
  - —Turn the radio, record player, or other appliance such as a vacuum cleaner on.
  - —Put socks or other article of clothing on the child or on a doll.
  - —Have the child stack blocks, one on another.
  - —Set dishes and silverware on the table.
  - —Turn water faucets on.
  - —Put jewelry on.
  - —Put lids or covers on containers.

Subskill 3: Learning "up" and "down"

Activities:

- Throw a balloon "up" in the air and watch it come "down." You may also use balls. Exaggerate this by starting in a crouched position and slowly moving up as you throw the ball or balloon "up" in the air.
- Ask the child if he wants to come "up" before picking him up. Tell him, "Let's put you 'down'" before doing so. Encourage the child to vocalize an approximation of "up" before lifting him up.
- Move a puppet "up, up, up" or walk a doll "up" a block staircase. Have the child imitate both actions and words.
- Build a block tower, telling the child, "I'm stacking them 'up,'" Encourage the child to imitate. "You stacked them 'up.'"
- Knock your blocks "down," telling the child, "I knocked them 'down.'" Exaggerate this by falling over on your side as you knock the blocks down.
- Teach through natural usage in such phrases as, "You fell down," "Let's pick you up," "Up we go!" etc.

Subskill 4: Learning "under" and "behind" (for the older child)

Activities:

- Teach through natural usage (e.g., "Where's your shoe? Look, its under your bed," etc.)
- Place toy animals behind a barn or under a glass jar.
- Place a ball under or behind a box. Talk about it. Let the child place the ball in the same position.
- Take pictures of the child in, on, under, or behind a box. Talk about where the child is relative to the box. Reenact the situation.

Goal 5. Understanding of simple commands and carry-through with appropriate behavior

Subskill 1: Conditioned response to voice

Activities:

- Using standard play audiometry techniques, have the child:
  - —Stack blocks or rings at the verbal command "put it on."
  - —Drop beads or buttons into a container at the command "put it in."

—Push a toy car into a small garage upon hearing a verbal command, such as "push it in."
—Go down a slide on hearing the verbal command "slide down," "go," etc.
—Release a small car down an inclined board on hearing "let it go."
—Jump off a low platform after hearing verbal command such as "jump."
—Throw beanbag into box at the verbal command "throw it."

Subskill 2: Imitation of body movements

Activities:

- Have the child imitate gross body movements in the game: "This is the way I . . ."
  —clap my hands,"
  —raise my arms,"
  —pat my head,"
  —close my eyes,"
  —open my mouth," etc.
- Encourage the child to follow verbal requests by moving her through the actions and, using gestures appropriately, asking her to—
  —wave "bye-bye,"
  —stand up,
  —come here,
  —throw a kiss,
  —play peek-a-boo, etc.
- Encourage the child to follow simple commands with a doll by telling him to—
  —kiss the baby,
  —brush her hair,
  —wash her face,
  —rock the baby, etc.
- Using real objects, demonstrate housekeeping with the child. Ask her to imitate you as you do different actions and name them for her (e.g., mop, sweep, wash, stir, mix, etc.). Request that she perform the actions on verbal cue.
- While using Playdough, show the child two or three different actions. Name the actions for the child (e.g., roll, pat, squeeze) and request that he perform the actions on verbal cue.

- Repeat the above activity during ball play, performing such actions as throwing, rolling, bouncing, kicking, etc.

Subskill 3: Learning "no" with cessation of activity

Activities:

- Say the word "no" firmly while shaking your head and finger to indicate "no" when undesirable behavior or dangerous situations occur.
- Remove the child from an undesirable situation, saying "no" and shaking your head, and provide a distraction to change the child's focus of attention.

Subskill 4: Learning "come here"

Activities:

- Teach through natural usage, gesturing or moving the child through the action if necessary.
- Using two adults, have the child and one adult sit about 3 feet apart on one side of the room, with the second adult about 10 feet away. The second adult gestures and says "come here" to first adult (or older child) who walks across the room and is immediately rewarded. Next, it is the child's turn to "come here"; he may need guidance for the first few times. The gesture should be eliminated when teaching recognition of the word.

Subskill 5: Learning "stand up" and "sit down"

Activities:

- Teach through natural usage.
- Play with bendable dolls, making them stand up or sit down on toy furniture. These flexible dolls may also be used to teach other action verbs such as walk, run, jump, lie down, or fall down. Have the child perform these actions with the doll.
- Take pictures of the child standing and sitting. Talk about them. Reenact the situation.
- Find pictures in magazines of people standing and sitting. Talk about them and have the child imitate the action.

Subskill 6: Learning "open"

Activities:

- Hold a box or plastic egg by your face. Wait until the child makes eye contact and say, "Open the (egg)." Let the child open the container and remove the "surprise," e.g., a tiny toy animal, cotton ball, jelly bean, etc. When she looks again at your face, say, "It's open." To encourage expressive language development, have the child vocalize or attempt to say "open" before the adult opens the box or egg or gives it to the child to open.
- Teach through natural usage, opening doors, windows, containers, drawers, the child's toy chest, etc. Encourage vocal imitation before opening.
- Use bottles or jars with lids that come off easily.
- Use large boxes, with a doll or toy in each box.
- Use smooth-edged coffee cans with plastic lids and put a crayon in each can.
- "Open" little Japanese paper parasols.

Subskill 7: Learning "push" or similar action verb

Activities:

- Push toy cars one at a time across the floor, saying "push the car" before each car is released.
- Push the child in a box across the kitchen or other smooth floor. Stop and repeat "push me" as the child indicates she wishes to do it again. Encourage verbal imitation.
- Let the child push chairs around a room. Play with him and repeat "push the chair" many times.
- Say "push" in a phrase each time you push the child in a swing.

Subskill 8: Learning "point to," "show me," "give me," etc.

Activities:

- Encourage the child to give you a toy or object by holding out your hand and asking for the object. "Give me the (ball)."
- When playing guessing games, such as "Where's (the picture of) Daddy?" (as in Goal 1, Subskill 1) or "Show me the ball" (as in Goal 1, Subskill 13), give the child a chance to respond and if she doesn't

seem to understand, gently guide the child through the desired response.

- Remember, when asking questions of the child, look to her expectantly for a response, even if she is not yet ready. Then help her "answer" your question.

Subskill 9: Imitating actions in pictures (for the older child)

Activities:

- Adult draws stick-figure representations of several different actions with written directions under them on several cards. Child selects a card, looks at the picture, then shows the card to the adult who says the whole command: "Go get the book," "Open the door," "Go to Mommy," etc. Child and adult take turns selecting and following commands.
- Vary the above game by hiding a "prize" that the player finds after following the command.

Goal 6. Comprehension of simple question forms

Subskill 1: Where?

Activities:

- Use a mirror and ask, "Where's (Johnny)?" while pointing to the child. Encourage him to point to himself.
- When the child is holding a (ball), ask him, "Where is your (ball)?" If he looks at it, raises it, or hands it to you, reward him. If not, point to it and say, "Here it is." "Here is your (ball)."
- Repeat this procedure when the toy is nearby.
- Play hide-and-seek with the child. Pretend to look for the child, repeating, "Where's (Andy)?" "There's (Andy)! There you are!"
- Play the "shell game" by placing three small boxes or cups on the table. Put a small toy under one of the boxes and move them all around. Ask the child, "Where's the (dog)?" and encourage her to lift each box. Respond with either, "It's not there" or "There's the (dog)!"
- Use puzzle pieces with each piece picturing an object. Talk about each object as pieces are taken out. Then point to each hole and ask, "Where's the (cat)?" and have the child put the appropriate piece in.

- Using the same formboard, hold up each piece and ask, "Where does the (cat) go?"
- Going through a family scrapbook, ask, "Where's (Daddy)?" or "Who is this?" Model answer for the child until she is able to answer independently.

Subskill 2: Who?

Activities:

- Look through a family album. Ask the child, "Who's this?" while pointing to a particular person. If that person is present, encourage the child to look at, point to, or go to the person in the picture. Otherwise, model the answer for the child until he can answer independently.
- Have someone stand behind a door, out of the child's sight, and knock on the door. If the child cannot hear the knock, let her place her hand on the door to feel it. Ask, "Who's there? " looking expectantly at the child. Open the door, saying, "It's (Daddy)!"

Subskill 3: What?

Activities:

Note: Encourage early in the child a response "readiness" or "posture." Your attitude of expecting him to try to respond, or try to vocalize a word when it is called for, will do more than anything else to motivate the child to attempt it. Wait, with an encouraging, expectant look on your face. He may come forth with some attempt, say, at the word. If so, respond at once. Your response will be the way to encourage the child's response, or to encourage him to go on saying the particular word, in appropriate situations.

- Ask the child, "What's that?" when pointing to or showing him something. Hesitate expectantly and then say, "It's (an airplane)." Do this with several objects or pictures. As the child gets older and becomes more familiar with these words, you may ask "Where is the (airplane)?" or "Show me the (airplane)."

B. Expressive Language

Goal 1. Control of tongue, lip, and facial muscles

Subskill 1: Control of tongue

Activities:

Note: The tongue is the chief organ of speech. It possesses great mobility due to its structure. It has unlimited capacity for motion and should be moved with great freedom. Without tongue control, the child will have difficulty making the proper tongue placements to produce vowels and consonants correctly. Control of the tongue can be gained by directed exercises. These exercises, when mastered, should enable the child to place the tongue in any position required to produce a given sound. The following is a list of exercises designed for full control of the tongue. The young child should not necessarily be expected to complete all of these.

- Sit the child in front of you in front of a mirror.
  - —Thrust the tongue out quickly.
  - —Thrust the tongue far out quickly. Draw it back slowly.
  - —Put the tongue far out slowly. Draw it back quickly.
  - —Put the tongue far out slowly. Draw it back slowly.
  - —Turn the point up and apply tip to different points on the lips, teeth, and roof of the mouth.
  - —Turn point down over the lower lip, as far as possible.
  - —Turn point down over the lower teeth.
  - —Thrust the tongue into the cheek.
  - —Rotate around the lips, beginning at the right and going up.
  - —Reverse above.
  - —Extend the tongue a little over the lower lip and groove it.
  - —Flap the point as in saying "la, la, la."
  - —Shut the point of the tongue against the upper teeth. Open it. Repeat.
  - —Shut the back of the tongue against the roof of the mouth at the point where the hard palate ends and the soft palate begins.
  - —Open the mouth, narrow the tongue, and move it rapidly from side to side.
  - —The tongue may be widened and narrowed in eight positions:
    - = with the point on the upper lip
    - = with the point on the upper teeth

= with the point on the gum behind the upper teeth
= with the tongue extended beyond the lips
= with the point on the roof of the mouth just beyond the gum, widen and narrow it until it touches the teeth on either side
= with the point on the lower lips
= with the point on the lower teeth
= with the point well within the mouth

—With the mouth open but not too wide, let the tongue lie soft and flat in the mouth. Draw the back of the tongue flat within itself until it becomes thick and bulky.
—With the mouth open about the width of two fingers, keep the tongue flat and still

Note: The preceding activities are listed in sequential order according to difficulty. Encourage the child to imitate whatever exercises he can. To make these activities more interesting, use a puppet with a tongue to demonstrate the various tongue movements and positions, or play peek-a-boo in conjunction with the specific target tongue movements. Discontinue mirror use after the child can imitate you without watching himself in the mirror.

- Put peanut butter, honey, or chocolate syrup on various parts of the child's mouth and lips. Demonstrate licking it off. Encourage the child to imitate.
- Place peanut butter, honey, or chocolate syrup on a spoon far enough out in front of the child's mouth so that she will have to stick out her tongue to get a taste.
- Place some Cheerios in a bowl. Demonstrate eating the cereal out of the bowl, using your tongue. Encourage the child to imitate.

  Note: The test to ascertain whether the tongue is under complete control is to place it in any position and hold it perfectly still for several seconds. During tongue gymnastics, observe the following guidelines:

—Breathe quietly.
—Do not move the lips or muscles of the cheeks.
—Repeat each exercise several times.
—Practice often, until control has been gained.
—Do not carry the exercise to the point of fatigue.
—During the first four exercises, open the mouth wide enough so that the tongue does not touch the lips.

Subskill 2: Control of lip and facial muscles

Activities:

- Sit the child in front of you in front of a mirror:
  - —Wrinkle your nose.
  - —Frown or smile.
  - —Raise your eyebrows.
  - —Blink your eyes.
  - —Blow out your cheeks.
  - —Suck in your cheeks.
  - —Pucker your lips.
  - —Blow a kiss.
  - —Make "raspberries" on your arm.
  - —Open your mouth wide, then close it back up quickly.
  - —Round your lips, producing the /oo/ sound.
  - —Spread your lips, producing the /ee/ sound.
- Encourage the child to imitate all of the above exercises. To make the exercises more interesting, use a puppet to demonstrate the various lip and facial movements or play peek-a-boo with the target lip and facial movements. Discontinue mirror use after the child can imitate you without watching himself in the mirror.

Goal 2. Control of breath stream and blowing

Note: Without specific work on breathing, many hearing-impaired children will tend to become shallow breathers and thus will not have enough breath to complete a phrase or sentence. Interrupting a phrase in order to draw a breath disrupts the normal rhythm of speech and thus decreases speech intelligibility.

Subskill 1: Production of breath stream

Activities:

- Blow out a lit candle. Encourage the child to imitate.
- Place a tissue over your mouth and blow it up in the air. Encourage the child to imitate.
- Blow seeds off a dandelion. Encourage imitation.
- Hold a bubble wand and demonstrate blowing. Encourage imitation.
- Blow cotton, Styrofoam chips, or Ping-Pong balls across a table. Encourage imitation.

- Blow through a straw into a glass of water. Encourage imitation.
- Blow up balloons. Encourage imitation.
- Blow a feather up in the air or off a table. Encourage imitation.
- Blow Styrofoam chips or cotton out of a L'Eggs container. Encourage imitation.
- Blow party horns. Encourage imitation.
- Blow soap bubbles out of a bowl. Encourage imitation.
- Build a card tower and demonstrate blowing it over.
- Blow Ping-Pong balls across water. Encourage imitation.
  Note: Other materials can be used in blowing exercises, such as Easter grass, pinwheels, paper strips, and mobiles. Use the appropriate language in combination with the above activities, e.g., "Blow," "Blow it," "You blew it," "You blew it out," etc. In addition, all of the above activities can be done in front of a mirror so that the child can see himself blowing.

Subskill 2: Control of breath stream

Activities:

- Stand in front of a mirror and produce a continuous breath stream, fogging up the mirror. Call the child's attention to the breath mark. Encourage imitation.
- Stand in front of a mirror. Take deep breaths (be very dramatic) and blow out. Encourage the child to imitate. Take another deep breath. Modify and control exhalation of breath. Encourage child to imitate. To make this activity more interesting, use a puppet. Facing the mirror, start with your head down and the puppet's head down. As you inhale deeply, slowly raise your head until you and the puppet come to a full upright position. Open your eyes wide. As you exhale, slowly lower your head and eyes. Do the same with the puppet. Repeat this, increasing the speed of inhalation and exhalation. Later, vary the speed of inhalation and exhalation (e.g., inhale rapidly, exhale slowly). Give the child a puppet and encourage imitation.
- Modify and control the breath stream, using any of the materials listed under Subskill 1. Encourage the child to imitate.
  Note: The child should be capable of producing a breath stream prior to engaging in the preceding exercises. Thus, success in Subskill 1 is a necessary prerequisite to the activities in Subskill 2. Discontinue mirror use after the child can imitate you without watching herself in the mirror.

Goal 3. Imitation of meaningful gestures and actions

Examples of meaningful gestures and actions that could be used for imitation are shaking head "yes" and "no," waving "hi" and "bye-bye," and blowing kisses.

Activities:

- Hold the child in front of you. Get him to look at you and make one of the above actions several times. Wait for him to imitate you, then repeat the action again. Reward the child with a smile or verbal praise if he attempts to imitate you.
- When the child does imitate an action several times, switch to a different action and encourage him to make the new action.
- Each time you say "no" as a warning, as a denial, or as a no thank you, shake your head as well. Encourage the child to imitate.
- Do an activity similar to the one above, encouraging imitation of shaking the head "yes." In whatever situations you may find yourself saying "yes" (e.g., "Yes, you may have the toy," or "Yes, I want that"), shake your head up and down as well. Encourage the child to imitate.
- Ask the child what she wants. Offer her choices of food or toys. When she turns her head and pushes something away, establish eye contact with her and say, "No, you don't want it?" and shake your head "no." If she indicates she does want something, say, "Yes, you want it," shaking your head "yes." Require an imitation of the gesture before taking away or giving her something.
- Use a doll house and dolls. Have the dolls walk in and out of the front door to the house. Wave and say "bye-bye" as they walk out the door. Wave and say "hi" as they walk back in. Using toy cars, have the dolls drive away from the house, and then, later; drive back up in front of the house. Wave and say "hi" or "bye-bye" as you do so. Encourage the child to imitate your gestures.
- Play a game where the child stands at a door in the house waiting for you to knock. Have the mother or father call the child's attention to the sound of the knocking. As the child opens the door, wave and say "hi." Be enthusiastic. Leave again, waving and saying "bye-bye" as you shut the door. Repeat this several times. Reverse roles. Have the child knock at the door. Use gestures and vocalization of "hi" and "bye" appropriately. Encourage the child to imitate both your gestures and your words. To make this activity more interesting, bring a

doll or puppet with you as you walk in and out of the door. Have the doll wave and say "hi" or "bye."

- Pick up the receiver to a toy telephone. Wave and say "hi" as you pick it up. Wave and say "bye" as you hang it up. Hand the child the phone. Encourage imitation.
- "Hi" and "bye" can be used incidentally throughout all therapy sessions. For example:
  - —Wave and say "hi" whenever the child comes to therapy. Wave and say "bye-bye" when he leaves.
  - —Wave and say "bye" as you put the toys away.
- After numerous presentations of waving and saying "hi" and "bye," say the words without using the gestures at an appropriate time (e.g., as the child is leaving). See if the child responds by waving his arm. Reward appropriately.
- Blow kisses to the child as she leaves therapy or drives away in a car with her parent(s).

Goal 4. Vocalization through imitation and spontaneity

Note: Ling (1976) states that "there appear to be five broad, mainly sequential stages through which children must—and normally do—pass as they develop speech production skills" (p. 113). He describes these stages as (1) production of undifferentiated vocalization; (2) production of nonsegmental voice patterns varied in duration, intensity, and pitch; (3) production of a range of distinctly different vowel sounds; (4) production of simple consonants releasing, modifying, or arresting syllables; and (5) production of consonant blends (p. 113). For our purposes, we will be focusing primarily on the first four stages.

Ling points out that the patterns produced in these stages may or may not have communicative significance, depending on whether they are produced at a phonetic level (simply as sounds) or a phonological level (within a meaningful system). The skills acquired at each stage have hierarchical and cumulative importance, since the acquisition of control over production serves to supply the foundation for adequate development in the next and subsequent stages. He adds that some overlapping in these stages does occur.

Ling further states that the first step in therapy should be to determine what sound patterns, if any, there are already in the child's phonetic repertoire. Once this has been determined, we should work toward extending that repertoire at both the phonetic and phonological levels.

According to Ling's developmental schema of speech and language, our first goal would be to develop freely elicited vocalizations from the child if they are not already present. Once vocalizations has been established, duration, loudness, and pitch should be successively brought under control. He points out that continued attention should be given to suprasegmental structure at each stage of spoken language development. In developing the production of vowel sounds, Ling stresses that our primary concern should be the development of tongue control. He suggests that tongue control can best be developed by presenting the child with highly contrasting vowel sounds to imitate. An example of this would be the high-front /i/, a low-central /a/, and a high-back /u/.

Ling feels that imitation of the neutral vowels should not be stressed in therapy because a wide range of vowels can be produced with neutral or central tongue placement and because lip rounding alone can reproduce a sufficient lowering of all formants. He points out that "this is not to say that sounds such as /i/ and /u/ should be taught first, but . . . that the child should not be allowed to develop the concept that vowel production involves only central or near-central tongue movement" (p. 117).

According to Ling, three factors must be considered when choosing consonant sounds to develop through therapy activities. We must look at the sensory cues the consonant provides (auditory, visual, and tactile), their relative organic difficulty, and what consonant sounds there are already in the child's repertoire. However, the importance of continuous development and expansion of sounds spontaneously produced by the child must be stressed. Ling emphasizes the need to present all consonants, with the possible exception of certain nasals (Ling, 1976), in the context of units of at least syllabic size (e.g., C–V combinations).

Activities for the stimulation of vocalization:

- Give the child a noisemaker (rattle, bell, music box, etc.). Imitate the sound yourself. Reward her when she makes any sound by patting her, smiling, and talking.
- Make pleasurable sounds when dressing, feeding, or bathing the child. Encourage the child to make sounds of any type.
- Sing or hum to the child in simple sounds, such as "mmmm" or "la-la-la." Encourage attempts to make any type of sound.
- When diapering, bathing, holding the child, or just watching him, if he makes a sound like a coo or a gurgle, respond to him by stroking his stomach, moving your head close enough so that you're sure that he sees you, and repeat the sound that he makes.

- Imitate the child's vocalizations as exactly as you can. Praise him when he repeats them. Play an echo game.

Activities to encourage vocalization for the expression of needs:

- When the child pulls at you or fusses for attention, ask her what she wants. If she does not point or vocalize, point to several locations you think are appropriate (e.g., refrigerator, toy chest, water faucet), using simple language to express what she might want. "You want milk?" "More milk?" Wait for the child to point and vocalize before giving her what she wants. If the child says one of the sounds in the word or vocalizes, smile and say the complete word for her and give her the thing she wants.
- Put three or four toys or items of food in front of the child. Before she can play with or taste any of these items, require that she point to the item she wants and vocalize. Have Mom or Dad set an example for the child by vocalizing her desires and pointing to the object named.
- Use all opportunities to combine the word "come" with the gesture to indicate "come." When the child tugs at your arm to indicate that she wants you to come, say, "You want me to come. Come." Encourage the child to imitate your vocalizations.
- Encourage the child to vocalize and shake her head "no" rather than throwing a toy or piece of food. When you see that she doesn't want something, require vocalization combined with head-shaking before you take that thing away.

Activities to encourage imitation and spontaneous production of vowels and babbling sets:

- Imitate the child's vocalizations as exactly as you can. Praise him when he repeats them. Play an echo game.
- Direct the child's attention toward your face. Say a consonant-vowel combination several times (e.g., ma-ma-ma, or da-da-da). Encourage the child to imitate.
- Switch from one consonant-vowel combination to another after an immediate imitation (e.g., ba-ma ba-ma). Encourage the child to imitate.
- Show the child a realistic animal toy. Name the animal and make the sound that the animal makes (e.g., woof woof, meow, moo) while holding the animal up by your mouth (this calls attention to your lips). Place the animal by the child's mouth. Encourage the child to imitate.
- Produce the vowel sound /oo/ while engaging in various blowing activities. Encourage imitation.

- Thumb through a picture book and name the animals. Produce the animal sound while holding a picture of the animal up by your face. Encourage the child to imitate. Repeat with other animal pictures.
- Run cars along the floor, producing one or two vowel sounds. Give the child a car and encourage him to imitate your vocalizations. (Note: A variety of toys can be used in this activity, such as cars, trucks, airplanes, boats, etc. Increase and vary the vowel sounds as the child progresses.)
- Combine a vowel sound that the child is imitating with one or two consonants that he is already producing. If he is not producing any consonant sounds, use consonants that can be seen and felt easily (e.g., the front consonants /m/ and /b/). Repeatedly produce one of the C–V combinations as you move a car along the floor. Give the child a car and encourage him to imitate you. Later, try combining the same vowel with another consonant. Next, try varying the consonants used in combination with the vowel as you push the car along the floor. Encourage the child to imitate. If the child succeeds in imitating you, vary the vowels used in combination with the consonants chosen for stimulation. (Note: Increase and vary the consonants used as the child progresses.)

Activities to develop suprasegmental features of speech (pitch, rhythm, intensity, etc.):

- Sing and say nursery rhymes to the child with exaggerated rhythm.
- When babbling or talking to the child, use exaggerated pitch patterns. Reward the child with a kiss or smile when she talks back.
- Use words such as "oh-oh," "all gone," and "bye-bye" with exaggerated pitch changes. Encourage the child to imitate.
- Push cars along the floor using one or two vowel sounds. Vary the rhythm and intonation of the sounds as you roll the cars along the floor. Use Mom or Dad as a model. Push the car to (Dad). Instruct (him) to push the car back while imitating your vocalizations. Push the car to the child while vocalizing. Tell her to "roll it back." Encourage imitation of your vocalizations. Vocalize for the child if she fails to vocalize on her own.
- Combine a vowel sound that the child is imitating with one or two consonants that she is already producing spontaneously. If she is not producing any consonant sounds, use consonants that can be seen and felt easily (e.g., /m/ or /b/). Repeatedly produce one of the C–V combinations while moving a car along the floor. Vary the rhythm and intonation of your vocalizations. Push the car to Mom or Dad as you

vocalize. Instruct (Dad) to push the car back while imitating your vocalizations. Push the car to the child while vocalizing. Encourage imitation of your vocalizations. Vocalize for the child if she fails to vocalize on her own.

Note: A variety of toys can be used in the two preceding activities—cars, trucks, airplanes, etc. Use any toy that can be used in such a manner as to exaggerate the rhythm and intonation of your vocalizations (e.g., jerky for "ba' ba' ba" or smooth for "ahhh. . ."). Instruct Mom and Dad to do the same. Increase and vary the vowels and consonants used as the child progresses.

- Vocalize vowels or C–V combinations while drawing on a mirror with shaving cream. Make the movement of drawing match the rhythm of your vocalizations. Encourage the child to imitate your vocalizations.
- Vocalize vowels or C–V combinations while making crayon marks on paper. Make the movement of drawing match the rhythm of your vocalizations. Encourage the child to imitate your vocalizations.
- Vocalize in front of a mirror with the child facing the mirror and leaning against your body. Sway body rhythmically or clap your hands to match the vocal pattern. Encourage the child to match the rhythm of your vocalizations.
- Push large toys such as a truck, train, or small chair around the room making an appropriate vocalization such as "choo-choo" or "putt-putt-putt." Give the toys or chair to the child. Guide her in imitating your motions and vocal patterns.
- Put several toys in a sack (e.g., boat, train, or car). Take out one toy and tell the child, "Here is a (boat). The (boat) goes (putt putt putt)." Move rhythmically to match your vocalizations. After you move the (boat) across the table, give the toy to the child to move across the table. Encourage the child to imitate your movements and vocalizations. Associate different vocalizations with the other toys, following the same procedure.
- Play singing games in which the adult sings in a very high voice and changes to low, and encourages the child to imitate.
- Use four puppets. The adult and the child have one puppet on each hand. The adult makes one puppet talk in a high voice and encourages the child to make his corresponding puppet use a high voice. Do the same with the other puppet, using a low voice.
- Make a proper chart with a vertical slot and attach a paper airplane that moves up and down in the slot. Have the child sit by the chart

and move the airplane up to the top of the slot when high-pitched vocalizations are heard, and move the airplane to the bottom of the slot when low-pitched vocalizations are heard. Reverse roles. The child produces high- and low-pitched vocalizations as the adult moves the airplane up and down.

- Demonstrate long or short duration on a toy whistle or with your voice. Have the child imitate the sound. After several practices, sit behind the child and make either a long or short noise. Instruct the child to imitate the sound heard.
- Construct a cardboard face with a small hole in the mouth and through it put a long, thin piece of licorice. The child pulls the licorice through the hole in the mouth as the adult vocalizes. When vocalization ceases, the child stops pulling and the licorice is cut off and given to the child. Adult and child reverse roles.
- Train the child to move a toy across the table or floor rapidly when she hears fast vocalizations and to move it slowly for slow vocalizations. Let the child take turns producing the vocalizations as the adult matches the movement of the toy to the rate of the child's vocalizations.
- Using either recorded music, a drum, voice, or piano:
  —Demonstrate hand-clapping in a rhythmic pattern in response to music. Encourage the child to imitate.
  —Demonstrate a rhythmic pattern of drumbeats. Encourage the child to imitate using his own drum.
  —Vocalize rhythmic patterns and encourage the child to imitate.

Goal 5. Vocalization of meaningful words

Subskill 1: Production of "more"

Activities:

- Use all possible opportunities to express verbally "more." "You want some more?" "More milk?" "More beads?" "There's more in here."
- Use any of the following: puzzles, blocks, shape sorter, beads, buttons, etc. Place the blocks, beads, or whatever you choose in a can. Wait for the child to establish eye contact and say, "There's something in here!" Take out a (block) and say, "It's a (block)." Hand the (block) to the child. Wait for her to look up at you or to hold out her hand to

indicate that she wants more. Tell her, "There's more in here." "Do you want more?" Demand an approximation of "more" before handing her another (block). Use Mom or Dad as a model. Instruct her to ask for "more." Hand her a (block).

- Choose a particular food that the child is fond of. Do a snack activity. Give the child a little bit of the food chosen. Wait for her to indicate that she wants more. Demand an approximation of "more" before giving her more. Use Mom or Dad as a model. (Note: Foods that the child can participate in making are particularly interesting (e.g., popcorn, orange juice, etc.).

Subskill 2: Production of "no"

Activities:

Note: When the child begins to shake his head "no," he will do it many times. This is a strong indication that this word has meaning for the child and thus would be a good word to work on for the production of meaningful words.

- Use all possible opportunities to express verbally "no." "No, you can't do that," "No, I don't want that," etc.
- Encourage the child to say "no," rather than throw a toy or piece of food. When you see that he doesn't want something, require an approximation of "no" before taking that thing away. (Note: The activities you use to stimulate the approximation of "no" will depend on the individual child. The idea is to approach the child with something you know he does not like or want at that particular moment.)

Subskill 3: Production of "hi" and "bye-bye"

Activities:

- These words can be used incidentally throughout the therapy session. For example: Say "hi" when the child comes to therapy. Say "bye" when she leaves. Say "bye-bye" as you put the toys away.
- Dress a doll in a coat. Say "bye" and take the doll out of the room. Give the doll to the child and encourage her to imitate your vocalizations.
- Use a doll house and dolls. Have the dolls walk in and out of the front door to the house. Say "bye-bye" as they leave the house; say "hi" as they enter. Have the dolls drive up to and away from the house in toy cars. Say "hi" and "bye" as you do so. Give the child a toy doll and car. Encourage her to imitate your vocalizations and actions.

- Have the child stand by a door in the house, waiting for you to knock. Say "hi" as the child opens the door. Be enthusiastic. Leave again, saying "bye." Repeat several times. Reverse roles. Have the child knock at the door. Reward any spontaneous production of "hi" or "bye."
- Pick up the receiver of a toy telephone. Say "hi" as you pick it up; say "bye" as you hang up. Hand the phone to the child. Encourage imitation. Immediately reward any spontaneous production of "hi" or "bye."

REFERENCES

Ling, D. *Speech and the hearing impaired.* Washington, D.C.: A.G. Bell Association for the Deaf, 1976.

Appendix C

Information and Service Agencies

Administration for Children; Youth, and Families
U.S. Department of Health and Human Services
Washington, D.C. 20201

Alexander Graham Bell Association for the Deaf
1537 35th Street, N.W.
Washington, D.C. 20007

American Speech and Hearing Association
10801 Rockville Pike
Rockville, Maryland 20852

Closer Look
National Information Center for the Handicapped
P.O. Box 1492
Washington, D.C. 20013

Conference of Executives of American Schools
for the Deaf and Convention of American Instructors of the Deaf
5034 Wisconsin Avenue, N.W.
Washington, D.C. 20016

Council on Education of the Deaf
Clark School for the Deaf
Northampton, Massachusetts 01060

Council for Exceptional Children
1920 Association Drive
Reston, Virginia 22091

Council of Organizations Serving the Deaf
4201 Connecticut Avenue, N.W.
Suite 210
Washington, D.C. 20008

Deafness Research Foundation
366 Madison Avenue
New York, New York 10017

ERIC (Educational Resource Information Center)
Clearinghouse on the Handicapped and Gifted
1920 Association Drive
Reston, Virginia 22091

International Association of Parents of the Deaf
814 Thayer Avenue
Silver Spring, Maryland 20910

National Association of the Deaf
814 Thayer Avenue
Silver Spring, Maryland 20910

National Association of Hearing and Speech Agencies
919 18th Street, N.W.
Washington, D.C. 20006

National Committee for Multi-Handicapped Children
239 14th Street
Niagara Falls, New York 14303

National Information Center for the Handicapped
Box 1492
Washington, D.C. 20013

Parenting Materials Information Center
Southeast Educational Development Laboratory
211 East Seventh Street
Austin, Texas 78701

Planned Parenthood Federation of America
810 Seventh Avenue
New York, New York 10019

Western Institute for the Deaf
215 East 18th Avenue
Vancouver 10, British Columbia
Canada

Index of Subjects

E

L

M

N

O

P

Q

R

S

U

V

Index of Names

G

H

I

J

K

L

M

T

U

V

W

Y

Z